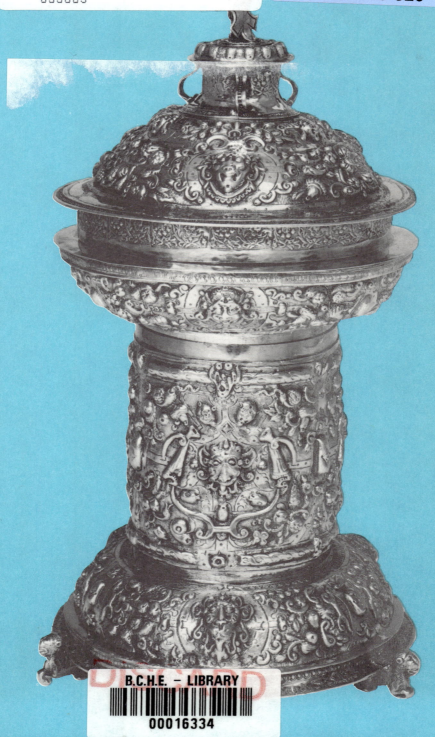

The Role of Salt in Cardiovascular Hypertension

THE NUTRITION FOUNDATION
A Monograph Series

The Role of Salt in Cardiovascular Hypertension

Edited by

Melvin J. Fregly

Department of Physiology
University of Florida
College of Medicine
Gainesville, Florida

Morley R. Kare

Monell Chemical Senses Center
University of Pennsylvania
Philadelphia, Pennsylvania

1982

ACADEMIC PRESS

A Subsidiary of Harcourt Brace Jovanovich, Publishers

New York   London
Paris   San Diego   San Francisco   São Paulo   Sydney   Tokyo   Toronto

ACADEMIC PRESS, INC.
111 Fifth Avenue, New York, New York 10003

United Kingdom Edition published by
ACADEMIC PRESS, INC. (LONDON) LTD.
24/28 Oval Road, London NW1 7DX

Library of Congress Cataloging in Publication Data
Main entry under title:

The Role of salt in cardiovascular hypertension.

    (A monograph series / the Nutrition Foundation)
    Includes bibliographies and index.
    1. Hypertension--Etiology. 2. Sodium--Physiological
effect. 3. Salt in the body. I. Fregly, Melvin J.
II. Kare, Morley Richard, Date. III. Series:
Monograph series (Nutrition Foundation)
RC685.H8R64   616.1'32071   82-6781
ISBN 0-12-267280-1   AACR2

PRINTED IN THE UNITED STATES OF AMERICA

83 84 85   9 8 7 6 5 4 3 2

Contents

v

22   The Loop of Henle Is the Nephron Site Responsible for Escape from the Sodium-Retaining Effects of Mineralocorticoids
JOHN A. HAAS AND FRANKLYN G. KNOX

23   Is a Circulating Sodium Transport Inhibitor Involved in the Pathogenesis of Essential Hypertension?
GRAHAM MACGREGOR AND HUGH DE WARDENER

24   Abnormal Erythrocyte Na^+, K^+ Cotransport System: A Proposed Genetic Marker of Essential Hypertension
RICARDO P. GARAY, PATRICK HANNAERT, GEORGES DAGHER, CORINNE NAZARET, ISABELLE MARIDONNEAU, AND PHILLIPE MEYER

List of Contributors

Numbers in parentheses indicate the pages on which the authors' contributions begin.

Philip Aaronson (425), Department of Pharmacology, University of Miami School of Medicine, Miami, Florida 33101

Arline McDonald Allen[1] (63), Department of Community Health and Preventive Medicine, Northwestern University Medical School, Chicago, Illinois 60611

Frederic C. Bartter (207), Research Service, Audie L. Murphy Memorial Veterans Hospital, San Antonio, Texas 78284

Harold D. Battarbee (155), Department of Physiology and Biophysics, Louisiana State University Medical Center, Shreveport, Louisiana 71130

Gary K. Beauchamp (145), Monell Chemical Senses Center, and Department of Otorhinolaryngology and Human Communication, University of Pennsylvania, Philadelphia, Pennsylvania 19104

Gerald S. Berenson (49), Department of Medicine, and Specialized Center of Research—Arteriosclerosis, Louisiana State University Medical Center, New Orleans, Louisiana 70112

Mary Bertino (145), Monell Chemical Senses Center, University of Pennsylvania, Philadelphia, Pennsylvania 19104

Rosemary D. Bevan (355), Department of Pharmacology, University of California School of Medicine, Los Angeles, California 90024

Mordecai P. Blaustein (417), Department of Physiology, University of Maryland School of Medicine, Baltimore, Maryland 21201

David F. Bohr (221), Department of Physiology, University of Michigan School of Medicine, Ann Arbor, Michigan 48109

Thomas B. Bolton (359), Department of Pharmacology, St. George's Hospital Medical School, University of London, London SW 17 ORE, England

[1]Present address: Department of Nutrition and Medical Dietetics, College of Associated Health Professions, University of Illinois Medical Center, Chicago, Illinois 60612

Edward J. Calabrese (33), Division of Public Health, School of Health Sciences, University of Massachusetts, Amherst, Massachusetts 01003

David Clough (403), Department of Physiology, Uniformed Services University of The Health Sciences, School of Medicine, Bethesda, Maryland 20014

David M. Cohen (221), Department of Physiology, University of Michigan School of Medicine, Ann Arbor, Michigan 48109

Richard Cooper (63), Department of Community Health and Preventive Medicine, Northwestern University Medical School, Chicago, Illinois 60611

Georges Dagher (345), Institut National de la Santé et de la Recherche Medicale (INSERM U7), Centre National de la Recherche Scientifique, Hôpital Necker, Paris 75015, France

John W. Dailey (155), Department of Pharmacology, Louisiana State University Medical Center, Shreveport, Louisiana 71130

Catherine S. Delea (207), Audie L. Murphy Memorial Veterans Hospital, San Antonio, Texas 78209

Hugh de Wardener (331), Department of Medicine, Charing Cross Hospital Medical School, London W6 8RF, England

Stephen P. Dybus (221), Department of Physiology, University of Michigan School of Medicine, Ann Arbor, Michigan 48109

Karl Engelman[2] (145), Department of Medicine, Hospital of the University of Pennsylvania, Philadelphia, Pennsylvania 19104

Gail C. Frank (49), Department of Medicine, and Specialized Center of Research—Arteriosclerosis, Louisiana State University Medical Center, New Orleans, Louisiana 70112

Marilyn S. Fregly (3), College of Journalism and Communications, University of Florida, Gainesville, Florida 32611

Melvin J. Fregly (3, 103, 293), Department of Physiology, University of Florida College of Medicine, Gainesville, Florida 32610

Sydney M. Friedman (385), Department of Anatomy, University of British Columbia, Vancouver, British Columbia V6T 1W5, Canada

Edward D. Frohlich (313), Alton Ochsner Medical Foundation, New Orleans, Louisiana 70121

Toshiro Fujita (207), Institute of Clinical Medicine, University of Tsukuba, Niiharigun, Ibaraki 305, Japan

Ricardo P. Garay (345), Institut National de la Santé et de la Recherche Medicale (INSERM U7), Centre National de la Recherche Scientifique, Hôpital Necker, Paris 75015, France

Flora Gosch (63), Department of Community Health and Preventive Medicine, Northwestern University Medical School, Chicago, Illinois 60611

---

[2]Present address: Clinical Research Center, Hospital of the University of Pennsylvania, Philadelphia, Pennsylvania 19104

Roger J. Grekin (221), Department of Physiology, University of Michigan School of Medicine, Ann Arbor, Michigan 48109

Mary D. Grigorian (221), Department of Physiology, University of Michigan School of Medicine, Ann Arbor, Michigan 48109

John A. Haas (323), Department of Physiology and Biophysics, Mayo Medical School, Rochester, Minnesota 55901

Francis Haddy (403), Department of Physiology, Uniformed Services University of The Health Sciences, School of Medicine, Bethesda, Maryland 20014

Charles E. Hall (233), Department of Physiology and Biophysics, University of Texas Medical Branch, Galveston, Texas 77550

John E. Hall (247), Department of Physiology and Biophysics, University of Mississippi Medical Center, Jackson, Mississippi 39216

Patrick Hannaert (345), Institute National de la Santé et de la Recherche Medicale (INSERM U7), Centre National de la Recherche Scientifique, Hôpital Necker, Paris 75015, France

David P. Henry (267, 281), Department of Medicine, Indiana University School of Medicine, Indianapolis, Indiana 46223

Shirley Hungerford (233), Department of Physiology and Biophysics, University of Texas Medical Branch, Galveston, Texas 77550

James C. Hunt (453), Center for the Health Sciences, University of Tennessee, Memphis, Tennessee 38163

Stephen Huot (403), Department of Physiology, Uniformed Services University of The Health Sciences, School of Medicine, Bethesda, Maryland 20014

Morley R. Kare (145), Monell Chemical Senses Center, University of Pennsylvania, Philadelphia, Pennsylvania 19104

Michael J. Katovich (293), Department of Pharmaceutical Biology, College of Pharmacy, University of Florida, Gainesville, Florida 32610

Franklyn G. Knox (323), Department of Physiology and Biophysics, Mayo Medical School, Rochester, Minnesota 55901

Michael Kolber (425), Department of Pharmacology, University of Miami, School of Medicine, Miami, Florida 33101

Lewis H. Kuller (89), Department of Epidemiology, Graduate School of Public Health, University of Pittsburgh, Pittsburgh, Pennsylvania 15261

Kiang Liu (63), Department of Community Health and Preventive Medicine, Northwestern University Medical School, Chicago, Illinois 60611

Thomas E. Lohmeier (247), Department of Physiology and Biophysics, University of Mississippi Medical Center, Jackson, Mississippi 39216

Friedrich C. Luft (267, 281), Department of Medicine, Indiana University School of Medicine, Indianapolis, Indiana 46223

Robert E. McCaa (191), Department of Physiology and Biophysics, University of Mississippi Medical Center, Jackson, Mississippi 39216

Graham MacGregor (331), Department of Medicine, Charing Cross Hospital Medical School, London W6 8RF, England

Allan A. MacPhee (313), Alton Ochsner Medical Foundation, New Orleans, Louisiana 70121

D. D. Makdani (19), Human Nutrition Research Laboratory, Lincoln University, Jefferson City, Missouri 65101

Isabelle Maridonneau (345), Institut National de la Santé et de la Recherche Medicale (INSERM U7), Centre National de la Recherche Scientifique, Hôpital Necker, Paris 75015, France

George R. Meneely (155, 175), Department of Medicine and the Department of Physiology and Biophysics, Louisiana State University Medical Center, Shreveport, Louisiana 71130

Phillipe Meyer (345), Institut National de la Santé et de la Recherche Medicale (INSERM U7), Centre National de la Recherche Scientifique, Hôpital Necker, Paris 75015, France

Olaf Mickelsen[3] (19), Department of Food Science and Human Nutrition, University of Delaware, Newark, Delaware 19711

Sanford A. Miller (441), Bureau of Foods, Food and Drug Administration, Washington, D.C. 20204

John Mitchell (221), Department of Physiology, University of Michigan School of Medicine, Ann Arbor, Michigan 48109

Corinne Nazaret (345), Institut National de la Santé et de la Recherche Medicale (INSERM U7), Centre National de la Recherche Scientifique, Hôpital Necker, Paris 75015, France

Motilal Pamnani (403), Department of Physiology, Uniformed Services University of The Health Sciences, School of Medicine, Bethesda, Maryland 20014

Yi-jen Pan (247), Department of Physiology and Biophysics, University of Mississippi Medical Center, Jackson, Mississippi 39216

Carol Perfetti (89), Department of Epidemiology, Graduate School of Public Health, University of Pittsburgh, Pittsburgh, Pennsylvania 15261

M. Ian Phillips (127), Department of Physiology, University of Florida College of Medicine, Gainesville, Florida 32610

Laura I. Rankin (267), Department of Medicine, Indiana University School of Medicine, Indianapolis, Indiana 46223

Efrain Reisin (313), Hypertension and Research Division, Alton Ochsner Medical Foundation, New Orleans, Louisiana 70121

Joseph Schachter (89), Department of Epidemiology, Graduate School of Public Health, University of Pittsburgh, Pittsburgh, Pennsylvania 15261

Rachel Schemmel (19), Department of Food Science and Human Nutrition, Michigan State University, East Lansing, Michigan 48824

Jeremiah Stamler (63), Department of Community Health and Preventive Medicine, Northwestern University Medical School, Chicago, Illinois 60611

[3]Present address: Route 1, Lula, Georgia 30554

Rose Stamler (63), Department of Community Health and Preventive Medicine, Northwestern University Medical School, Chicago, Illinois 60611

Robert A. Stewart[4] (79, 449), Gerber Products Company, Fremont, Michigan 49412

Daniel H. Suarez[5] (313), Alton Ochsner Medical Foundation, New Orleans, Louisiana 70121

Maurizio Trevisan (63), Department of Community Health and Preventive Medicine, Northwestern University Medical School, Chicago, Illinois 60611

Robert W. Tuthill (33), Division of Public Health, School of Health Sciences, University of Massachusetts, Amherst, Massachusetts 01003

Cornelis van Breemen (425), Department of Pharmacology, University of Miami School of Medicine, Miami, Florida 33101

Antonie W. Voors (49), Department of Preventive Medicine, and Specialized Center of Research—Arteriosclerosis, Louisiana State University Medical Center, New Orleans, Louisiana 70112

Larry S. Webber (49), Department of Biometry, and Specialized Center of Research—Arteriosclerosis, Louisiana State University Medical Center, New Orleans, Louisiana 70112

Myron H. Weinberger (267, 281), Department of Medicine, Indiana University School of Medicine, Indianapolis, Indiana 46223

Thomas C. Westfall (371), Department of Pharmacology, University of St. Louis School of Medicine, St. Louis, Missouri 63104

Charles F. Whitten (79), Department of Pediatrics, Wayne State University School of Medicine, Detroit, Michigan, and Gerber Products Company, Fremont, Michigan 49412

David B. Young (247), Department of Physiology and Biophysics, University of Mississippi Medical Center, Jackson, Mississippi 39216

[4]Present address: Fremont, Michigan 49412
[5]Present address: Military Hospital, Buenos Aires, Argentina

List of Participants

International Conference on The Role of Salt In Cardiovascular Hypertension, Monell Chemical Senses Center, March 25–27, 1981

Dr. Arline Allen
Dr. Frederic C. Bartter
Dr. Harold D. Battarbee
Dr. Gary K. Beauchamp
Dr. Gerald S. Berenson
Dr. Mary Bertino
Dr. John Bevan
Dr. Rosemary D. Bevan
Dr. Mordecai P. Blaustein
Dr. Thomas B. Bolton
Dr. Edward J. Calabrese
Dr. William J. Darby
Dr. Karl Engelman
Dr. Marilyn S. Fregly
Dr. Melvin J. Fregly
Dr. Constance L. Friedman
Dr. Sydney M. Friedman
Dr. Toshiro Fujita
Dr. Ricardo P. Garay
Dr. Roger J. Grekin
Dr. Francis Haddy
Dr. Charles E. Hall
Dr. George A. Hayden

Dr. James E. Hunt
Dr. Morley R. Kare
Dr. Michael J. Katovich
Dr. Franklyn G. Knox
Dr. Friedrich C. Luft
Dr. Graham MacGregor
Dr. Robert E. McCaa
Dr. George R. Meneely
Dr. Olaf Mickelsen
Dr. Sanford A. Miller
Dr. M. Ian Philips
Dr. Efrain Reisin
Dr. Armando Sandoval
Dr. Joseph Schachter
Dr. Robert A. Stewart
Dr. Mary K. Stiedeman
Dr. Andrew J. Sullivan
Dr. Louis Tobian
Dr. Cornelis van Breemen
Dr. Myron H. Weinberger
Dr. Thomas C. Westfall
Dr. David B. Young

Foreword

In recent years, a cavalier appraisal of the roles of food and nutrition in health and diseases (particularly chronic diseases) has led to wide acceptance of "conclusions" that often are based on narrow and superficial knowledge of basic physiologic and nutrition science. Not infrequently, popularization of such inadequately examined concepts has led to premature induction of efforts to promote changes in food habits, composition of foods, and regulatory matters. Responsibility for this situation lies not only with those writers without scientific knowledge or training whose zeal for solving major riddles of causes of disease far exceeds their understanding of either science or human needs, but also with many members of the scientific and medical community whose rifle-barreled vision leads to making facile generalizations in areas in which they, too, are ignorant.

In no field is such a state better illustrated than the current controversies regarding the roles of nutrition and foods in cardiovascular diseases and cancer. Professionals frequently are unaware of the complexities of phenomena in fields outside their training and expertise and have insufficient opportunity to relate to scientists with expert knowledge that they lack.

To balance and broaden an understanding of the complex aspects of food, nutrition, and health, The Nutrition Foundation initiated this series of carefully planned monographs to bring to each subject knowledge from a broad spectrum of related sciences. In developing each monograph, an opportunity for displaying information and discussing it has been provided through the medium of an international symposium preceding the final editing of the individual chapters.

This volume is the second monograph in the series that specifically deals with aspects of salt. It addresses the complex scientific aspects of the physiologic and metabolic effects of salt with full appreciation of the neuroendocrinologic phenomena that so often are ignored by those whose depth in modern physiologic science is limited.

The first volume, "Biological and Behavioral Aspects of Salt Intake," uniquely probes those factors that alter man's appetite for salt and summarizes observations from comparative physiology that may assist in understanding the physiologic and pathologic significance of levels of salt intake and the behavioral patterns that determine or result from the intake.

The comprehensive scope of these two monographs was made possible by collaboration of scientists identified with and knowledgeable in the many perspectives from which one must view the panorama of the use of salt and its roles in health, especially cardiovascular hypertension. Both volumes have resulted from cooperative efforts of The Nutrition Foundation, the Monell Chemical Senses Center, the National Institutes of Health, and the University of Florida. As President of The Nutrition Foundation, I express the appreciation of this Foundation for the opportunity to contribute to a better understanding of the basic scientific information relating to the unresolved issue of the most desirable intake levels of the essential nutrient, sodium chloride, in health and disease.

William J. Darby
President
The Nutrition Foundation, Inc.
New York and Washington, D.C.

Preface

This book is based on the proceedings of a symposium on ''The Role of Salt In Cardiovascular Hypertension,'' which was held at the Monell Chemical Senses Center of the University of Pennsylvania on March 25–27, 1981. The convening of this symposium represented the twentieth anniversary of an earlier symposium of identical title which was held at the College of Medicine of the University of Florida. Thirty-five investigators who were actively engaged in all aspects of the role of salt in cardiovascular hypertension participated in that symposium. The Foreword introducing the volume containing the proceedings of that symposium states the following:

> It was the aim of this symposium to cover thoroughly a restricted area of the field of cardiovascular hypertension. The time seemed propitious for a discussion of the role played by salt in hypertension because a number of investigators has been able to induce hypertension when salt is given in excess quantities to experimental animals. Others have demonstrated that salt ''sensitizes'' rats to the hypertensive effects of certain pressor agents such as desoxycorticosterone acetate or to the hypertension induced by a regenerating adrenal gland. Salt may or may not be a common denominator among the various types of hypertension but it cannot be denied that this agent alone is capable of producing hypertension whether administered in excess in food or in drinking water. It seems certain that a better understanding of the physiologic function of sodium, and the other inorganic ions of the body, is necessary before an understanding of the etiology of hypertension will be possible.
>
> Fregly, M. J. (1961). *Am. J. Cardiol.* **8**, 526.

In the twenty years that have passed since this Foreword was written, the contribution of the renin–angiotensin–aldosterone system to the control of sodium excretion and, more recently, to sodium intake has been clarified. Contributors to this volume will review current knowledge in these areas. During the intervening years, pharmacologic agents that can inhibit the renin–angiotensin–aldosterone system at strategic levels have also been developed and used to treat hypertension clinically. Some of these, e.g., the inhibitors of the angiotensin I-converting enzyme, are also discussed. More recently, a role for catecholamines in the control of sodium excretion, and perhaps sodium intake, is emerging. Further, our knowledge of the interaction of sodium at the level of the smooth muscle cell has expanded greatly, and recent developments in this area, particularly with respect to the presence of a circulating inhibitor of Na^+,K^+-ATPase activity in hypertensives, are discussed in this volume.

It is apparent that the awareness of the public regarding a potential role for sodium in the development of hypertension has heightened during the past twenty years. The culmination of this awareness is the proposal under consideration by the Federal Government for the labeling of the sodium content of processed foods. The current status of this proposal and the response of industry to it are included.

Indeed, I believe the time is propitious for a reconsideration of the role played by salt in cardiovascular hypertension.

Some participants of the earlier symposium who attended this one include Drs. Sydney Friedman, Francis Haddy, C. Erich Hall, George Meneely, and Louis Tobian. I would like to pay tribute to those who attended the earlier symposium and are now deceased. They include Drs. Lewis K. Dahl, Dwight J. Ingle, Arthur Grollman, Floyd R. Skelton, Arthur Corcoran, and Howard G. Swann. It is to their memory that this book is dedicated.

We were fortunate in the planning of the symposium to have the advice and counsel of Drs. Frederick Bartter, Rosemary D. Bevan, Francis Haddy, and Myron Weinberger. I would like to acknowledge their generous help and encouragement, and to express our deep appreciation and thanks to them. I would also like to acknowledge the major support of the National Heart, Lung, and Blood Institute and the Nutrition Foundation. Additional support for the symposium was provided by the CIBA-Geigy Corporation and the Squibb Corporation. Administrative support was given at every level by the Monell Chemical Senses Center. I would like to express my thanks to the staff of the Center for their important contribution to the success of the symposium and this treatise.

Melvin J. Fregly

The Role of Salt in
Cardiovascular Hypertension

I

Sodium Intake and the Factors Affecting It

1

The Estimates of
Sodium Intake by Man

MARILYN S. FREGLY AND MELVIN J. FREGLY

I. INTRODUCTION

Sodium chloride is the most abundant salt occurring naturally in the food of man. It is also added to processed foods for a variety of reasons: to enhance flavor, to season, and to preserve. In addition, it is used by the food processing industry for certain technical reasons, e.g., as a curing agent, as a formulating and processing aid, and as a conditioner of dough by the baking industry. In addition to the sodium naturally present in food and to that added by the food

3

processor, man customarily adds NaCl both during cooking and to the food presented at the table.

The total daily intake of sodium chloride (NaCl) in American and other cultures has been the subject of a number of studies. Attempts have been made to arrive at estimates of both discretionary (consumer controlled) and nondiscretionary (commercially controlled and/or naturally occurring) daily NaCl intakes. Among these are the National Research Council (NRC) Survey of Industry (Subcommittee on Review of GRAS List, 1972; Committee on GRAS List Survey, 1978), the Food and Drug Administration's (FDA) Selected Minerals in Food Survey (Food and Drug Administration, 1977; Shank, 1980), data on the production and sale of salt (Wood, 1970; Bowen *et al.*, 1973; Dickinson, 1980), the Health and Nutrition Examination Survey (HANES I) (Abraham and Carroll, 1981), and data on daily urinary excretion of sodium (Dahl and Love, 1957; Coatney *et al.*, 1958; Altman and Dittmer, 1974; Mickelson *et al.*, 1977).

II. ESTIMATES OF NONDISCRETIONARY SODIUM INTAKE

A. National Research Council Survey of Industry

In 1970 a subcommittee of the NRC surveyed the food industry regarding the quantity of NaCl and other sodium salts added to food both to improve the taste of the food and to produce certain desired technical effects important in processing the food (Subcommittee on Review of GRAS List, 1972). This survey revealed that as much as 1 g of sodium accrued to the average total daily sodium intake as a result of the addition of sodium salt other than NaCl.

The amount of NaCl present in processed food in 1970 was estimated by NRC to be about 60% of the total quantity used by the food processing industry. A portion of the NaCl used by industry does not appear in the final food product. It is used in various stages of processing but is discarded prior to packaging of the product, e.g., brines. Based on this estimate and on the tonnage of salt sold to the food processing industry in 1970, the estimated per capita NaCl consumption was calculated to be 18 g/day. A resurvey of the food processing industry carried out in 1975 revealed a nondiscretionary daily intake of NaCl amounting to 8.4 g/day (Committee on GRAS List Survey, 1978). This large difference in intakes estimated by the two studies could be related to a reduction in the amount of sodium used in food processing during the five year interval but it is more likely to be related to errors of estimation by the 1970 survey.

B. Food and Drug Administration Selected Minerals in Food (Market Basket) Survey

A second attempt to assess daily intake of NaCl was made by the FDA. Food (consisting of 117 individual food items of 12 food composites) was purchased retail to make up a 3900-kcal daily diet such as might be consumed by a typical 15- to 20-year-old American male (Food and Drug Administration, 1977; Shank, 1980). The food was purchased at markets in northeastern, southeastern, western, and central locations in the United States during 1976, 1977, and 1978. The foods were then prepared as they would be for home consumption but without the addition of NaCl during preparation. Table I lists the food composites and their sodium content for market basket collections in 1976, 1977, and 1978. A discretionary average intake of 1.9–2.0 g sodium (4.8–5.1 g NaCl)/day is included in Table I to account for the sodium normally used in home food preparation and seasoning at the table. The 1976, 1977, and 1978 analyses reveal that about 6.8 g of sodium (17.2 g NaCl) was ingested daily with the 3900-kcal diet. Since the minimal daily requirement for vitamins and nutrients is now customarily expressed per 1000 kcal, Table I provides this information for the sodium content in the various food composites of the three separate market basket collections. The

TABLE I

Sodium Content by Food Composite of 3900-kcal Daily Diet Collected in FDA Selected Minerals in Food Survey

Food composite	1976 sodium[a] (mg)	1976 sodium[a] (mg/1000 kcal)	1977 sodium[b] (mg)	1977 sodium[b] (mg/1000 kcal)	1978 sodium[c] (mg)	1978 sodium[c] (mg/1000 kcal)
Nondiscretionary						
Dairy products	717	184	704	180	792	203
Meat, fish, poultry	1000	256	952	244	921	236
Grain and cereal products	2036	522	2005	514	2002	513
Potatoes	65	17	75	19	82	21
Leafy vegetables	18	5	22	6	22	6
Legume vegetables	224	57	243	62	258	62
Root vegetables	16	4	18	5	17	4
Garden vegetables	264	68	285	73	284	73
Fruits	74	19	66	17	75	19
Oil and fats	380	97	387	99	406	104
Beverages	9	2	17	4	24	7
Total nondiscretionary	4803	1232	4774	1224	4886	1252
Discretionary						
Sugar, salt, and adjuncts[d]	1970	505	1923	493	2042	524
Total intake	6773	1737	6697	1717	6928	1776

[a] Mean value of 20 to 25 market basket collections.
[b] Mean value of 25 market basket collections.
[c] Mean value of 8 market basket collections.
[d] Includes the salt normally used in home food preparation and for seasoning at the table.

values for the 3 years are quite similar and average approximately 1740 mg of sodium/1000 kcal (4.39 g of NaCl/1000 kcal). The assumption used in this calculation is that the salt intake of adults consuming less than 3900 kcal/day is proportionately less.

C. Estimation of Sodium Intake from Production and Sale of Sodium Chloride

Additional estimates of daily intake of NaCl have been made from the total amount of table salt purchased for the year 1968 (275,000 tons) (Wood, 1970). For a population estimated at 200 million, this amounts to a usage of 3.42 g/person/day. This was assumed to represent an estimate of the discretionary use of salt and was not adjusted for amounts that were not actually ingested.

Data from the Bureau of Mines for 1970 to 1973 on production and usage of NaCl in all aspects of food production and processing were used by Bowen et al. (1973) to calculate daily per capita NaCl consumption. The manufacture of NaCl for all purposes, of which food processing was one, averaged 23.6 g/person/day. Bowen et al. estimated that the total daily usage of NaCl for food processing and production to be 8 g/person/day with an additional 6.5 g/person/day used for discretionary purposes. This amounts to a total daily NaCl intake of 14.5 g/day. This figure was adjusted for an estimated amount of NaCl used in food processing but not present in the final product. The Salt Institute estimates that 4.1 percent of total sales is for food grade NaCl (Dickinson, 1980). Their estimate of *total* daily per capita consumption of NaCl calculated from the sale of food grade NaCl to both food processors and consumers in 1977 is 8–10 g.

D. Health and Nutrition Examination Survey (HANES I)

An estimate of nondiscretionary daily sodium intake was also made in the first Health and Nutrition Examination Survey (HANES I)(Abraham and Carroll, 1981). This survey sampled 20,749 persons aged 1–74 years during 1971–1974. Information regarding food intake was obtained on the basis of the 24 hr recall method for the day, midnight to midnight, preceding the interviews and included all regular meals as well as foods and snacks eaten between meals. Only week days were used. Foods were grouped into 18 separate categories many of which do not overlap with the categories chosen by the FDA market basket survey (Table I). The daily nondiscretionary NaCl intake for males 1–74 years of age was 6.8 g while that for females was 4.6 g (Table II). The results of this study also showed that intake of NaCl varied with age; the maximum (7.6 g) was ingested by males in the age range of 18–44 years. In the case of females, the maximum (5.6 g) was ingested in the age range 6–11 years. These are the first data to suggest that intake of NaCl is a function of age and sex and that the

TABLE II

Mean Daily Nondiscretionary Sodium Chloride Intake by Sex and Age: United States, 1971–1974[a]

Sex	Age (years)	Mean sodium chloride intake (g/day)
Male	1–5	4.7
	6–11	6.3
	12–17	7.4
	18–44	7.6
	45–64	6.4
	65–74	5.6
Mean	1–74	6.8
Female	1–5	4.3
	6–11	5.6
	12–17	5.0
	18–44	4.7
	45–64	4.3
	65–74	3.8
Mean	1–74	4.6

[a] Adapted from Abraham and Carroll (1981).

maximal intake occurs at a considerably younger age for females than for males (Table II).

III. NONDISCRETIONARY INTAKES OF SODIUM NOT INCLUDED IN THE ABOVE STUDIES

A. Sodium in Drinking Water

Sodium ion occurring in drinking water must also be taken into account when estimating nondiscretionary sodium intake. Although sodium ion ingested with food is substantially greater than that ingested with drinking water, the latter may represent from 0.5 to 10% of the total daily intake of sodium ion by normal individuals (Laubusch and McCammon, 1955). The concentration of sodium ion in drinking water varies considerably from state to state, within states, and even within a given city (Bills *et al.*, 1949; Cech *et al.*, 1979; Cooper and Heap, 1967; Corley, 1965; Elliott and Alexander, 1961; Elton *et al.*, 1963; Gonzales *et al.*, 1979; Laubusch and McCammon, 1955).

A study by White *et al.* (1967) which sampled water supplies from 2035 municipalities revealed that 41.8% had a sodium ion concentration exceeding 20 mg/liter. This is the maximal concentration of sodium considered permissible for use with the 500 mg sodium restricted diet developed by the American Heart Association (1957). Corley (1965) listed 53 communities in Nebraska where he found a sodium ion concentration greater than 50 mg/liter in the drinking water. Bills *et al.* (1949) surveyed 150 municipal water supplies that provide an estimated 28% of the population of continental United States with their water. They reported sodium ion concentrations of 1–340 mg/liter. Assuming a daily water intake of 2.5 liters for an adult, a water supply containing sodium ion at a concentration of 200 mg/liter would provide 500 mg of sodium ion per day. This is approximately the daily requirement of normal individuals for sodium as suggested by Meneely and Battarbee (1976b). For those individuals with cardiac decompensation who conscientiously follow their low sodium ion diet, the sodium ion ingested with drinking water may represent a hidden danger (Cooper and Heap, 1967; Elliott and Alexander, 1961).

The amount of sodium ion ingested by individuals within a given community may also differ, and depends on the sources of water supplied to inhabitants. A recent study of the city of Houston, Texas, whose municipal water system is very complex and involves both surface and ground water sources, has shown a sodium ion concentration varying from 19 to 235 mg/liter in various portions of the city (Gonzales *et al.,* 1979). The water was sampled from 50 different locations within the city limits. Those sections of the city supplied by deep wells had the highest sodium ion concentration in their drinking water. For patients on a 500 mg sodium restricted diet, only the water containing the lowest sodium ion concentration could be used.

The long-term effect of ingestion of drinking water that contains high concentrations of sodium ion was studied by Calabrese and Tuthill (1977) and Tuthill and Calabrese (1979). Three hundred high school sophomores living in a community in which the drinking water contained a sodium ion concentration of 107 mg/liter had a blood pressure frequency distribution curve that was shifted upward for both systolic and diastolic blood pressures when compared with high school sophomores (300) from a nearby, appropriately matched community with drinking water that contained 8 mg sodium/liter. Females from the community with the elevated sodium concentration in drinking water exhibited a blood pressure frequency distribution pattern characteristic of females 10 years older whereas the males from this same community had a pattern characteristic for males 2 years older. These results are the first to implicate the sodium content of drinking water as a potential factor in the etiology of hypertension.

B. Sodium from Water Softeners

In those areas where home water softeners are used, additional sodium ion is added to the water (Cole, 1951). The generally used cation exchange process depends on the ability of an exchanger to give up its sodium for other cations in the water (usually calcium and magnesium ions). The higher the concentration of these cations, the higher the sodium ion concentration in the drinking water. Information is not readily available to the citizens of a community regarding either the concentration of sodium in the drinking water of their community or the use of water softening processes by municipal water authorities within that community.

C. Sodium in Drugs

Although few prescription drugs contain sodium, a large number of nonprescription, over-the-counter (OTC) drugs may contribute significantly to the daily sodium intake (Bennett, 1980; Expert Panel on Food Safety and Nutrition, 1980). Sodium is present in many of these medications both as an active ingredient and as an excipient. Some common sodium containing excipients include sodium alginate, sodium bisulfate, sodium caprylate, sodium carboxymethyl cellulose, sodium chloride, sodium hexametaphosphate, and sodium saccharin.

It was noted recently that some OTC antacids can supply a total daily sodium intake of at least 1200 mg (equivalent to 3 g NaCl) (Expert Panel on Food Safety and Nutrition, 1980). Of the pain relievers, only aspirin (sodium salicylate) may present a potential problem to patients on a sodium restricted diet. Approximately 49 mg of sodium (125 mg NaCl) are contained in each dose. Certain antacids, e.g., Sal Hepatica (1000 mg/dose) and Brioschi (710 mg/dose), and sleep aids, e.g., Miles Nervine Effervescent (544 mg/dose), also contain significant amounts of sodium. Although it is difficult to estimate the amount of sodium ingested daily with the drugs used by the average American, it is clear that this source must be taken into consideration in the estimation of total sodium intake.

D. Estimates of Discretionary Intake

Mickelson et al. (1977) carried out a 28-day study on 10 healthy men fed "carefully controlled low-sodium" foods but permitted to add table salt to their food. The basal diet provided 2500 kcal. Total intake of sodium ion by the men amounted to 5.55 ± 0.85 (SD) g/day (14.0 g NaCl/day). Of this, the nondiscretionary intake was 3.71 ± 0.33 g/day (9.1 g NaCl/day) whereas the discretionary intake was 2.18 ± 0.33 g/day (5.5 g NaCl/day). Others have estimated the discretionary intake of NaCl to be 3–6.5 g/day (Select Committee on GRAS Substances, 1979).

E. Estimates of Total Intake from Daily Urinary Sodium Excretion

Daily intake of sodium has also been estimated by the daily urinary excretion of this ion. Dahl and Love (1957) studied employees at the Brookhaven National

Laboratories. Twenty-four hour urine collections were made on 1124 males over a 3-year period. Calculating from these urine analyses, they estimated daily intake of NaCl to be 10 g (range 4–24 g). The Handbook of Biological Data lists daily sodium excretion to be 60 mg/kg/day and urinary chloride excretion to be 100 mg/kg/day (Altman and Dittmer, 1974). This amounts to 3.6 g sodium and 6 g chloride excreted per day for a 60-kg adult. If all of the sodium ion excreted is the result of ingestion of sodium chloride, the total intake would amount to 9 g/day. Coatney *et al.* (1958) studied the 24 hr urinary sodium excretion of 16 healthy subjects of military age on 2 to 8 occasions during a period of 5 months. They estimated the average daily NaCl intake at 11 g/day.

Table III summarizes the estimates of daily NaCl intakes as discussed above and attempts to separate the total intake into nondiscretionary and discretionary intakes. As can be seen, the total NaCl intakes estimated in the variety of ways discussed above are roughly comparable, varying from 10 to 14.5 g/day. The discrepant value of 17.1 g/day estimated by the 1976–1978 FDA Selected Minerals in Food Survey is based on a total dietary intake of 3900 kcal which accounts, in part at least, for this high value. No estimate has been made in Table III of the amount of sodium ion ingested by way of drugs.

The weighted means of the levels of NaCl added to foods are shown in Table IV by the category of the processed food. The values listed do not mean that all manufacturers processing food of a given category have the same level of NaCl in their product. Using these weighted mean values and data on the mean portion or amount of each of these categories consumed daily per person, as determined by the U.S. Department of Agriculture, an estimate of the daily NaCl intake was made. The NRC Subcommittee cautioned that this method overstates the average intake of NaCl.

The figures given in Table IV, representing responses from more than 20 food processors, suggest a possible nondiscretionary daily intake of 6.9 g of NaCl for humans 2 years and older in 1970. These data suggest that the baked goods, breakfast cereals, and grain products categories combined account for 32% of the total daily nondiscretionary NaCl intake. The HANES I data indicate that the grain products category (including bread, rolls, biscuits, muffins, cornbread, crackers, and unsalted pretzels) contributes 20–27% of the daily nondiscretionary NaCl intake in all age and sex subgroups. This is a somewhat lower estimate than that of the FDA market basket survey from which Table IV is derived, but the HANES data do not include in the grain products category the NaCl ingested with cereal products. The meat, fish, and poultry category contributed 20.8% to the total nondiscretionary intake in the FDA survey while the mixed protein dishes and meat categories contributed 21 and 18% of the nondiscretionary intake of males and females, respectively, in the HANES report. The milk and milk products category was the third major source of nondiscretionary NaCl intake contributing 14.9 and 14.0% to the total for the FDA and HANES surveys,

TABLE III

Sources of Dietary Sodium and Estimates of Total Sodium Intake[a]

	Sodium intake (expressed as sodium chloride) (g/day)	Comments
A. Nondiscretionary sources of sodium		
1. Naturally occurring sodium in foods	2.5–4.5	Estimated food composition
	3.0	Chemical analysis (institutional diet)
2. Sodium added by industrial processing		
a. salt	6.9	1970 NRC estimate (3200-kcal diet)
	8	Bowen et al. (1973)
	8.4	Total 1975 usage by food industry
b. Other sodium-containing ingredients	1.0	Calculated from 1970 NRC survey
3. Total nondiscretionary sodium	12–12.5	Calculated from 1976–1978 FDA Selected Minerals in Food Survey (3900-kcal diet)
	4.6–6.3	HANES I Data, Abraham and Carroll (1981)
	9.1	Mickelson et al. (1977)
B. Discretionary addition of salt to foods by the consumer	3.4	1968 retail sales
	4.4–6	1965 USDA survey
	6.5	Bowen et al. (1973)
	5.5	Mickelson et al. (1977)
C. Total salt usage	8–10	Dickinson (1980)
	10	Urinary excretion, Dahl and Love (1957)
	11	Urinary excretion, Coatney et al. (1958)
	14.5	Bowen et al. (1973)
D. Total sodium intake	12	Estimated from review of literature, Meneely and Battarbee (1976b)
	17.1	1976–1978 FDA Selected Minerals in Food Survey (3900-kcal diet)
	14.0	Mickelson et al. (1977)

[a] These values are not necessarily additive; see text for discussion. Adapted from report of Select Committee on GRAS Substances (1979).

TABLE IV

Calculation of a Possible Average Daily Intake Based on Level of Addition of Sodium Chloride to Food by Food Category[a]

Food category	Level of addition to processed food (weighted mean %)	Possible average daily intake (g) 2–65+ yr
Baked goods, baking mixes	1.31	1.8
Breakfast cereals	1.09	0.2
Grain products such as pastas or rice dishes	0.74	0.2
Fats and oils	1.43	0.2
Milk products	0.45	0.2
Cheese	1.00	0.1
Frozen dairy desserts, mixes	0.04	[b]
Processed fruits, juices, and drinks	0.48	0.6
Meat products	2.49	1.9
Poultry products	0.83	0.1
Egg products	0.64	[b]
Fish products	0.96	0.1
Processed vegetables, juices	0.68	0.6
Condiments, relishes, and salt substitutes	3.18	0.3
Soft candy	0.42	[b]
Sugar, confections	0.51	[b]
Sweet sauces, toppings, syrups	0.47	[b]
Gelatins, puddings, fillings	0.41	0.1
Soups, soup mixes	1.02	0.3
Snack foods	2.08	[b]
Beverages, nonalcoholic	0.04	[b]
Beverages, alcoholic	0.02	[b]
Nuts, nut products	1.12	0.1
Reconstituted vegetable proteins	7.27	[b]
Gravies, sauces	1.17	0.1
Dairy product analogs	0.64	[b]
Hard candy	0.41	[b]
Seasonings and flavorings	50.53	[b]
Calculated possible average daily intake of added sodium chloride for the age group, 2–65+ years		6.9

[a] Adapted from Report of Select Committee on GRAS Substances (1979).

[b] Less than 0.05 g.

respectively. These data suggest that two categories, grain and cereal products and meat products, account for about 50% of the total daily nondiscretionary NaCl intake. Thus, these two food categories, as well as milk and milk products, should be given special consideration in attempts to reduce sodium intake. It must be cautioned, however, that individuals vary considerably in the quantities of food ingested from each of the categories listed in Table IV. It is for this reason that labeling of the sodium content of processed food should be undertaken. This has also been recommended by the Salt Institute (1980) and is under consideration by the FDA (Shank, 1980). The consumer interested in reducing sodium intake could then make rational choices both between the same processed food products of different food processors and among the various food composites listed in Table IV.

The long-term effects on the American population of ingestion of NaCl at levels of 10–14.5 g/day, or greater, are not known with certainty. This subject has been reviewed by a number of investigators, committees, and task forces (Battarbee and Meneely, 1977–1978; Chapman and Gibbons, 1950; Dahl and Love, 1957; Dustan and Frohlich, 1949; Freis, 1976; Grollman, 1961; Meneely and Battarbee, 1976a,b; Salt Institute, 1980; Select Committee on GRAS Substances, 1979; Tobian, 1974; National Academy of Sciences, 1980). It is clear, however, that the levels of NaCl ingested by Americans are 10–20 times the minimal level compatible with health in man (Dahl, 1972; Meneely and Battarbee, 1976b). Although hypertension develops in certain species of animals fed high levels of dietary NaCl chronically (Corbett *et al.*, 1979; Dahl *et al.*, 1972; Meneely and Ball, 1958; Meneely *et al.*, 1957), the level of intake that can induce hypertension in man has not been established.

Dahl (1972) reported a positive correlation between dietary intake of NaCl and the percentage of the population that was hypertensive in a series of different populations. Others have been unable to verify a relationship between the level of dietary sodium intake and the incidence of hypertension within given populations (Battarbee and Meneely, 1977–1978; Dawber *et al.*, 1967; Schlierf *et al.*, 1980). Battarbee and Meneely (1977–1978) have concluded that attempts to correlate the incidence or degree of hypertension with sodium consumption in subsets of a given population ''are almost futile'' since the dynamic range of sodium consumption is not likely to be large enough to bring out a clear correlation. An additional factor that must be taken into account is the simultaneous dietary potassium intake. A number of studies has shown that potassium can ameliorate some of the toxic effects of ingestion of sodium in excess (Battarbee and Meneely, 1977–1978; Meneely and Battarbee, 1976a,b). In spite of the difficulty in assigning NaCl a role in the development of hypertension, a number of investigators, clinicians, committees, and task forces feel that it is appropriate to recommend a reduced consumption of NaCl for the U.S. population (Battarbee and Meneely, 1977–1978; Dahl, 1972; Freis, 1976; National Academy of Sciences, 1980). However, others argue that a reduction in NaCl intake is neither appropriate nor necessary for those who do not have an elevated blood pressure (Salt Institute, 1980).

Recently, Senator McGovern stated that the 5 g of NaCl per day recommended by his Dietary Goals Committee was intended to represent salt added to the diet by individuals or processors and did not include salt that occurs naturally in food (American Dietetic Association, 1979; McGovern, 1979). This would increase the daily total recommended salt level from 5 to 8 g. The Food and Nutrition Board of the National Academy of Sciences favors even greater restriction of intake to 3 g/day (National Academy of Sciences, 1980). The controversy is not likely to end between those who believe that present evidence is sufficient to recommend limitations of salt intake for the general population and those who believe that such limitations should be recommended only by an individual's physician. The Surgeon General of the United States suggests "that the prudent approach, given present knowledge, would be to limit salt consumption by cooking with only small amounts, refraining from adding salt to food at the table, and avoiding salty prepared foods" (Office of the Assistant Secretary for Health and Surgeon General, 1979).

The necessity of salt for health and the potential consequences of its overuse were recognized more than a thousand years ago. The Code of Health of the School of Salerum, purported to be the first Christian medical school and founded about 900 A.D., had the following to say about the role of salt in health and disease:

> Salt-cellars ever should stand at the head
> of dishes, whereso'er a table's spread.
> Salt will all poisons expurgate with haste
> And to insipid things impart a taste.
> The richest food will be in great default
> Of taste without a pinch of sav'ry salt.
> Yet of salt meats, the long protracted use
> Will both our sight and manhood, too, reduce;
> And above all, let none express surprise,
> To loathsome psora and to cramps give rise.   (Ordronaux, 1870).

It is our hope that the results of this symposium will help to bridge this thousand year gap.

ACKNOWLEDGMENT

This research was supported by grant HL 14526-09 from the National Heart, Lung and Blood Institute.

REFERENCES

Abraham, S., and Carroll, M. D. (1981). "Fats, Cholesterol and Sodium Intake in the Diet of Persons 1–74 years: United States," Advance Data 54, Reissue. USDHEW, Washington, D.C.

Altman, P. L., and Dittmer, D. S., eds. (1974). "Handbook of Biological Data," p. 1496. Fed. Am. Soc. Exp. Biol., Bethesda, Maryland.

American Dietetic Association (1979). Commentary. Dietary goals for the United States. *J. Am. Diet. Assoc.* **74,** 529–533.

American Heart Association (1957). "Your 500 Milligram Diet." Am. Heart Assoc., New York.

Battarbee, H. D., and Meneely, G. R. (1977–1978). Toxicity of salt. *CRC Crit. Rev. Toxicol.* **5,** 355–376.

Bennett, D. R. (1980). Sodium content of prescription and nonprescription drugs. *In* "Sodium and Potassium in Foods and Drugs" (P. L. White and S. C. Crocco, eds.), pp. 65–75. Am. Med. Assoc., Chicago, Illinois.

Bills, C. E., McDonald, F. G., Niedermeir, W., and Schwartz, M. C. (1949). Sodium and potassium in foods and waters: Determination by flame photometer. *J. Am. Diet. Assoc.,* **25,** 304–314.

Bowen, R. E., Reid, E. J., and Moshy, R. H. (1973). Designing formulated foods for the cardiac concerned. *Prev. Med.* **2,** 366–377.

Calabrese, E. J., and Tuthill, R. W. (1977). Elevated blood pressure and high sodium levels in the public drinking water. *Arch. Environ. Health* **32,** 200–202.

Cech, I., Smolensky, M. H., and Gonzales, E. A. (1979). Excessive sodium in drinking water. *South. Med. J.* **72,** 639–641.

Chapman, C. B., and Gibbons, T. B. (1950). The diet and hypertension. *Medicine (Baltimore)* **29,** 30–69.

Coatney, G. R., Mickelson, O., Burgess, R. W., Young, M. D., and Pirkle, C. I. (1958). Chloroquin or pyrimethamine in salt as a suppressive against sporozoite-induced vivax malaria (Chesson strain). *Bull. W.H.O.* **19,** 56–67.

Cole, S. L. (1951). Sodium in southern California water. *Ann. West. Med. Surg.* **5,** 177–180.

Committee on GRAS List Survey (Phase III) (1978). "1975 Resurvey of the Annual Poundage of Food Chemicals Generally Regarded as Safe (GRAS)," pp. 1–26. Prepared under DHEW Contract No. FDA 223-77-2025 by the Food and Nutrition Board, Division of Biological Sciences, National Academy of Sciences—National Research Council, Washington, D.C.

Cooper, G. R., and Heap, B. (1967). Sodium ion in drinking water. II. Importance, problems and potential applications of sodium-ion-restricted therapy. *J. Am. Diet. Assoc.* **50,** 37–41.

Corbett, W. T., Kuller, L. M., Blaine, E. H., and Damico, F. J. (1979). Utilization of swine to study the risk factor of an elevated salt diet on blood pressure. *Am. J. Clin. Nutr.* **32,** 2068–2075.

Corley, W. D. (1965). Sodium content of drinking water in Nebraska. *Nebr. State Med. J.* **50,** 164–166.

Dahl, L. K. (1972). Salt and hypertension. *Am. J. Clin. Nutr.* **25,** 231–244.

Dahl, L. K., and Love, R. A. (1957). Etiological role of sodium chloride intake in essential hypertension in humans. *JAMA, J. Am. Med. Assoc.* **164,** 397–400.

Dahl, L. K., Leitl, G., and Heine, M. (1972). Influence of dietary potassium and sodium/potassium molar ratios on the development of salt hypertension. *J. Exp. Med.* **136,** 318–330.

Dawber, T. R., Kannel, W. B., Kagan, A., Donabedian, R. K., McNamara, P. M., and Pearson, G. (1967). Environmental factors in hypertension. *In* "The Epidemiology of Hypertension" (J. Stamler, R. Stamler, and N. Pullman, eds.), pp. 255–265. Grune & Stratton, New York.

Dickinson, W. E. (1980). Salt sources and markets. *In* "Biological and Behavioral Aspects of Salt

Intake'' (M. R. Kare, M. J. Fregly, and R. A. Bernard, eds.), pp. 49–52. Academic Press, New York.

Dustan, H. P., and Frohlich, E. D. (1979). ''Report of The Hypertension Task Force,'' Vol. 8, NIH Publ. 79-1630, pp. 1–182. U.S. Dept. of Health, Education and Welfare, Bethesda, Maryland.

Elliott, G. B., and Alexander, E. A. (1961). Sodium from drinking water as an unsuspected cause of cardiac decompensation. *Circulation* **23**, 562–566.

Elton, N. W., Elton, W. J., and Nazareno, J. P. (1963). Pathology of acute salt poisoning in infants. *Am. J. Clin. Pathol.* **39**, 252–264.

Expert Panel on Food Safety and Nutrition (1980). ''Dietary Salt,'' pp. 1–7. Inst. Food Technol., Chicago, Illinois.

Food and Drug Administration (1977). ''Preliminary Data: FY77 Selected Minerals in Food Survey/Total Diet Studies.'' USDHEW, Washington, D.C.

Freis, E. D. (1976). Salt, volume and the prevention of hypertension. *Circulation* **53**, 589–595.

Gonzales, E. A., Cech, I., and Smolensky, M. H. (1979). Sodium in drinking water: Information for clinical application. *South. Med. J.* **72**, 753–755.

Grollman, A. (1961). The role of salt in health and disease. *Am. J. Cardiol.* **8**, 593–602.

Laubusch, E., and McCammon, C. S. (1955). Water as a sodium source and its relation to sodium restriction therapy patient response. *Am. J. Public Health* **45**, 1337–1343.

McGovern, G. (1979). Salt and our health. *Congr. Rec.* **125**(144), 1–4.

Meneely, G. R., and Ball, C. O. T. (1958). Experimental epidemiology of chronic sodium chloride toxicity and the protective effect of potassium chloride. *Am. J. Med.* **25**, 713–725.

Meneely, G. R., and Battarbee, H. D. (1976a). High sodium-low potassium environment and hypertension. *Am. J. Cardiol.* **38**, 768–785.

Meneely, G. R., and Battarbee, H. D. (1976b). Sodium and potassium. *Nutr. Rev.* **4**, 225–235.

Meneely, G. R., Ball, C. O. T., and Youmans, J. B. (1957). Chronic sodium chloride toxicity: The protective effect of potassium chloride. *Ann. Intern. Med.* **47**, 263–273.

Mickelson, O., Makdani, D., Gill, J. L., and Franck, R. L. (1977). Sodium and potassium intakes and excretions of normal men consuming sodium chloride or a 1:1 mixture of sodium and potassium chloride. *Am. J. Clin. Nutr.* **30**, 2033–2040.

National Academy of Sciences (1980). ''Toward Healthful Diets,'' Publ. No. 0-309-03077-3. Food and Nutrition Board, Div. Biol. Sci., Assembly of Life Sciences, National Academy of Sciences—National Research Council, Washington, D.C.

Office of the Assistant Secretary for Health and Surgeon General (1979). ''Healthy People: The Surgeon General's Report on Health Promotion and Disease Prevention,'' DHEW Publ. No. (PHS) 79-55071. US Govt. Printing Office, Washington, D.C.

Ordronaux, J. (1870). ''Regimen Sanitatis Salernitarium, Code of Health of the School of Salernum,'' p. 89. Lippincott, Philadelphia, Pennsylvania.

Salt Institute (1980). ''Salt in the Diet, A Common Sense Approach. A Position Paper,'' pp. 1–4. Salt Institute, Alexandria, Virginia.

Schlierf, G., Arab, L., Schellenberg, B., Oster, P., Mordasini, R., Schmidt-Gayk, H., and Vogel, G. (1980). Salt and hypertension: Data from the Heidelberg study. *Am. J. Clin. Nutr.* **33**, 872–875.

Select Committee on GRAS Substances (1979). ''Evaluation of the Health Aspects of Sodium Chloride and Potassium Chloride as Food Ingredients,'' SCOGS-102, pp. 1–69. Fed. Am. Soc. Exp. Biol., Bethesda, Maryland.

Shank, F. R. (1980). Recent data on the amounts of sodium and potassium being consumed and future considerations for food labeling. *In* ''Sodium and Potassium in Food and Drugs'' (P. L. White and S. C. Crocco, eds.), pp. 23–32. Am. Med. Assoc., Chicago, Illinois.

Subcommittee on Review of the GRAS List (Phase II) (1972). ''A Comprehensive Survey of Industry on the Use of Food Chemicals Generally Regarded as Safe (GRAS).'' Prepared under DHEW

Contract No. FDA 70-22 by the Committee on Food Protection, Division of Biology and Agriculture. National Academy of Sciences—National Research Council, Washington, D.C.

Tobian, L. (1974). Current status of salt in hypertension. *In* "Epidemiology and Control of Hypertension" (Q. Paul, ed.), pp. 131–146. Stratton Intercontinental Medical Book Co., New York.

Tuthill, R. W., and Calabrese, E. J. (1979). Elevated sodium levels in the public drinking water as a contributor to elevated blood pressure levels in the community *Arch. Environ. Health* **34,** 197–203.

White, J. M., Wingo, J. G., Alligood, L. M., Cooper, G. R., Gutridge, J., Hydaker, W., Benack, R. T., Dening, J. W., and Taylor, F. B. (1967). Sodium ion in drinking water. I. Properties, analysis and occurrence. *J. Am. Diet. Assoc.* **50,** 32–36.

Wood, F. O. (1970). Present usage of iodized salt in the United States–Geographical differences. *In* "Summary of Conference: Iodine Nutriture in the United States," pp. 30–33. Food and Nutrition Board, National Academy of Sciences—National Research Council, Washington, D.C.

2

The Intake of Salt and a One-to-One Mixture of Sodium and Potassium Chlorides by Normal Young Men

OLAF MICKELSEN, RACHEL SCHEMMEL, AND
D. D. MAKDANI

I. CARBOHYDRATES AND HYPERTENSION

There are a few things that should be mentioned when considering the possible role of sodium in the etiology and treatment of hypertension. The first of these

19

THE ROLE OF SALT IN
CARDIOVASCULAR HYPERTENSION

relates to the interaction of the diet fed experimental animals and the sodium compound used to produce the hypertension. A causal relation between diet and hypertension probably influenced Kempner (1948) to use the rice–fruit diet in treating hypertensive patients. That premise likely was sparked by Snapper who, in his book (1965), describes his earlier work emphasizing the rarity of hypertension among the rice-eating people in eastern Asia. Subsequent work took the emphasis off the nature of the diet and put it on the low sodium content of the rice–fruit diet as being the important factor explaining its therapeutic efficacy (Dole *et al.*, 1950).

Although Kempner (1948) originally felt that rice, a carbohydrate-rich food, was of therapeutic value in treating hypertension, it was not until some years after his original work that the nature of the dietary carbohydrate was shown to influence the blood pressure of experimental animals. In one of those studies (Hall *et al.*, 1972), hypertension was produced in rats by providing one group with the sole source of water as a sucrose solution of dilute sodium chloride; another group received a similar solution except that an equal amount of glucose replaced the sucrose. The rats offered the sucrose–saline solution developed more severe hypertension than those fed the glucose–saline solution.

That the carbohydrate in the diet does influence the development of hypertension produced in experimental animals by a high intake of sodium chloride was demonstrated by Beebe *et al.* (1976). They fed different groups of weanling rats nutritionally complete rations containing either sucrose or corn starch as the carbohydrate source. These rations were the same in proximate composition as the control, grain ration. All rats were provided with a 1% sodium chloride solution for the first 9 weeks of the study; for the next 9 weeks, the salt concentration was increased to 1.5%. Throughout the study, the only fluid available to the rats was one of these salt solutions. Blood pressure increased more rapidly in the rats fed the sucrose ration than in the animals fed either the starch or grain ration. In week 18 of the study, the sucrose-fed rats had slightly higher blood pressures than the animals in the other two dietary groups. The increased blood pressure associated with large amounts of sucrose in the diet was also evident in the experiments where only distilled water and no sodium chloride therein was available to the rats, as well as in the study when the rats were offered a 2% sodium chloride solution to drink.

The absence of sodium chloride from the drinking water was associated with blood pressures which were within the normal range. However, the blood pressure of the rats fed the sucrose ration was higher ($p < 0.01$) than that of the grain-fed animals (127 ± 9 versus 109 ± 14 mm Hg). When other groups of rats were offered a 2% solution of sodium chloride for drinking purposes, the blood pressure at the end of 10 weeks again was higher among those animals fed the sucrose (178 ± 14 mm Hg) than among those fed the starch ration (150 ± 20 mm Hg). Both of these values were higher than the blood pressure of rats fed the grain ration (127 ± 20 mm Hg). Perhaps of greater significance than the actual blood pressures attained by the rats fed the different rations and receiving a 2% sodium chloride solution to drink was the mortality experience. Of the eight weanling rats initially in each group, six died in the sucrose ration group, four in the starch ration group, and only one in the grain ration group. All rats that died, in the week prior to their death, had blood pressures exceeding that of the remaining animals in the group.

These results indicate that not only does the nature of the carbohydrate in the ration influence both blood pressure and survival of hypertensive animals fed extra sodium chloride but that some other dietary component plays a very important role in protecting animals from the dire consequences of a high salt intake. This was obvious in that the blood pressure of the animals fed the purified-type rations had higher blood pressures and greater mortality than those in the group fed the grain ration. These differences occurred despite the fact that in all possible respects the proximate composition of the purified-type rations simulated that of the grain ration.

Confirmation for the observation that sucrose in the ration, with no change in sodium intake, increases the blood pressure of spontaneously hypertensive rats comes from the work of Young and Landsberg (1981). Within 1 week of adding sucrose to a "chow" ration, the blood pressure of their rats increased by an average of 14 mm Hg. An isocaloric substitution of fat for the sucrose had no effect on blood pressure.

II. FIBER AND ITS POSSIBLE ASSOCIATION WITH HYPERTENSION

At first glance, one might suggest that the purified-type rations used by Beebe *et al.* (1976) differed from the grain ration in fiber content. However, cellulose was added to the purified-type rations at a level equal to the listed fiber content of the grain ration. Despite this, there is the possibility that the fiber added to the purified-type rations might not have been added at the proper concentration and might not have had the same physiological properties as the fiber in the grain ration. The amount of fiber added to the purified-type rations may have been too low since the newer methods of fiber analyses suggest that the old method for determining crude fiber in plant foods may have underestimated the true fiber content by a factor of four to six. Under those circumstances one might suggest that the differential effects of the grain and purified-type rations might have been due to an inadequate amount of fiber in the purified-type rations.

Perhaps of equal importance is the possibility that the cellulose added in the dry state to the dry ingredients in the purified-type diets might not have had the same physiological properties as the fiber in the grain ration. The basis for that suggestion is the observation we made with a bread containing added purified cellulose. The rats that were fed a complete ration with about 85% of a high fiber bread gained only two-thirds as much weight as the animals fed a similar ration but in which ordinary bread was incorporated. Adding dry cellulose to the ordinary bread ration resulted in the same weight gain for those animals as for those fed the ordinary bread ration to which no cellulose was added. This similarity in weight gain occurred despite the fact that the ordinary bread ration contained the same kind and concentration of purified cellulose as the high fiber bread ration. Apparently, the incorporation of the cellulose into the dough, which is baked into bread, alters the physicochemical properties of the cellulose in such a way that it has different physiological properties. Only the bread made with the cellulose as an integral ingredient of the dough prior to baking increased the satiety value of the diet. That reduced the feed intake of those rats so that they gained much less weight than the animals fed the same kind of ration except that the dry cellulose was added to the dried bread after it was baked.

III. DIET AND HYPERTENSION: HUMAN OBSERVATIONS

Suggestive evidence that the components of the diet other than sodium chloride play an important role in the development of hypertension comes from a study of the diet consumed by the Japanese in Hawaii. Those individuals who had migrated from Japan to Hawaii had a high incidence of hypertension and other cardiovascular diseases (Hilker *et al.,* 1965). That observation led to a study in which weanling rats, fed a Japanese-type diet, developed more severe hypertension than the animals fed a grain-type ration which provided them with the same amount of sodium (Hilker *et al.,* 1965). The rats fed the grain-type ration received slightly more sodium than the animals fed the Japanese-type diet. Despite this, they had a lower blood pressure throughout the study year than their littermates fed the Japanese-type diet (131 $\pm$ 3.2 versus 158 $\pm$ 6.9 mm Hg; average $\pm$ standard error of the mean). The results of this study can be considered to be no more than suggestive evidence for the premise that the nature of the diet plays an important role in determining an animal's blood pressure response to the sodium chloride in the ration. This limitation stems from the fact that too many factors were varied in each experiment. One of the more important of these was the ratio of sodium to potassium, which, in the four diets used in that study, ranged from 0.9 to 7.2.

Additional suggestive support for the concept that the nature of the diet, apart from its sodium content, may play a role in the treatment of hypertension comes from work with hypertensive outpatients. They were advised to follow a diet that provided 30–50 g of fiber per day, a small amount of sodium (1.5 g per day) and, on a molar basis, about twice as much potassium (Dodson *et al.,* 1981). Of the

32 patients in the 9-month study, 25 showed such a reduction in blood pressure that they either "ceased anti-hypertensive therapy" or reduced the dose they used. Although the investigators (Dodson *et al.,* 1981) attributed the beneficial effects seen among their hypertensive patients primarily to the fiber addition, the validity of that conclusion must await further studies. Such a study should involve a control group with the only change in treatment the increase in fiber content of the diet.

IV. SODIUM AND POTASSIUM RATIO IN THE DIET

Another factor that frequently is overlooked in many epidemiological studies of hypertension is the ratio of sodium to potassium in the diets of the groups of people being studied. Individuals living in rural, predominantly agricultural areas of the southwestern Pacific probably follow a largely vegetarian-type diet made up, almost exclusively, of unprocessed plant foods. Such fare will provide the individual not only with a small amount of sodium but also with a fairly high intake of potassium. As we shall point out, potassium, to a large extent, is capable of overcoming the hypertensive effects of sodium. Furthermore, in the urban centers of the southwest Pacific area, for various reasons, the people are likely to consume more processed foods than their relatives who remain in the rural areas. Sodium chloride plays a very prominent role in many food processing techniques. That, associated with a possible increase in animal foods, at the expense of plant foods, will markedly alter the sodium to potassium ratio in the diets.

The epidemiological difference in blood pressure between rural and urban peoples in underdeveloped countries partially may be related to the nature of the salt used in seasoning their food. In many primitive cultures, as Trowell (1980) has pointed out, some peasant agricultural people with no access to sodium chloride frequently use plant ash as a condiment. The plant ash would contain a great deal more potassium than sodium and so alter, still more, the ratio of these two cations in such a way as to prevent the development of hypertension. The possible significance of an altered dietary sodium to potassium ratio in the development of hypertension was stressed by Meneely and Battarbee (1978). They stated that, "The high sodium–low potassium environment of civilized people, operating on a genetic substrate of susceptibility is the cardinal factor in the genesis and perpetuation of 'essential' hypertension."

It would appear premature to label the sodium chloride added to the diet as the primary etiological factor in hypertension, especially that occurring among people in the urban centers of underdeveloped countries. The elucidation of that problem must await answers to the role played by various dietary components in the development of hypertension. There is a possibility that the nature of the diet, as well as the stresses associated with urban living in those regions, are as important in the development of hypertension as dietary sodium or the sodium to potassium ratio.

V. HIGH SODIUM INTAKE AND DIABETES

Before leaving the subject of high levels of dietary sodium, it may be important to mention a beneficial effect of such a dietary practice. This was seen by Dr. McQuarrie and his colleagues (1936) among their juvenile diabetic patients. According to Dr. McQuarrie's version of that work, one of his nurses commented that some of their diabetic children were using very large amounts of salt on their food. Dr. McQuarrie's suggestion was to provide each child with his/her own salt shaker which should contain known amounts of sodium chloride. This would permit determining the amount of salt each patient used. Some of these diabetic children were adding as much as 90 g of sodium chloride per day to their food.

There were a number of consequences of this very high salt consumption. As one would expect, body weight increased due to the retention of salt and water. With the latter, blood pressure increased. The unexpected observation was that the glucose level in the blood and urine were restored almost to normal despite the fact there had been no change in the level of insulin injections. At that time, insulin levels were adjusted to maintain blood sugar approaching normal.

To illustrate the changes produced by such high salt intakes, it may be advisable to mention the practice of one of their subjects. This 15-year-old diabetic boy was consuming 60 g of sodium chloride per day. His body weight increased by 2.5 kg which was associated with the retention of 27 g sodium chloride during the first 2 days of the study. Thereafter, he was in equilibrium as far as the salt was concerned. His urine glucose decreased from an average control level of 73 g per day to 13 g by the end of the second day of the high salt intake. This was associated with a reduction in the fasting serum glucose from 290 to 131 mg per 100 ml of blood without any change in the insulin injections. Accompanying the high salt intake, the sodium level of the serum increased from 300 to 340 mg per 100 ml.

McQuarrie and co-workers wanted to find out whether it was the sodium or the chloride ion which was responsible for the effects related to carbohydrate metabolism. They found that both sodium bicarbonate and sodium citrate produced similar effects but their action was slightly less than that of an equivalent amount of sodium chloride. On the basis of results similar to these, it was reported that "sodium is the element which is responsible in large part for the effects observed" (McQuarrie *et al.*, 1936, p. 88).

Insofar as blood pressure was concerned, they found that a nondiabetic boy showed no increase in either systolic or diastolic pressure when he consumed 20 g of salt while the regular hospital diet was served. However, as soon as the special, low potassium diet was started, his blood pressure increased. Throughout the 9 days of the high salt intake, there were no "signs of hypoglycemia."

The differential effect of the sodium chloride when the "low" and "high" potassium diets were fed and the antagonistic reaction of potassium chloride when it was substituted for sodium chloride led to a study of the interrelation between these two cations. As a result of these studies, they concluded that "1 milli-equivalent of K is capable of antagonizing the effect of at least 3 milli-equivalents of Na, as far as the carbohydrate metabolism and blood pressure are concerned" (McQuarrie et al., 1936, p. 90).

The effect of the sodium on carbohydrate metabolism appeared to be associated with the need for insulin injections. That became evident when a diabetic girl whose condition was controlled by diet was studied. Her diet was adjusted so she excreted over 30 g of glucose in the urine every day. Neither sodium chloride nor potassium chloride supplements to the diet reduced the urinary glucose. If anything, the 25 g of potassium chloride per day increased urinary glucose to a level of 120 g per day.

The possible relation of sodium to carbohydrate metabolism was further emphasized by the work of Crabtree and Longwell (1936). They reported that when "young male rats" were fed a purified-type ration, the addition thereto of either 6.25 or 9.09% sodium chloride for 10–15 days markedly increased the liver glycogen concentration ($0.18 \pm .01$ versus $0.31 \pm .03\%$ for the 6.25% NaCl addition and $0.30 \pm .03$ versus $0.75 \pm .03\%$ for the 9.09% NaCl addition). These increases in liver glycogen occurred despite the fact that there was no change in the glycogen content of the gastrocnemius muscles. Since that work, there has been little activity in this field other than the demonstration that the sodium ion is involved in the absorption of glucose from the intestinal tract (Riklis and Quastel, 1958; Crane, 1962).

VI. SODIUM AND CARBOHYDRATE METABOLISM IN ACUTE STARVATION

Another fact that links sodium to carbohydrate metabolism is the observation that individuals doing without food for periods of 24 or more hours experience an increased sodium excretion. This naturesis was terminated very abruptly by the ingestion of as little as 50 g of glucose (Gersing and Bloom, 1962). These investigators were able to show that this increased sodium loss from the body during starvation was not associated with the action of the adrenal cortex. Aside from that, these investigators had no explanation for the observed interrelation of sodium and glucose metabolism.

VII. SODIUM AND POTASSIUM RATIO IN TREATING HYPERTENSION

The relation between sodium and potassium in the treatment of hypertension stems from an observation made by Addison (1928). As early as 1923, he found that his hypertensive patients experienced a reduction in blood pressure when they were given daily supplements of potassium chloride. That work was extended by Priddle (1931, 1962) who treated his hypertensive patients with a low salt diet supplemented with potassium citrate. Such a therapeutic procedure according to Priddle (1962) resulted, not only in a reduction in blood pressure greater than could be attributed to the low salt ration, but also in an improvement in the clinical condition and well-being of his patients.

One of the major problems associated with the use of a low sodium diet in the treatment of hypertension is the tendency for many such patients to surreptitiously add extra salt to their food. Although there are no data on that score, a study of 132 hypertensive patients indicated a relatively poor compliance with a less stringent aspect of their therapy. In that evaluation of the extent to which hypertensive patients took their prescribed pills, Hershey and co-workers (1980) reported that only 50% followed their prescribed therapy consistently.

VIII. DEVELOPMENT OF A MIXTURE OF SODIUM AND POTASSIUM CHLORIDE AS A CONDIMENT

A mixture of equal parts of sodium and potassium chlorides was developed to assist patients with hypertension to restrict their salt intake and to provide a possible preventive condiment to those individuals who have a genetic and/or environmental tendency to hypertension. That work was started since most of the salt substitutes contain potassium chloride which, to most individuals, has a very bitter flavor. However, it was observed that the presence of sodium chloride together with the potassium chloride masked the bitter flavor of the potassium compound and enhanced the saltiness of the mixture to the point where it was as salty as the same weight of sodium chloride (Frank and Mickelsen, 1969).

That work was initiated by having a taste panel of normal individuals consume the same noon meal each day for a week. Each day of that period, the food was prepared with a condiment that had a different ratio of sodium chloride to potassium chloride. The salt on the table, available for seasoning the food, had the same ratio of these two salts as was used in the food preparation. The latter included the butter, which because it had a different salt mixture added to it each day, appeared slightly different in shape from packaged butter.

In a random manner, the condiments used during that week had sodium chloride at levels of 100, 80, 70, or 40%; in each case, the remainder was potassium chloride. The prepared food served each day contained the same amount of the mixture, assigned for that day, as was used when ordinary salt was the seasoning agent. The panelists consumed about 2.25 g of the condiment with no difference for the various mixtures. The foods incorporated into the menu were those that would likely be salted before eating such as celery stalks, radishes, lettuce, and chicken broth. Initially, the panelists were given no explanation as to the purpose of the study. On its completion, they were asked what might have been the object of the study. Since the butter served each day had a different shape than packaged butter and the investigator was interested in cardiovascular diseases, all panelists responded that different spreads were being tested. No one commented on the seasoning agents used throughout that week.

On the basis of the preceding study, extensive tests were performed with aqueous solutions of various mixtures of sodium and potassium chlorides. This procedure was chosen since the aqueous solutions of the salts should enhance any bitter or unpleasant taste to a greater extent than would be apparent when the mixture was incorporated into a food. Of the 72 panelists, 67% reported that a 0.064% potassium chloride solution tasted bitter. However, the addition of 0.1% sodium chloride to that solution eliminated the bitter flavor for all but 11% of the panelists.

The addition of the sodium chloride to the potassium chloride not only masked the bitter flavor of the latter but also enhanced the saltiness of the former. This was evident when solutions of 0.10, 0.15, or 0.20% sodium chloride were supplemented with potassium chloride. Most of the panelists rated the solutions containing the added potassium chloride saltier than the control solution. That was especially true as the concentration of the potassium chloride in the solution approached or exceeded that of the sodium chloride (Frank and Mickelsen, 1969).

The evidence suggests that about 10% of normal individuals can detect a slight, bitter flavor when the 1:1 mixture of sodium chloride and potassium chloride is used in or on foods. The most frequent comment has been that the bitter flavor is apparent when this mixture is used to season fried eggs. For other foods and for most people, this mixture can be used as ordinary salt both in preparing the food and in seasoning it to taste. The amount of the mixture that is needed for such purposes is exactly the same as the weight of ordinary salt. This means that for every gram of ordinary salt used, it can be replaced by an equal weight of the mixture, thus reducing the sodium chloride added to the diet to 0.5 g.

The physical properties of the two chlorides make them ideally suited for combination in such a mixture. By visual inspection, it is impossible to distinguish between ordinary salt and the mixture. The crystals of both salts are colorless, transparent, and cubic in form with similar refractive indices. The specific gravities of the two crystalline compounds are so close to each other that the mixture will not separate during storage or transportation. Both salts are soluble to almost the same extent in water. The same anticaking agents work equally well with the mixture and ordinary salt. The mixture can be iodized under the same conditions as ordinary salt (Frank and Mickelsen, 1969).

A. Hams Salted with Ordinary Salt or the Mixture

Foods that ordinarily contain large amounts of salt can be prepared with the 1:1 mixture, thus reducing the sodium content very appreciably. That became evident when fresh hams were cured in the one case with ordinary salt and in the other with the sodium chloride–potassium chloride mixture. A third group of hams was cured with potassium chloride. Those hams tasted so bitter that the panelists, using the triad technique of evaluating the food, complained of being unable to properly evaluate the hams when the very bitter sample was included (Smith *et al.*, 1970).

Although the taste panel results suggest that the hams cured with ordinary salt were superior to those prepared with the mixture, the panelists indicated after the study was over that if they were offered the hams as part of a meal, they would have difficulty in detecting any difference in their taste. When offered a choice of the two hams in the taste test, the panelists, on 71% of the occasions, preferred the ham cured with ordinary salt. On 23% of the occasions, they either preferred the ham prepared with the 1:1 mixture or rated the two hams as equally good. On 6% of the occasions, the two kinds of ham were rated equally bad.

It is impossible to explain why such a large percentage of the panelists detected a difference between the two hams. This becomes more difficult when it is appreciated that the overall ratings for the two hams were essentially the same. The panelists rated each sample tasted for color, aroma, moisture, tenderness, texture, flavor, and acceptability.

The only plausible explanation for the variation in the responses of the taste panelists is that the 1:1 mixture produced a slightly different flavor in the hams during curing than ordinary salt. This is based on the panelists' responses that they preferred the hams cured with ordinary salt because of flavor or taste (Smith *et al.*, 1970).

The hams made with the 1:1 mixture had only half as much sodium as those cured with ordinary salt. Analyses of samples from the three hams with ordinary salt indicated their sodium content as 1.35, 1.08, and 1.08%, with an average of 1.2%. Those hams cured with the 1:1 mixture had 0.54, 0.46, and 0.59%, for an average of 0.53% sodium. The mixture also increased the potassium content of the ham by a factor of 3.2, thus further increasing its tendency to provide a more favorable ratio in the diet of these two cations (Smith *et al.*, 1970).

B. Intake of Salt and the 1:1 Mixture by Normal Young Men

A number of years ago, the 1:1 mixture was mistakenly taken for a salt substitute by two cardiac patients for whom a low sodium diet had been prescribed. The crises that developed in them led to a hearing with the Food and Drug Administration. At that meeting, it was suggested that the label of the 1:1 mixture should indicate that it was not a salt substitute and should not be used by patients "on sodium or potassium restricted diets unless approved by a physician."

It was stated at that meeting that when the 1:1 mixture was used, twice as much of it as ordinary salt had to be used to produce the same degree of saltiness. This statement was based on the reported experience of a housewife. She had compared the 1:1 mixture with a brand of ordinary salt whose crystal size was markedly different from that of the mixture. The saltiness of sodium chloride is related to crystal size as is demonstrated by the large crystals of sodium chloride used on pretzels.

That claim resulted in another study to determine how much salt a group of normal college men use. For that, 26 men were fed a normal ration for 8 days. During that time each subject's salt usage at the table was measured. In addition, 24-hr urine samples were analyzed for sodium. From these data, the 20 subjects with the highest salt intake were chosen for further study. The subjects were paired on the basis of their salt usage and one of each pair was randomly assigned to either the regular salt or the 1:1 mixture group (Mickelsen et al., 1977).

During the 4-week diet study, unprocessed foods were used so as to reduce, as much as possible, the amount of sodium in the basal diet. Two different kinds of bread and butter were prepared: one with regular salt and the other with the 1:1 mixture. It was desired to decrease the sodium in the basal diet so that maximal usage of ordinary salt and the 1:1 mixture would be encouraged. Again, the seasoning used by each subject at the table was measured. Every subject had to eat all of the basal diet which provided about 2500 kcal. To maintain weight, the subjects could consume, ad libitum, salt-free cookies and candies.

The average condiment usage by the subjects for the 28-day period averaged 5.55 g for those in the ordinary salt group with a range from 1.52 to 14.89 g. Those subjects receiving the 1:1 mixture used an average of 4.97 g with a range from 2.45 to 7.43 g. Throughout the study, there was no consistent trend in condiment usage by the subjects in either group.

The similarity in condiment usage by the subjects in the two groups resulted in a marked reduction in total sodium intake for the group using the 1:1 mixture. Those subjects who used ordinary salt secured 1.53 g from their food and 2.2 g from their salt shakers for an average total intake of 3.7 g of sodium. That was 1.8 times as much sodium as the subjects using the 1:1 mixture. The latter received 1.0 g sodium from their diet and 1.0 g from the condiment used at the table for a total of 2.0 g. The lower sodium in their food resulted from the use of the 1:1 mixture in preparing their bread and butter. The total average potassium intake was 4.0 g/day for the subjects using the regular salt and 6.0 g for those using the 1:1 mixture.

Compared to the preliminary 8-day period, those subjects, who, during the main part of the study, were assigned to the ordinary salt group, used an average of 3.07 g salt for seasoning. That increased to 5.55 g/day when the low salt diet was fed. The corresponding values for the subjects who were transferred to the 1:1 mixture were 3.07 and 4.95 g. With the change in the diet, every subject but one increased his condiment usage. The higher condiment usage by the subjects during the 28-day period was due to the fact that, during that period, the foods were prepared without any added salt. The foods chosen for that dietary period were those that would ordinarily be associated with a reasonably high salt content but which could be purchased in the unprocessed form.

Thus, the 1:1 mixture is used by the average individual in no greater amount for seasoning food than ordinary salt. As a result, the sodium intake associated with the seasoning agent is reduced by 50% and the overall potassium in the diet increased by about 150%.

REFERENCES

Addison, W. L. T. (1928). Observations on the management of hypertension. *Can. Med. Assoc. J.* **18,** 281–285.

Beebe, C. G., Schemmel, R., and Mickelsen, O. (1976). Blood pressure of rats as affected by diet and concentration of NaCl in drinking water. *Proc. Soc. Exp. Biol. Med.* **151,** 395–399.

Crabtree, D. G., and Longwell, B. B. (1936). Effect of excessive dietary sodium chloride upon liver and muscle glycogen in the rat. *Proc. Soc. Exp. Biol. Med.* **34,** 705–707.

Crane, R. K. (1962). Hypothesis for mechanism of intestinal active transport of sugars. *Fed. Proc., Fed. Am. Soc. Exp. Biol.* **21,** 891–895.

Dodson, P. M., Humphreys, D. M., Patrick, O., and Cox, E. V. (1981). Dietary fibre, sodium, and blood pressure. *Proc. Nutr. Soc.* **40,** 42A.

Dole, V. P., Dahl, L. K., Cotzias, G. C., Eder, H. A., and Krebs, M. E. (1950). Dietary treatment of hypertension. Clinical and metabolic studies of patients on the rice-fruit diet. *J. Clin. Invest.* **29,** 1189–1206.

Frank, R. L., and Mickelsen, O. (1969). Sodium-potassium chloride mixtures as table salt. *Am. J. Clin. Nutr.* **22,** 464–470.

Gersing, A., and Bloom, W. L. (1962). Glucose stimulation of salt retention in patients with aldosterone inhibition. *Metab., Clin. Exp.* **11,** 329–336.

Hall, C. E., Ayachi, S., and Hall, O. (1972). Salt appetite and hypertensive response to salt and to deoxycorticosterone in Sprague-Dawley and Long-Evans rats. *Tex. Rep. Biol. Med.* **30,** 155–162.

Hershey, J. C., Morton, B. G., Davis, J. B., and Reichgott, M. J. (1980). Patient compliance with antihypertensive medication. *Am. J. Public Health* **70,** 1081–1089.

Hilker, D. M., Wenkam, N. S., and Lichton, I. J. (1965). Blood pressure elevation and renal pathology in rats fed simulated Japanese diets. *J. Nutr.* **87,** 371–384.

Kempner, W. (1948). Treatment of hypertensive vascular disease with rice diet. *Am. J. Med.* **4,** 545–577.

McQuarrie, I., Thompson, W. H., and Anderson, J. A. (1936). Effects of excessive ingestion of sodium and potassium salts on carbohydrate metabolism and blood pressure in diabetic children. *J. Nutr.* **11,** 77–101.

Meneely, G. R., and Battarbee, H. D. (1978). High sodium-low potassium environment and hypertension. *Am. J. Cardiol.* **38,** 768–785.

Mickelsen, O., Makdani, D., Gill, J. L., and Frank, R. L. (1977). Sodium and potassium intakes and excretions of normal men consuming sodium chloride or a 1:1 mixture of sodium and potassium chlorides. *Am. J. Clin. Nutr.* **30,** 2033–2040.

Priddle, W. W. (1931). Observations on the management of hypertension. *Can. Med. Assoc. J.* **25,** 5–8.

Priddle, W. W. (1962). Hypertension: Sodium and potassium studies. *Can. Med. Assoc. J.* **86,** 1–9.

Riklis, E., and Quastel, J. H. (1958). Effects of cations on sugar absorption by isolated surviving guinea pig intestine. *Can. J. Biochem. Physiol.* **36,** 347–362.

Smith, E. H., Mickelsen, O., Pearson, A. M., and Frank, R. L. (1970). Taste panel evaluation of hams cured with sodium chloride and a 1:1 mixture of sodium and potassium chlorides. Unpublished report.

Snapper, I. (1965). ''Chinese Lessons to Western Medicine,'' p. 170. Grune & Stratton, New York.

Trowell, H. C. (1980). Salt and hypertension. *Lancet* **2,** 88.

Young, J. B., and Landsberg, L. (1981). Effect of oral sucrose on blood pressure in the spontaneously hypertensive rat. *Metab., Clin. Exp.* **30,** 421–424.

3

The Influence of Elevated Levels of Sodium in Drinking Water on Elementary and High School Students in Massachusetts

EDWARD J. CALABRESE AND ROBERT W. TUTHILL

33

THE ROLE OF SALT IN
CARDIOVASCULAR HYPERTENSION

Copyright © 1982 by Academic Press, Inc.
All rights of reproduction in any form reserved.
ISBN 0-12-267280-1

I. INTRODUCTION

Attempts to derive a sodium standard as a result of the National Safe Drinking Water Act of 1974 have been hampered by a dearth of definitive human population studies demonstrating the effects on health of sodium in the drinking water. For this reason, the U.S. Environmental Protection Agency did not propose a maximal concentration limit for sodium in drinking water (Federal Register, 1975). The American Heart Association (1957) implied that a limit of 20 mg Na/liter be adopted as a standard in order to afford protection to those individuals with heart or kidney ailments who require a low sodium diet. Similarly, the EPA has recently recommended that a level of 20 mg Na/liter be a goal for public water systems when proposing a requirement for monitoring sodium levels in water supplies (Federal Register, 1979).

Nearly all of the previous studies of the relationship between hypertension and sodium intake have considered the contribution of sodium from food rather than from water. This is understandable in light of the fact that water contributes from less than 0.15% to 9.0% of the total sodium an individual consumes with the important exception of persons on a restricted salt diet (Schroeder, 1974; American Heart Association, 1957).

The present paper represents a summary of the past 3 years of research, which has been designed to assess whether elevated levels of sodium in the community drinking water could bring about an increase in the blood pressure (BP) levels of elementary (third grade) and high school (tenth grade) students.

II. TENTH GRADE STUDY

The authors compared BP distributions among students in two geographically contiguous Massachusetts communities markedly similar with regard to size, income, education, and recent rate of growth (Calabrese and Tuthill, 1977; Tuthill and Calabrese, 1979). One community had a low concentration of sodium (8 mg/liter) in the public drinking water while the other had a considerably higher level (107 mg/liter). These differences in sodium concentrations have existed for the past 17 years (Table I).

A. Methods

The tenth grade class of the public high schools in the two communities was chosen as the population to be surveyed. Of approximately 850 tenth grade students in the schools, 606 obtained permission to be screened, for an overall response rate of approximately 67 and 76% of the high and low Na groups,

TABLE I

Socioeconomic Comparisons of the High and Low Sodium Communities[a]

Characteristics	High sodium community	Low sodium community
1970 population	low 20,000s	low 20,000s
Percent population change 1960–1970	17.0	16.3
Median family income	$13,434	$13,281
Median school years	12.7	12.5
Percent black	0.4	0.7
Percent foreign born	6.0	5.7
Water sodium level (1976)	107 mg/liter	8 mg/liter

[a] 1970 U.S. Census data.

respectively. In the high sodium community 300 students participated and 306 participated in the low sodium community.

The screenings were scheduled such that 150 students were screened on each of the four days, two successive days in one community and on the same two days of the week the following week in the second community. Thus, the screenings were conducted equally on mornings and afternoons in each town.

Four highly skilled and carefully standardized nurses took the BP of the students, with three working at a time on a 45 min rotation. The same nurses took the BP readings at both schools on all 4 days. The aneroid manometers used were standardized twice each day. In order to minimize the effects of recent food intake and exercise on BP, the students were screened at least 45 min after a meal and they did not attend gym glasses at least 1 hr before being screened. The students were brought quietly to the screening area and spent at least 6 min seated, completing a questionnaire, before proceeding to the BP stations where they progressed to each of the nurses for a casual seated BP reading on the left arm. Each successive nurse was blind to the previous reading for each person. Thus, three readings were obtained for each student, and these measurements were averaged to provide an estimate of the BP for each individual. The pulse rate for each child was recorded by the nurse at the first station.

The questionnaire completed by each student was designed to provide information in regard to variables known to affect BP. If any of these factors differed significantly between the two communities they could then be controlled in the analysis. Thus, information was obtained on age, height, weight, length of residence in town, smoking history, length of time since last cigarette and last meal, recent excessive weight gain or loss, whether on a low sodium diet, eating habits in relation to salty items, amount of community water drunk either plain or

interpretation of the original study. However, the results indicated elevated concentration of sodium in drinking water to be the prime explanatory factor in the differences in BP distribution between the two towns.

III. THIRD GRADE REPLICATION STUDY

A third grade study in the same two communities was carried out to confirm the earlier findings by possibly replicating the tenth grade differences and to rule out potentially confounding variables in the first study, such as possible differential illicit drug use in the two high school populations.

A. Methods

There were seven elementary schools in each community with 384 third graders in the high sodium community and 301 third graders in the low sodium community. In the high sodium community 346 out of 384 children were screened, for a net participation rate of 90.1 and 87.0%, respectively.

The screenings were conducted in fourteen sessions over eight school days within a 2-week period. Careful attention was paid to ensure that the towns were screened equally on mornings and afternoons to eliminate diurnal variation in BP as a possible confounding variable. In each town, four schools were screened in the morning and three in the afternoon. This resulted in 65.2% of the high sodium community children being screened in the morning, compared to 69.7% in the low sodium community.

Five nurses whose blood pressure measuring technique had been carefully standardized were available to do the screening. The same four nurses did the screening at eleven of the sessions with the fifth nurse substituting for one of the other four during three of the sessions. Three children at a time were screened at three different stations, each child moving from station to station, so that three casual BP readings on the left arm using a mercury sphygmomanometer at eye level were recorded for each child. Each reading was taken by a different nurse who was blind to the readings of colleagues. The nurses rotated through the stations on a time schedule, with only three of the four working at a time, one at each station, with pulse rate recorded by the nurse working at the first station, procedures similar to those previously described.

The children were brought to the screening area (usually a gym, auditorium, extra room, or school nurse's office) slowly and quietly, and were seated quietly for several minutes before being screened. No gym classes were scheduled in the hour prior to the screening, and meals were consumed at least 45 min before the screening. Age, height, and weight were recorded from current school records. In both towns, height and weight had been measured in the immediately preceding months by the school nurses. The school scales were checked for accuracy at the time of screening, and all weighed to within 1 lb of a 40 lb weight (which approximated the weight of these children).

Additional information on factors related to BP was obtained for each child from a short questionnaire completed by the parents in conjunction with the permission slip. The questionnaire provided information on family history of high BP, source of drinking water, length of residence in town, medications being taken by the child which may affect BP, infant feeding habits, and the educational level and occupation of the main wage earner in the family. In addition, each child was asked to complete a 24-hr dietary diary to be used to assess sodium, potassium, and calcium intakes. Again, the three BP readings for each child were combined to form an average reading on which the following analyses were based.

As in the tenth grade study, a subset of 100 of the individuals from each community were asked to provide household water samples. In addition, each child was asked to fill out a 24-hr dietary diary which was begun in school after lunch with the teacher's help and completed at home with the parents' aid. The records indicated the portion size, whether the food was fresh, frozen, or canned, the quantity of salt added in cooking, and the amount and type of liquid consumed. The diaries were obtained several weeks after the blood pressures were recorded.

B. Results

The results for third graders have supported the original high school findings; there was a statistically significant difference in mean BP between the two communities, for both boys and girls, for systolic and diastolic BP. The mean systolic and diastolic BP for boys from the high and low sodium communities was 101.3/56.3 and 98.0/53.7 mm Hg, respectively. This represented a difference in systolic BP of 3.3 mm Hg ($p = 0.001$) and a 2.6 mm Hg difference in mean diastolic BP ($p = 0.032$). The difference in mean systolic and diastolic BP was also significant between the girls. The high sodium community girls' mean BP was 97.9/58.1 mm Hg, and it was 95.3/54.5 mm Hg among the low sodium community girls. The resulting systolic and diastolic BP differences were 2.6 and 3.6 mm Hg, which were statistically significant at $p = 0.023$ and $p = 0.002$, respectively.

As with the tenth graders, the upshifts occurred along the entire distribution of systolic and diastolic BP for the third graders from the high sodium community relative to the low sodium community third graders for both boys and girls (Fig. 2). The upshift was least marked for systolic BP for girls and more distinct for systolic BP for boys. However, the pattern was completely consistent for all four comparisons. When testing the statistical significance of the difference in the two

Edward J. Calabrese and Robert W. Tuthill

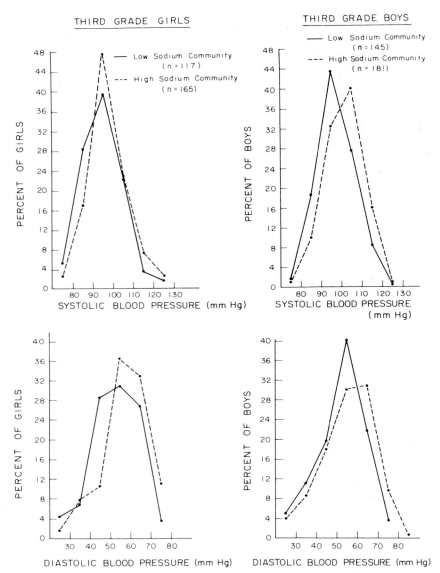

Fig. 2. Systolic and diastolic blood pressure distributions by sex for third grade students in communities with high versus low sodium levels in the drinking water.

distributions for each of the four comparisons, the female systolic distributions did not differ significantly between the two towns at $p = 0.14$. The female diastolic comparison and the male systolic and diastolic comparisons revealed statistically significant differences by community of at least $p = 0.008$.

These results are very similar in pattern to the differences found in the screening of the tenth grade populations of these two communities. Clearly the consistent pattern of the results for both sexes for both systolic and diastolic BP among the third graders, and their consistency with the earlier tenth grade findings, lends importance to these results in conjunction with their statistical significance.

The statistical assessment of these data upheld the initial findings. In fact, the statistical adjustment for differences in the confounding characteristics resulted in an adjusted difference in mean BP between the two towns which was even greater than when these factors were uncontrolled. That is, the net impact of adjusting for differences in height, weight, and socioeconomic status resulted in a larger difference in systolic and diastolic BP between the two towns, for both boys and girls.

The resultant adjusted differences were all statistically significant. The difference in diastolic BP between high and low sodium community boys had an associated significance level of $p = 0.014$. For the difference in systolic BP between both high and low sodium community boys and girls and for the difference in diastolic BP between high and low sodium community girls, the associated significance level was $p \leq 0.001$.

Dietary Diaries

Codable 24-hr dietary diaries were collected from 312 (90.2%) of the children in the high sodium community and 240 (91.6%) of those in the low sodium community. Table II indicates the mean dietary intake of sodium, potassium, and calcium and shows the sodium/potassium ratio for the four sex/community groups. The dietary sodium intake is about 13% higher and the potassium intake about 8% higher in the high sodium community compared to the low sodium community for both sexes. Calcium intake is about 20% higher for males and 16% higher for females, whereas the sodium/potassium ratio is 5% higher for the males and about 2–3% higher for females in the high sodium community.

In absolute terms, the high sodium community pupils' intake is about one-third of a gram more sodium per day, one-quarter of a gram more potassium, and one-fifth of a gram more calcium. These figures do not include the sodium in the drinking water consumed either directly or when mixed with orange juice concentrate, Kool Aid, etc. Data on liquid consumption collected at a later time indicated that the third grade high sodium pupils consumed about one liter of tap water per day, obtaining 120 mg of sodium per day from this source. Assuming a similar amount of water consumption in the low sodium community, the children there would receive 8 mg of sodium per day from their drinking water. If the

TABLE II

The Mean Dietary Intake of Sodium, Potassium, and Calcium

	High sodium community	Low sodium community	Difference		p value (2-tail)
			Amount	%	
Males[a]					
Sodium (mg)	2904	2557	347	13.6	0.004
Potassium (mg)	3239	2995	244	8.1	0.056
Calcium (mg)	1225	1023	202	19.7	0.001
Na/K ratio	0.958	0.914	0.044	4.8	0.366
Females[b]					
Sodium (mg)	2851	2523	328	13.0	0.015
Potassium (mg)	3036	2804	232	8.3	0.054
Calcium (mg)	1152	991	161	16.2	0.002
Na/K ratio	1.000	0.976	0.024	2.5	0.610

[a] High sodium community, $n = 160$; low sodium community, $n = 130$.
[b] High sodium community, $n = 152$; low sodium community, $n = 110$.

sodium obtained from water is added to both communities' total dietary intake, then about one-quarter of the excess sodium intake in the high sodium community is derived from this source: 24.4% for males (112/459 mg) and 25.5% for females (112/440 mg).

Evaluation of the drinking water for heavy metal constituents known to affect BP did not reveal any consistent difference of biological significance other than the originally defined differences in sodium values.

IV. BOTTLED WATER STUDY: PRELIMINARY FINDINGS

A. Methods

An experimental study was initiated to provide a more comprehensive test of the hypothesized relationship between the concentration of sodium in drinking water and BP. Specifically, the concentration of sodium in drinking water was reduced in a population of fourth graders for a 3-month period to see if this would result in a decrease in BP.

Participation was solicited from the families of the fourth grade children in the high sodium community whose parents had consented to their participation in the previous year's study among the third graders. For 3 months the cooperating families were instructed to use regularly the bottled water for all of the children's drinking water and for the preparation of foods and beverages. Additionally, bottled water was provided in the classrooms to serve the drinking needs of the children while at school. No control was exerted over the preparation of school lunches.

Children were matched by triads on the basis of sex, school, and baseline BP. The members of the triads thus formed were then randomly assigned to the three water groups with one member of each triad per water group. Participating children and their families, the school personnel, and the nurses recording BP were blind as to the type of bottled water being used by each child.

The three water groups were: (1) those receiving water taken directly from the public distribution system of their own high Na (110 mg/liter) community; (2) those receiving water taken directly from the public distribution system of the low Na community (8 mg/liter) with NaCl added to the 110 mg/liter level characteristic of the high Na community water; and (3) those receiving water taken directly from the public distribution system of the low Na community (8 mg/liter). These three groups made it possible to assess whether any reduction in BP was related to differences in sodium levels or to differences in other unknown characteristics of the waters.

The water was bottled and delivered to the individual homes and schools every 2 weeks during the study. Insuring a high standard of water quality was an important consideration throughout the study. The range of sodium concentrations in the water received by the three groups was monitored for every batch during the study and averaged 110, 110, and 9 mg/liter, respectively, with little variation.

Monitoring of BP occurred on a biweekly basis. A baseline BP was obtained the week before water use was changed and was used for the initial matching of triads. Six subsequent screenings followed, at 2-week intervals, for the 12-week duration of the project.

Screening procedures were standardized among the seven schools. As in the earlier studies, at each screening the children proceeded through three stations with his/her pulse being recorded by the nurse at the first station, and a casual seated BP on the left arm being taken at each station with a mercury sphygmomanometer. For purposes of statistical analysis, the three BP readings for each student were averaged.

In addition to regularly monitoring BP, first morning urine specimens and 2-day diet records were collected first before beginning the bottled water usage, and monthly thereafter for the 3 months. The urine specimens were analyzed for sodium and potassium levels. The diet records are being analyzed for levels of sodium, potassium, and calcium ingested at each meal.

Further data collected on each child included height and weight changes, changes in dietary habits (particularly salt use) over the study period, how frequently the child ate the school lunch, and the socioeconomic status of the family

as defined by education and occupation of the principal wage earner. The questionnaire information gathered during the previous year provided data on the
length of residence of the children in the town, family history of high BP, and the
infant feeding habits regarding breast milk versus a formula preparation, commercially or home prepared solid foods, and the age at which solid food intake
was instituted. In addition, parents were asked to complete a questionnaire at 2-
week intervals reporting the extent to which their children were adhering to the
bottled water regimen.

B. Results

Of the 353 eligible children, some 170 families (48%) agreed to participate in
the study. During the course of study, six of these 170 families (or 4.5%)
withdrew. The data analysis is based on 51 complete triads from the 56 original
triads (or 91%). Among these pupils there were 14 individuals missing one of
the six follow-up BPs for which a substitution was made of the mean of the BP

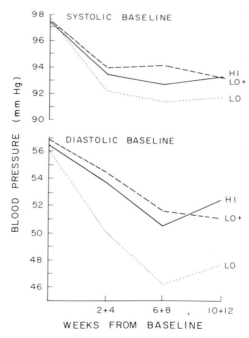

Fig. 3.   Systolic and diastolic blood pressure of 25 triads of girls at baseline and at combined
follow-up weeks, adjusted for weight and pulse, by treatment group. HI, high Na community water
(110 mg/liter); LO+, low Na community water plus Na (110 mg/liter); LO, low Na community water
(8 mg/liter).

readings on either side. For all analyses, individual BP was the average of the three BP's taken at each sitting.

Figure 3 illustrates the results for the 25 triads of girls. In this graph pairs of biweekly values were averaged as monthly values. For both systolic and diastolic BP the low (LO) sodium water group shows a consistently greater decline in BP when compared to the other two high Na groups. In contrast, the response of boys was nil as can be seen in Fig. 4 with monthly averages.

In Table III the experience of the girls is examined more completely showing the amount of difference in BP between the three water condition groups for the three monthly follow-up periods. The low sodium group had the consistently higher BP decline in all follow-up periods, ranging from 1.7 to 2.3 mm Hg for systolic BP and from 3.4 to 4.6 mm Hg for diastolic BP. All the p values for the difference of means test were significant at $p \leq 0.10$. In the case of the six follow-up periods over half the p values were significant at $p \leq 0.10$. But the likelihood of all six follow-up period readings being consistently lower was 0.0156.

The final statistical procedure was a two-way analysis of covariance for re-

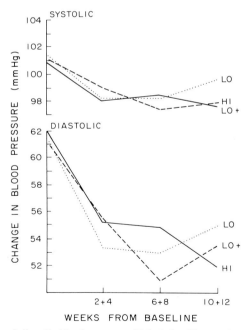

Fig. 4. Systolic and diastolic blood pressure of 26 triads of boys at baseline and at combined follow-up weeks, adjusted for weight and pulse, by treatment group. HI, high Na community water (110 mg/liter); LO+, low Na community water plus Na (110 mg/liter); LO, low Na community water (8 mg/liter).

TABLE III

Mean Decline in Systolic and Diastolic Blood Pressure (mm Hg) of the Treatment Groups for the Follow-Up Periods Combined (Girls)

Group	Baseline	Follow-up period (weeks)		
		2 + 4	6 + 8	10 + 12
Systolic				
High	97.5	−3.9	−4.7	−3.8
Low[+]	97.6	−3.5	−3.4	−4.2
Low	97.7	−5.4	−6.3	−5.9
Diastolic				
High	56.4	−2.6	−5.8	−3.9
Low+	56.9	−2.3	−5.2	−5.7
Low	56.1	−5.3	−9.8	−8.4

peated measures controlling for the confounders weight and pulse for girls. If six follow-up periods are used, the p for systolic BP was .05 and diastolic BP 0.01. For the combined three follow-up periods the p for systolic BP was 0.08 and for diastolic BP 0.01.

In regard to other potential confounders, there were no significant differences between boys and girls or among water groups within sex categories. Dietary data are still being coded and are not yet available.

In summary, the female data seem to indicate a sensitivity of BP to reduction of small amounts of Na in the drinking water. However, the male data do not show a similar effect. In the tenth grade study females in the high Na community showed a higher shift in BP than males did. Yet the relatively large reduction in BP for the small reduction in Na in drinking water in this study still seems somewhat surprising.

C. Future Studies

Subsequent investigations have continued to examine in several ways the link between the elevated levels of sodium in drinking water and increased BP. Recent findings in our laboratory have revealed that low sodium vegetables cooked in drinking water with elevated levels of sodium showed a marked increase in total sodium content. Consumption of the three vegetables in common amounts per day after being soaked in water with 100 ppm or 250 ppm would contribute an additional 40 and 96 mg Na/day, respectively. If a commonly recommended cooking method of adding salt to the water were followed, the total amount of sodium taken up would be 1000 mg.

We are presently evaluating whether consumption of sodium from drinking water differentially affects BP in adolescents as compared with a similar quantity of sodium from food.

Finally, the original "high" sodium community is planning to reduce their current sodium levels of approximately 110–120 mg/liter to about 30 mg/liter. This offers a truly unique opportunity to evaluate the effects on the community of such an intervention and should provide extremely valuable information concerning the effects of elevated levels of sodium in drinking water on human health.

V. SUMMARY

Epidemiologic investigations in Massachusetts have revealed that the BP of third and tenth grade students from a community with 110 mg Na/liter in the drinking water was significantly upshifted as compared to similarly aged students from a closely matched, geographically contiguous control community with only 8 mg Na/liter. In addition, preliminary findings of the bottled water study in the high sodium community revealed that reducing the sodium content from 110 to 10 mg/liter over a 12 week period significantly reduced the BP of fourth grade girls but did not affect the boys similarly. In light of the multifactorial origins of differential blood pressure levels between individuals and groups, one must be cautious in the interpretation of these findings even though careful statistical analysis has effectively eliminated many of the potentially confounding variables in these studies. It is hoped that ongoing studies addressing the relationships of dietary sodium consumption and exposure to sodium via drinking water will provide more definitive conclusions in this area.

ACKNOWLEDGMENTS

The preliminary findings of the original Tenth Grade study were published by Calabrese and Tuthill (1977) followed by a more comprehensive report (Tuthill and Calabrese, 1979). A brief summary of the Tenth and Third Grade reports were published in the Proceedings of the Annual Conference of the American Water Works Association held in June, 1979. A detailed presentation of the Third Grade study will be published in the American Journal of Public Health, May, 1981. Preliminary findings from the bottled water study were presented at the June 1980 meeting of the Society for Epidemiologic Research. A similar version of this paper is included in the proceedings of the *Drinking Water and Supply* Conference held in Amsterdam, August 1980, and which will be published in *Science and the Total Environment*.

We would like to acknowledge the overall efforts of our Research Associates, Janelle Klar and Thomas Sieger, who have been crucial to the success of this project. This research was supported by the Health Effects Research Laboratory of the United States Environmental Protection Agency, Cincinnati, Ohio (Grant #R-805612).

REFERENCES

American Heart Association (1957). "Your 500 Milligram Diet." Am. Heart Assoc., New York.

Calabrese, E. J., and Tuthill, R. W. (1977). Elevated blood pressure and high sodium levels in the public drinking water. *Arch. Environ. Health* **32**, 200–202.

Calabrese, E. J., and Tuthill, R. W. (1978). Elevated blood pressure and community drinking water characteristics. *J. Environ. Sci. Health, Part A* **A13**(10), 781–802.

Code of Federal Regulations (1979). Standards of quality bottled water. Title 21, Part 103. *Fed. Regist.* **35**, 50–54.

Federal Register (1975). National interim primary drinking water regulations. *Fed. Regist.* **49**, 59576–59577.

Federal Register (1979). Proposed regulations. *Fed. Regist.* **44**, 140.

Fries, E. D. (1976). Salt, volume, and the prevention of hypertension. *Circulation* **53**, 589–595.

National Center for Health Statistics (1977). Blood pressure levels of persons 6–74 years, United States. *Vital and Health Statistics, Ser. II. No. 203.* DHEW Publ. No. (HRA) 78-1648.

National Heart, Lung, and Blood Institute (1977). Task force on blood pressure control in children. *Pediatrics* **59**(5), Suppl., Part II.

Oberman, A., Lane, N. E., and Harlan, W. R. (1967). Trends in systolic blood pressure in the thousand aviator cohort over a twenty-four year period. *Circulation* **26**, 812–828.

Schroeder, H. A. (1974). The role of trace elements in cardiovascular diseases. *Med. Clin. North Am.* **58**, 381–396.

Silverburg, D. S., Van Nostrand, C., Juchli, B., Smith, E. S. O., and Van Dorsser, E. (1975). Screening for hypertension in a high school population. *Can. Med. Assoc. J.* **113**, 103–108.

Smith, W. M. (1977). Epidemiology of hypertension. *Med. Clin. North Am.* **61**, 467–486.

Swartz, H., and Leitch, C. J. (1975). Differences in mean adolescent blood pressure by age, sex, ethnic origin, obesity and familial tendency. *J. Sch. Health* **45**(2), 76–82.

Tuthill, R. W., and Calabrese, E. J. (1979). Elevated sodium levels in public drinking water as a contributor to elevated blood pressure levels in the community. *Arch. Environ. Health.* **34**(4), 197–203.

4

Studies of Blood Pressure and Dietary Sodium Intake in Children in Semirural Southern United States: The Bogalusa Heart Study

GERALD S. BERENSON, ANTONIE W. VOORS,
GAIL C. FRANK, AND LARRY S. WEBBER

49

THE ROLE OF SALT IN
CARDIOVASCULAR HYPERTENSION

It is generally recognized that the current high incidence of coronary heart disease, cerebrovascular accidents, and congestive heart failure in the United States is caused in part by essential hypertension. Evidence is increasing that control of hypertension will reduce such morbid events by the early recognition and regular treatment of mild hypertension (Hypertension Detection and Follow-Up Program Cooperative Group, 1979). It is logical to assume that prevention of these serious complications would be even more successful if hypertension could be controlled in its earlier phases. We have learned from necropsy studies that coronary artery disease begins in early childhood. From our clinical studies, along with others, we also believe essential hypertension begins early in life (Voors et al., 1977a). The early onset of essential hypertension is indicated by the high order of "tracking" of blood pressure levels; that is, children tend to remain in their ranks of blood pressure levels relative to their peers (Voors et al., 1980). All of these findings support the idea that early cardiovascular disease prevention is important. Although we know a great deal about both the effects and the clinical, physiological, and biochemical parameters of essential hypertension, as well as its end stage, we really know little of the early phase of essential hypertension—the subclinical, silent phase.

Concepts about the nature of hypertension in children are changing. Earlier reports held that hypertension in childhood is secondary with essential hypertension occurring only rarely (Loggie, 1975; Dustan, 1976). More recent studies, including our own observations, indicate that hypertension in children often does not show an underlying cause and that children ranking high in blood pressure among their peers are likely to continue this high ranking. Studies of young adults in the United States Navy (Harlan et al., 1973), and adolescents from Evans County (Heyden et al., 1969) who were followed for many years, indicated that high levels of blood pressure in adolescence are closely related to hypertension in adulthood. These observations contribute to the concept that essential hypertension begins in childhood.

In the general population, blood pressure levels rise with age during childhood until an adult stature is reached (18–20 years). Blood pressure then levels off, but in later years systolic pressure increases with age following an exponential curve.

As part of a comprehensive program to assess cardiovascular risk factor variables in children, the Bogalusa Heart Study was begun as a prospective investigation of the distributions, interrelationships, and course-over-time of risk factor variables in children (Berenson et al., 1980). Particular attention is given to methods for obtaining reproducible blood pressure levels and their changes over time. In order to study relationships of genetic and environmental factors contributing to the development of cardiovascular disease, a dietary study was incorporated into the program (Frank et al., 1978).

I. METHODS

A. Population Sample and General Methods

Our studies are being conducted in a semirural community, Bogalusa, Louisiana, with a biracial population of approximately 22,000. There are 5000 children, one-third of whom are black. The children are given a general examination for cardiovascular risk factors, which includes selected anthropometric measurements, serum lipid and lipoprotein analyses, and observations of blood pressure. The collection of information follows a rigid protocol and the measurements are obtained by trained observers, registered and licensed nurses. Additional observations include dietary studies, smoking behavior, and certain personality traits including Type A versus Type B behavior. The study is a mixed epidemiologic design with both cross-sectional surveys and longitudinal cohorts of children covering ages from birth to 17 years. Selected substudies of risk factor variables have been conducted with special objectives, for example, an in-depth blood pressure study (Berenson *et al.*, 1979a,b; Voors *et al.*, 1979). The general details of the study have been described in "Cardiovascular Risk Factors in Children" (Berenson *et al.*, 1980).

The methods and special studies pertinent to hypertension and dietary sodium intake in children will be presented briefly.

B. Blood Pressure Measurements

Blood pressure measurements are obtained from the right arm while the child is in a sitting position. Both the mercury sphygmomanometer and an automatic blood pressure recorder are used to obtain indirect blood pressure measurements, noting the first, fourth, and fifth Korotkoff phases. The children are randomized through a team of three nurses, each nurse recording three blood pressures. At the end of the examination, a random sample of the children is re-examined.

C. Dietary Studies

The 24-hr dietary recall has been adapted for use with children in the Bogalusa Heart Study. The accuracy for studying dietary intakes for groups of children has been improved by inserting various quality controls (Frank *et al.*, 1977). Briefly, these include using a standardized protocol for the interview dialogue and employing graduated food models for quantitation. A Product Identification Notebook was developed for completeness of recall of snack foods. Food items on representative school lunch trays are weighed for verification of serving size and for comparison to reported values in the recall interview. School lunch and home recipes are collected and entered onto a computerized nutrient data base, the Extended Table of Nutrient Values, prior to recall analysis (Moore *et al.*, 1974). Salt added at the table is entered as a separate food item and each "shake" or "pinch" is recorded as 0.05 g NaCl. Parents verify information on the use of salt and fat in cooking and supplementary vitamins. Duplicate recalls are obtained on a 10% random sample of each study group. Details of the methods used for younger children have been published previously (Frank *et al.*, 1982a; Berenson *et al.*, 1978a).

II. RESULTS AND DISCUSSION

For this presentation, three areas related to the relationship of NaCl, blood pressure, and potential hypertension are discussed in light of our studies of the early natural history of essential hypertension: (1) quantitation of the amount and

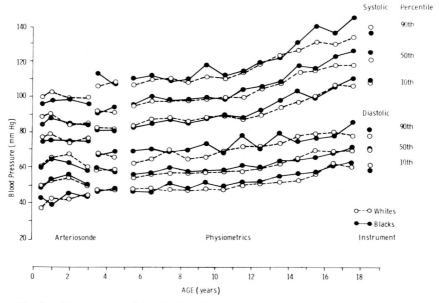

Fig. 1. Selected percentiles of indirect blood pressure levels for boys in a total community study. The observations shown here were recorded by an automatic instrument for some consistency of values across the age span of 6 months to 17 years. Similar levels are obtained with the mercury sphygmomanometer for ages 5–17. Although similar through childhood, levels for boys become slightly higher around 14 years of age. For diastolic pressure fourth Korotkoff phase is used.

nature of foods providing NaCl in the diets of children; (2) observation of a racial difference in the excretion of electrolytes; and (3) beginning studies to develop a model to prevent essential hypertension in early life.

It is now possible to provide considerable information on blood pressure levels of children, essentially from infancy through adolescence to young adulthood. Summary data are shown in Fig. 1 as selected percentiles related to age. Further analyses of the levels indicate a considerable variation as a result of height and weight for any given age. When blood pressure levels are controlled for height and weight, age appears to have little effect on the variability of the levels (Voors *et al.*, 1977b). Consequently, our data indicate it is more appropriate to express blood pressure levels in the growing child according to height, as in Fig. 2. Height is probably a better parameter to use during growth, considering the uncertainty of what normal weights really are in the general population. We also note that blood pressures obtained on children in Bogalusa are considerably lower than those reported in the NIH Task Force Report (Blumenthal *et al.*, 1977). The difference very likely is attributable to methodology and technique of acquiring blood pressures on children (Berenson *et al.*, 1978b). This observation is extremely important, since the use of a percentile grid to follow a child's blood

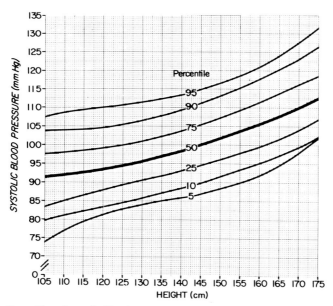

Fig. 2. Percentiles of systolic blood pressure levels are shown related to height of child rather than age. Because of variability of body size with developmental influences, level of blood pressure/ height is suggested as a reference. (Reprinted from Berenson *et al.*, 1980, with permission.)

pressure over time or to study the distribution of levels within a population requires comparable methodology. Further, it is not possible to provide precise definitions of hypertension in children. Cutpoints such as 135/85 are not satisfactory and selected percentiles or the use of standard deviations are arbitrary. From our data, however, the 95th percentile for a child age 14 with 128/78 may be comparable to an adult at age 40 years with 170/110. For practical purposes,

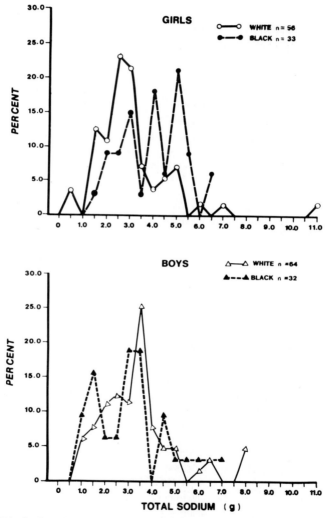

Fig. 3.   Distribution of a day's sodium intake for children reported by the 24-hr recall. The mean level is about 3.5 g. (Reprinted from Frank *et al.*, 1978, with permission.)

selected percentiles are probably better measures with which to follow children, provided that methods of obtaining blood pressure are comparable.

A. Dietary Studies of NaCl Intake in Children

Data on the quantity of dietary salt intake were obtained by 24-hr diet recalls. As shown in Fig. 3, there is a large variation of reported sodium intake for 10-year-old children with approximately 8.5 g NaCl consumed daily. On a weight basis, this is equivalent to an adult consuming 15 g/day. Table I shows mean sodium intake from several studies conducted at age 6 months and 12 months; two independent samples at 10 years of age; and 10-year-olds restudied at the age of 13. As might be expected, on a weight basis infants are consuming much more sodium than the older children. It is of interest to know what food groups are supplying sodium in the diet. Table II provides a list of the major food groups and the percent of the dietary sodium along with other components being obtained from each food group. For example, the bread, vegetable, meat, and milk groups provide considerable amounts of the daily sodium intake. It might be noted that the salt added to bread and cooked pastries or desserts accounts for a major portion of the daily sodium intake. In our local food preparation, the high content of salt in vegetables is primarily a result of the use of salted meats for seasoning.

It is also of interest to know the contribution of specific meals and snack foods to sodium intake and this is shown in Table III. Snacks account for approximately 20% of the sodium intake in the school-age child. In general, children are on a high sodium intake from infancy and through the school-age years.

B. Studies of Urinary Electrolyte Excretion

A special study was conducted on children selected by levels of blood pressure (high, middle, and low) taken from our cross-sectional survey of 4000 children. A sample of 272 children was chosen by a design with weighting of the extremes. They were then given an in-depth study to observe multiple parameters related to blood pressure. These studies included 24-hr urine collections for electrolyte and creatinine excretion and blood samples for a variety of analyses such as serum electrolytes, renin, dopamine-β-hydroxylase, and a series of hemodynamic studies. Details of in-depth blood pressure study have been reported (Berenson *et al.*, 1979a,b; Voors *et al.*, 1979), but an interesting observation on urinary electrolyte excretion is pertinent to this discussion. Although our studies suggest dietary intake of sodium is comparable in both black and white children, we note, as in Table IV, approximately equal amounts of sodium were excreted, and essentially equal amounts at the different blood pressure levels. Significant differences were noted, however, in urine potassium excretion. Black children

TABLE I

Sodium Intake (Mean) by Age of Infants and Children—Bogalusa Heart Study

	Age				
Dietary Component	6 months $n = 125$	12 months $n = 99$	10 years 1973 $n = 185$	10 years 1976 $n = 158$	13 years 1976 $n = 148$
Sodium, mg	881	1847	3330	3414	3395
Sodium, mg/kg	116	191	100	100	73
Recommended daily dietary allowance in 1980, mg	115– 350	250– 750	600– 1800	600– 1800	900– 2700

excreted approximately 10 mEq less in their urine (Table IV). Mechanisms accounting for this difference are not known at this time but the observation has been repeated in our more current studies being conducted on another sample of children. Although such differences might be explained by dietary intake, our 24 hr recalls suggest essentially comparable potassium intake between the races. We have not as yet had an opportunity to study electrolyte excretion in stools, which might account for a greater excretion of potassium in blacks and the difference in distribution in urine. This observation is presented as an interesting epidemiological finding that needs further investigation, but which may have significant

TABLE II

Dietary Studies in 10-Year-Old Children ($n = 185$): Percent of Dietary Components from Common Food Groups—Bogalusa Heart Study, 1973–1974

Food group	Calories	Protein	Saturated fat	Cholesterol	Sucrose	Sodium
			%			
Beef	6	15	9	13	0	7
Pork	5	7	9	6	0	5
Milk	15	23	26	16	3	7
Cheese	1	2	2	1	0	2
Egg	2	3	4	26	0	1
Bread	18	14	6	5	4	31
Vegetables/soups	8	9	7	4	1	17
Desserts	12	6	13	11	19	6
Candy	8	1	5	0	25	1
Snacks	3	1	3	0	0	3
Beverages	7	0	0	0	37	0
Other	15	19	16	18	11	20

TABLE III

Daily Sodium Intake by Meal and Snack Period for Different Ages of Children—Bogalusa Heart Study

Age	Breakfast		Lunch		Dinner		Snack	
	n	$\%^a$	n	$\%$	n	$\%$	n	$\%$
6 months	123	17	119	28	110	28	122	23
12 months	98	20	99	32	99	28	99	22
10 years, 1973	170	14	184	30	177	37	182	20
10 years, 1976	135	15	153	32	154	32	158	20
13 years	119	19	113	31	139	43	143	20

[a] Percent of daily sodium intake from meal for those (n) children eating the meal.

bearing on the capability of renal handling of electrolytes by the different races and susceptibility to hypertension from the high salt diet in our general population.

C. A Model of Intervention on High Blood Pressure Levels in Children

Eventually decisions have to be made as to when to begin intervention, prevention, or therapeutic measures in the early phases of hypertension. Unfortunately, no set rules or guidelines can be established at present. The observations of significant tracking and predictability of blood pressure levels are highly consistent with the concept that essential hypertension has its origin in youth and likely is existing already in a significant number of children who are presumed healthy

TABLE IV

24-Hr Urine Sodium and Potassium by Race and Blood Pressure Stratum in Children ($n = 249$), Ages 7–15 Years—Bogalusa Heart Study, 1975–1976

Electrolyte	Race	Blood pressure stratum		
		Low	Medium	High
		mEq (mean ± 2 SE)		
Na^+	White	106 ± 13	98 ± 17	109 ± 14
	Black	97 ± 12	103 ± 17	115 ± 18
K^+	White[a]	39 ± 4	34 ± 7	42 ± 7
	Black[a]	26 ± 3	27 ± 4	29 ± 5

[a] $p < 0.0001$.

and heretofore, according to adult standards, recognized as having normal blood pressure levels.

In an effort to investigate approaches to prevent the occurrence of essential hypertension, we undertook a program to develop a community model of intervention in a defined population of children. Since studies of children in Bogalusa are descriptive of the early natural history of coronary artery disease and essential hypertension, we do not want to tamper with the base population. Therefore, we selected a neighboring rural community, Franklinton, Louisiana, some 20 miles from Bogalusa. Franklinton has a population of about 9000; one-half are black. The program was developed largely as a feasibility study and a first approximation of how children whom we project to have a high risk of developing adult essential hypertension might be treated (Berenson et al., 1982).

Several major questions were posed for the study. Can we lower or modulate levels of blood pressure by usual clinical measures? Can we alter sodium intake and perhaps reduce the weight of the overweight children? The study was designed in three phases: The first phase was a survey of all children in the community to determine the distribution and percentiles of blood pressure levels for that population. Essentially, these were found to be similar to those obtained earlier in Bogalusa and described above. The second phase included performing serial examinations on a sample of children at or above the ninetieth percentile selected to be followed for repeat study. An additional group in the midrange of blood pressure levels was selected as a comparison group. These children were then re-examined on three separate occasions. The group of children persisting at or above the ninetieth percentile ($n = 100$) and at the midrange ($n = 50$) were selected for further examination or treatment. The third phase comprised the treatment phase and research on intervention.

From an original 1604 children representing 90% of the total population of children, 8 to 18 years of age, 150 children were selected to be followed in the third phase, 50 at the midrange level, and 100 persisting at the high level of blood pressure at or above the ninetieth percentile. The latter 100 children were randomized into two groups, and one group of 50 children was treated as will be discussed. An extensive examination was given to all 150 children, including physical examination, midstream clean-catch urines for sediment and bacteria, 24-hr urine samples, and laboratory blood analyses.

The treatment phase for the 50 selected children in the high range consisted of both primary and secondary treatment. Treatment included the use of drugs at a low dosage level. In order to accomplish this program, especially the treatment phase, it was necessary to approach various factions of the community as shown in Table V. Cooperation with the physicians, school staff (especially school lunch staff), grocery stores, and restaurants in the community was essential. The parents of the children were involved and those found to have high blood pressure were referred to their physician while indigent patients were provided medi-

TABLE V

Franklinton Blood Pressure Intervention—Total Community Approach

Physicians
Community structure
  Advisory group
  Organizational
  Newspapers
Parents
  Private-resource
  Indigent care
School staff
  Lunch, snacks, curriculum
Grocery stores
Restaurants

cal treatment. Various foods, salt-free products, and medications were given to the parents and to the children.

A Dietary/Exercise Alteration Program Trial (ADAPT) was developed as the basis for the primary therapy (Frank *et al.,* 1928b). This program organized both dietary and exercise management. A "Sodium-kcal Counter Booklet" and a "Low-Sodium Movin' On Recipe Book," were developed and adapted to our local food preparations. In addition, an educational and physical activity curriculum for both students and parents was developed and implemented.

The drug therapy consisted of a low dosage (approximately one-fourth of an adult dose based on the weight of each child) of propanolol and chlorthalidone in combination. The drugs were given to the children in the morning or divided into a morning and evening dosage according to the weight of the child.

The children were followed in a clinical setting, using our Mobile Research Unit and facilities of the school, at 2-week intervals initially, and later at monthly intervals.

Participation in the study was excellent, with cooperation at all levels. Our observations after 6 months following initial treatment indicated that approximately three-fourths of the treated children responded by decreasing their blood pressure to the midrange level (Table VI). One of the most difficult problems we observe is the resistance to change of lifestyles and dietary habits. To conduct such a study obviously involves many aspects within a total community and the need for obtaining cooperation from a great number of people.

A similar program could be approached in different ways, but any modification of that described for research purposes would require a complete community and 1 to 2 years to conduct. The Franklinton Blood Pressure Intervention Study described here is an initial effort for blood pressure intervention. It should provide others with an opportunity to improve the approach, and eventually to

TABLE VI

Franklinton Blood Pressure Intervention Results[a] after 6 Months in Children Ages 6–18 Years—Bogalusa Heart Study, 1980

Study group	n	Baseline, April[b] (mm Hg, mean ± 1 SD)	6 Months, Oct.[c] (mm Hg, mean ± 1 SD)
Systolic			
Low BP Control	45	103 ± 8.4	103 ± 7.9
High BP Control	44	118 ± 10.0	114 ± 8.6
Treated	44	117 ± 8.7	109 ± 9.1
Diastolic (fourth phase)			
Low BP Control	45	66 ± 4.6	66 ± 5.0
High BP Control	44	79 ± 6.4	74 ± 6.9
Treated	44	78 ± 4.8	71 ± 6.2

[a] Preliminary.

[b] Mean of five examination days for each child.

[c] Mean of all clinic visits except the first.

develop methods useful for a physician's care of a single child or for development of public health community-wide programs. It is our impression that without the capability of rigid reduction of sodium in our diets, the use of drugs will be required for the initial reduction of blood pressure levels in individuals sensitive to sodium and prone to develop hypertension. The long-term effects obviously are not possible to describe at this time. Yet, these studies are exciting and could have considerable impact on the prevalence of essential hypertension in adults.

III. SUMMARY

Studies being conducted in well-defined populations of children in rural United States indicate blood pressure levels have an approximately normal distribution. In the growing child, levels of blood pressure should be related to their height rather than their chronological age. Infants and children are exposed to a high sodium intake that likely is a major factor in the high prevalence of essential hypertension. Black individuals may have an even greater intolerance to high dietary sodium contributing to the greater morbidity from this disease. The observation of tracking and persistence of levels within given ranks relative to peers is good evidence essential hypertension begins early in life.

In an attempt to develop a model of intervention on a total population of children, it was possible to reduce blood pressure levels of children tracking at or above the ninetieth percentile to the midrange levels, fifty to sixtieth percentile, by a combination of primary and secondary treatment. A program of this type requires support and cooperation from many factions within the community. It is important to begin to explore models of intervention in an effort to prevent hypertensive disease in adulthood.

ACKNOWLEDGMENT

The Bogalusa Heart Study is a joint effort of many people. A special thanks is given to the Bogalusa staff and to the children of Bogalusa and Franklinton and their parents without whose cooperation this study would not be possible.

This research was supported by funds from the National Heart and Lung Institute of the U.S. Public Health Service and the Specialized Center of Research-Arteriosclerosis (HL 15103) at Louisiana State University Medical Center in New Orleans.

REFERENCES

Berenson, G. S., Foster, T. A., Frank, G. C., Frerichs, R. R., Srinivasan, S. R., Voors, A. W., and Webber, L. S. (1978a). Cardiovascular disease risk factor variables at the preschool age—The Bogalusa Heart Study. *Circulation* **57,** 603–612.

Berenson, G. S., Voors, A. W., Webber, L. S., and Frerichs, R. R. (1978b). Blood pressure in children and its interpretation. Task Force Report. (Letter to the editor.) *Pediatrics* **61,** 333–336.

Berenson, G. S., Voors, A. W., Dalferes, E. R., Jr., Webber, L. S., and Shuler, S. E. (1979a). Creatinine clearance, electrolytes and plasma renin activity related to the blood pressure of white and black children—The Bogalusa Heart Study. *J. Lab. Clin. Med.* **93,** 535–547.

Berenson, G. S., Voors, A. W., Webber, L. S., Dalferes, E. R., Jr., and Harsha, D. W. (1979b). Racial differences of parameters associated with blood pressure levels in children—The Bogalusa Heart Study. *Metab., Clin. Exp.* **28,** 1218–1228.

Berenson, G. S., McMahan, C. A., Voors, A. W., Webber, L. S., Srinivasan, S. R., Frank, G. C., Foster, T. A., and Blonde, C. V. (1980). "Cardiovascular Risk Factors in Children—The Early Natural History of Atherosclerosis and Essential Hypertension." Oxford Univ. Press, London and New York.

Berenson, G. S., Voors, A. W., Webber, L. S., Frank, G. C., Farris, R. P., Tobian, L., and Aristimuno, G. G. (1982). A model of intervention for prevention of early essential hypertension in the 1980's. *Hypertension* (submitted for publication).

Blumenthal, S., Epps, R. P., Heavenrich, R., Lauer, R. M., Lieberman, E., Mirkin, B., Mitchell, S. C., Naito, V. B., O'Hare, D. W., Smith, W. McF., Tarazi, R. C., and Upson, D. (1977). Report of the task force on blood pressure control in children. *Pediatrics* **59,** 797–820.

Dustan, H. P. (1976). Evaluation and therapy of hypertension—1976. *Mod. Concepts Cardiovasc. Dis.* **45,** 97–100.

Frank, G. C., Berenson, G. S., Schilling, P. E., and Moore, M. C. (1977). Adapting the 24-hr. recall for epidemiologic studies of school children. *J. Am. Diet. Assoc.* **71,** 26–31.

Frank, G. C., Berenson, G. S., and Webber, L. S. (1978). Dietary studies and the relationship of diet to cardiovascular disease risk factor variables in 10-year-old children—The Bogalusa Heart Study. *Am. J. Clin. Nutr.* **31,** 328–340.

Frank, G. C., Farris, R. P., Major, C. R., Webber, L. S., and Berenson, G. S. (1982a). Infant feeding patterns and their relationship to cardiovascular risk factor variables in the first year of life. (Submitted for publication.)

Frank, G. C., Farris, R. P., Ditmarsen, P., Voors, A. W., Mellert, H., and Berenson, G. S. (1982b). An approach to primary preventive treatment for children with high blood pressure in a total community. *Hypertension* (submitted for publication).

Harlan, W. R., Oberman, A., Mitchell, R. E., and Graybiel, A. (1973). A 30-year study of blood pressure in a white male cohort. *In* "Hypertension: Mechanisms Management" (G. Onesti, K. E. Kim, and J. H. Moyer, eds.), p. 85. Grune & Stratton, New York.

Heyden, S., Bartel, A. G., Hames, C. G., and McDonough, J. R. (1969). Elevated blood pressure levels in adolescents, Evans County, Georgia. *J. Am. Med. Assoc.* **209,** 1683–1689.

Hypertension Detection and Follow-Up Program Cooperative Group (1979). Five year findings of the hypertension detection and follow-up program. *J. Am. Med. Assoc.* **242,** 2562–2572.

Loggie, A. (1975). Hypertension in children and adolescents. *Hosp. Pract.* **10**(6), 81–92.

Moore, M. C., Goodloe, M. H., and Schilling, P. E. (1974). "Extended Table of Nutrient Values (ETNV)." International Dietary Information Foundation, Atlanta, Georgia (Data tapes at Louisiana State University Computer Center).

Voors, A. W., Webber, L. S., and Berenson, G. S. (1977a). A consideration of essential hypertension in children. *Pract. Cardiol.* **3,** 29–40.

Voors, A. W., Webber, L. S., Frerichs, R. R., and Berenson, G. S. (1977b). Body height and body mass as determinants of basal blood pressure in children—The Bogalusa Heart Study. *Am. J. Epidemiol.* **106,** 101–108.

Voors, A. W., Berenson, G. S., Dalferes, E. R., Webber, L. S., and Shuler, S. E. (1979). Racial differences in blood pressure control. *Science* **204,** 1091–1094.

Voors, A. W., Webber, L. S., and Berenson, G. S. (1980). Time course study of blood pressure in children over a three-year period—Bogalusa Heart Study. *Hypertension* **2,** Suppl. 1, 102–108.

5

Observational and Interventional Experiences on Dietary Sodium Intake and Blood Pressure

ARLINE McDONALD ALLEN, JEREMIAH STAMLER,
ROSE STAMLER, FLORA GOSCH, RICHARD COOPER,
KIANG LIU, AND MAURIZIO TREVISAN

This chapter presents an overview of the work of our research group on sodium and hypertension, with a focus on recent studies and investigations in progress. These include observational epidemiological studies and randomized controlled trials.

For at least a quarter of a century, it has been the basic judgment of the senior

63

THE ROLE OF SALT IN
CARDIOVASCULAR HYPERTENSION

members of our research group that ingestion of a habitual diet high in sodium plays a key role in the etiology and pathogenesis of hypertension in modern man (Stamler *et al.,* 1955). It is this conclusion that has stimulated our recurrent investigative efforts on this matter.

I. ANTHROPOLOGICAL CONSIDERATIONS

Recently, one of our central concerns has been to review the anthropological aspects of the relationship of man to dietary sodium. Contemporary concepts of primate evolution as it has occurred over the last 70 million years indicate that the earliest predecessors of man in the primate line can be traced back about 12 million years (Leakey and Lewin, 1977, 1979). It is also widely agreed at present that the critical evolutionary developments leading to man took place in sub-Saharan Africa. A decisive step was, after tens of millions of years of arboreal primate evolution, the descent to earth and the development of a nomadic food gathering and hunting means of subsistence. Estimates based on several sources of anthropological evidence indicate that throughout the millions of years of hominoid and hominid evolution, an average of about 30% of calories came from animal sources, the rest from vegetables. This yielded a daily sodium intake of as little as 10 mEq (230 mg), when the diet was primarily herbivorous, to as high as 60 mEq (1380 mg) with a heavily carnivorous fare from a successful hunt (Meneely and Battarbee, 1976). Neither the archeological record about fossil man nor the anthropological record about isolated gatherer–hunter societies in the modern world yields any evidence of *addition* of salt to food. It is probably a point of crucial importance that the need of the gatherer–hunter to be continuously on the move precluded any concern for accumulation of a food surplus, thereby precluding any concern for food preservation, since the worldly goods of the group had to be toted from place to place (Swartz and Jordan, 1976).

If it be accepted that the immediate predecessors of *Homo sapiens sapiens* can be traced back at least a million years, then this basic generalization about man and sodium holds true until shortly before the dawn of recorded history. Over hundreds of thousands of years, first and foremost in the crucial evolutionary milieu of Africa, man evolved under circumstances requiring the careful *conservation* of sodium as a vital aspect of the preservation of the physiological internal environment. The evolutionary experience conditioned the species primarily to be a very efficient *retainer* of sodium, capable of maintaining body levels of this decisive ion on a low intake in a hot climate. It did *not* condition the species primarily to be an efficient excretor of a sizable excess of ingested sodium.

With the invention of agriculture about 10,000 years ago, all this changed relatively rapidly (Childe, 1951). Man ended his nomadic existence. Both the possibility and the need arose to produce a food surplus (Leakey and Lewin,

1977, 1979). A wide range of food products became available on a regular basis for the first time (Fig. 1). Some of these, e.g., the all-important grains and legumes, could readily be preserved in their seed form. Others, however, required special treatment for preservation, e.g., dairy products, meats, poultry, fish, and vegetables. The earliest historical record indicates universally the use of added salt for this purpose (Tannahill, 1973; Wilson, 1974). That is, the evidence indicates that the sizable addition of salt to food, i.e., the widespread consumption of a relatively high salt diet by the human species, occurred for the first time late in human evolution as an essential by-product of the Neolithic agricultural revolution and its profound effects on the human food supply. So important was salt for ancient man, and so hard to come by, that slabs of salt or bags of salt were an early form of money. This indeed is the origin of our modern word salary, from the Roman *salis* for salt and *salarium* for salt money paid the Roman soldiers.

For centuries in the ancient and feudal world, this essential food preservative was in widespread use, albeit in relatively scarce supply. With the Industrial Revolution, the long-term trend was accentuated, since the technological and economic prerequisites became available to make salt plentiful and cheap (Multhauf, 1978). These are the anthropological and socioeconomic bases for the modern situation, e.g., the ingestion throughout the world, except for a few nonacculturated isolated populations, of a diet more or less high in sodium, based on addition of salt and other sodium-containing additives to foods. The findings in the Solomon Islands, absence of hypertension and of rise of blood pressure with age in five of six populations, with the one exception being the group

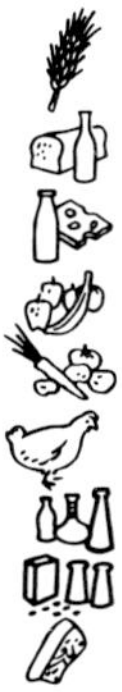

1. Cereals: wheats, barley, and later rye, rice and oats.
2. Fermented bread and beer with their yeast components.
3. Dairy foods: milk, cheese, soured whole milk, butter.
4. Fruits of many kinds.
5. Vegetables of many kinds, and root crops.
6. Poultry and eggs (hens introduced later from India).
7. Edible oils.
8. Spices, savoring agents for acceptability.
9. Beef, pork, mutton, and eventually poultry became regular supplies, economics permitting. (Meat supplies and fish and shellfish had been available in Paleolithic and Mesolithic times, but usually after a hand-to-mouth economy.)

Fig. 1. New foods made available by the Neolithic transition from food gathering to food producing.

TABLE I

Solomon Island Study: Prevalence of Elevated Blood Pressure (>140/>90), Adults Age ≥ 20

Tribe	Number of men	BP > 140/> 90 Number	%	Number of women	BP > 140/> 90 Number	%
Nasioi	59	2	3.4	63	0	0.0
Nagovisi	109	3	2.7	101	0	0.0
Lau	77	6	7.8	101	10	9.9
Baegu	126	1	0.8	109	0	0.0
Aita	81	0	0.0	88	0	0.0
Kwaio	128	1	0.8	114	1	0.9
U.S. White[a]	6504	1469	23.5	3358	383	11.6
U.S. Black	634	193	31.6	977	158	18.5

[a] U.S. data are from the Chicago Heart Association Detection Project in Industry, ages 25–44, diastolic pressure ≥ 90 mm Hg.

cooking food in brackish inlet water, are seminal in terms of the significance of dietary sodium (Table I) (Page *et al.*, 1974).

II. METHODOLOGICAL PROBLEMS

Many reports are in the literature indicating that nonacculturated populations habitually consuming low sodium diets show no rise in blood pressure with age and virtual absence of hypertensive disease (Chapman and Gibbons, 1950; Dahl and Love, 1954; Freis, 1976; Meneely and Dahl, 1961; Page *et al.*, 1974; Page, 1976). Interpopulation comparisons also indicate an association between habitual level of average sodium intake and of prevalence rates of hypertension, although the breadth and depth of such data are limited.

A major unsolved problem has been the within population situation: Is there a relationship between the habitual sodium intake of individuals and their risk of hypertensive disease? The available epidemiological data do not yield a clear and consistent answer to this question. Recent work has delineated at least two likely explanations for the difficulties in this area. First, human beings almost certainly differ, for genetic reasons not as yet defined biochemically, in their susceptibility to the effects of a diet habitually high in sodium. Within almost all human populations (excepting the aforementioned isolates) the exposure to high sodium is virtually universal for all individuals. That is, research on this question does not have the convenience afforded by a distinction of kind (yes or no), but instead must contend with making a distinction of degree.

To make this point abundantly clear, consider how the link was made between cigarette smoking and lung cancer. In every population studied, there was always a sizable proportion of people who had never smoked, so that the nonsmoker versus smoker contrast could readily be made, with the added fillip of dividing the smokers into amounts habitually smoked. Consider what a problem it would have been to make the connection between this habit and lung cancer if everyone had smoked cigarettes. Consider further the relative ease of determining how many cigarettes individuals habitually smoke per day, in contrast to the marked difficulty of quantitating the amount of sodium ingested daily. Consider further the additional difficulty arising from the fact that, in contrast to cigarette use, in modern societies sodium intake of individuals varies markedly from day to day. These are the methodological problems, formidable ones indeed, as research has only recently come to appreciate.

The matter of the intraindividual variability in daily sodium intake, as compared with the interindividual variability in habitual ingestion, has in the last years been one of the focuses of our research work. Years ago, Ancel Keys pointed out that when the intraindividual variation of a trait is greater than the interindividual variation, it is extremely difficult properly to classify individuals within a population with respect to that trait. Perhaps because it was not given detailed quantitative expression, this truism has not been widely appreciated. The result has been that several of the studies on the relationship of habitual sodium intake of individuals to their blood pressures are faulted because too few measurements of sodium were made to achieve valid classification of the individuals.

Kiang Liu and colleagues in our group have submitted this problem to systematic quantitative assessment, in both children and adults. Their findings are summarized in Table II (Liu *et al.,* 1979a,b,c). The ratios of the intra- to interindividual variances are high, much in excess of unity, for both children and adults (in contrast to such variables as serum cholesterol and blood pressure, for which they are about 1:3 so that a single measurement suffices to distinguish one person from another with a small error rate). As a consequence of the high ratio for dietary sodium, if only one or a few measurements are used to characterize an individual with respect to sodium intake, a sizable probability of misclassifica-

TABLE II

Individual Variation in 24-Hr and Overnight Sodium Excretion

Variable	Ratio of intra- to interindividual variances	
	Adult	Children
24-Hr Na excretion	3.20	1.94
Overnight Na excretion	3.26	2.50
Number of persons	142	73

TABLE III

**Chicago School Children Study on Sodium and Blood Pressure
Regression Coefficients for Single Day Sodium Excretion on Systolic
Blood Pressure**[a]

Day	Coefficient	Significance level (p)
Sunday	0.032	0.142
Monday	0.018	0.453
Tuesday	0.028	0.231
Wednesday	0.041	0.046
Thursday	0.032	0.096
Friday	0.015	0.362
Saturday	0.019	0.205
Average	0.059	0.045

[a] Other variables include height, weight, age, sex, race, and heart rate.

tion into a particular group and a sizable diminution of possible correlation coefficients between sodium intake and biological measures could result.

On the basis of the ratio of intra- to interindividual variances in sodium excretion among children, it was calculated that seven measurements are needed to assess the relationship between sodium excretion and systolic blood pressure, to achieve a diminution of the true correlation coefficient of no more than 10%. The data in Table III show that for any single measure with the exception of one (possibly due to chance) the p values for the regression coefficients for sodium excretion on systolic blood pressure adjusting for height, weight, age, sex, race, and heart rate did not achieve significance. However, the average of the seven 24-hr urinary sodium excretion measures was significant (Cooper *et al.*, 1980).

III. OBSERVATIONAL STUDIES

Based on this demonstration that under American conditions multiple measurements of sodium intake are essential to minimize error in classifying individuals with respect to sodium intake, a series of population studies was undertaken among Chicago school children age 10–15 to re-explore the entire problem. With the science class as the base for the attempt to win informed and dedicated cooperation of the students, seven consecutive days of 24-hr urine collection were carried out in student groups in seven schools. Relevant anthropometric measurements were also made, and standardized blood pressures were recorded as well. The findings for the first two schools are summarized in Tables III and IV (Cooper *et al.*, 1980). The 24-hr sodium excretion was significantly related to systolic blood pressure with both weight and height included as measures of body

TABLE IV

Dietary Sodium and Blood Pressure Study, 73 Chicago School Children Age 11–14, 1978

Variable	Multiple linear regression coefficient[a]	p
7-Day mean 24-hr Na excretion (mEq)	$0.0587 \pm .0286$[a]	0.045
Weight (lb)	$0.1587 \pm .0609$	0.011
Height (inches)	$0.3083 \pm .3272$	0.350
Age (years)	-1.5274 ± 1.8160	0.403
Sex	-1.2386 ± 2.4735	0.618
Race	0.6704 ± 3.4162	0.845
Heart rate (per min)	$0.1013 \pm .1242$	0.418
Constant	61.4247 ± 26.5262	0.024

[a] Systolic pressure is the dependent variable.

[b] Standard error.

size. The only other statistically significant variable was weight. No additional contributions were made by height, age, sex, race, or heart rate.

If these positive findings on the relationship between habitual sodium intake and blood pressure within a population can be confirmed, they are clearly of great importance. Analyses are still in progress of our more recent data collected in five additional schools in a similar fashion. At present, it is not possible to state whether the findings are confirmatory. A key problem in this work is the independent and objective assessment of the completeness of 24-hr urine collection, based on 24-hr creatinine excretion. The literature does not give quantitative criteria for this. Our group is currently addressing this problem.

Maurizio Trevisan and colleagues in our group are involved in evaluating measurements of intracellular sodium metabolism through assays of red blood cell sodium concentration (RBC [Na]) and sodium-stimulated lithium efflux (Li efflux) (Trevisan et al., 1982). Table V gives the technical error for these methodologies. They are low order. This is also true for the ratio of the intra- to interindividual variances. Thus, these measurements are suitable for use in epidemiological studies. In two of the schools where the children had collected 7-day food records and seven 24-hr urine samples, blood samples were drawn from a subgroup of 26 to determine RBC sodium concentration and Na-stimulated lithium efflux. The correlation coefficients between these aspects of intracellular sodium metabolism and related variables are shown in Table VI. RBC [Na] was negatively but not significantly correlated with urinary sodium excretion in this subgroup. No significant relationship was shown between urinary sodium excre-

TABLE V

Technical Error of Red Blood Cell Sodium Assays

Assay	n	Mean	Error	Percent error[a]
RBC Na$^+$ concentration (mEq/liter RBC)	13	7.73[b]	0.197	2.5%
Lithium efflux moles/RBC/hr	6	4.73[c]	0.303	6.4%

[a] Technical error divided by mean multiplied by 100.
[b] Mean of 26.
[c] Mean of 12.

tion and systolic or diastolic blood pressure. Urinary potassium excretion was positively and significantly related to diastolic blood pressure ($r = 0.343$, $p < 0.05$). Li efflux was positively and significantly related to systolic blood pressure in both simple correlation analysis and with cross-classification by tertiles. This correlation persisted after controlling for weight, height, age, and sex. No significant relationship was found between Li efflux and either RBC [Na], urinary sodium excretion, or urinary potassium excretion.

When the sample from the subgroup of school children was increased from 26 to 39, the inverse relationship between RBC [Na] and urinary sodium excretion reached significance (Table VII). This finding was confirmed with cross-classification by tertiles.

TABLE VI

Dietary Sodium and Blood Pressure Study, 26 Chicago School Children Age 11–14, 1980

Variable	RBC [Na]	Li efflux
Li efflux	−0.053[a]	—
Systolic BP	−0.098	0.532[b]
Diastolic BP	−0.081	0.191
7-day mean 24-hr excretion		
Sodium	−0.255	0.090
Potassium	0	0.176
Creatinine	0.076	0.174
Weight	0.094	0.304
Height	0.062	0.246
Age	−0.169	0.016

[a] Correlation coefficient.
[b] $p < 0.01$.

TABLE VII

Red Blood Cell Sodium Concentration and Urinary Sodium Excretion,[a]
39 Chicago School Children, 1980

Mean RBC [Na] by tertile (mEq/liter RBC)	Number of children	Urinary Na (mEq/24 hr, mean ± SD)
6.9	12	113.6 ± 46.7[b]
8.4	13	84.8 ± 21.7
10.8	14	80.7 ± 26.9[b]

[a] $r = 0.338$; $t = -2.31$.
[b] t, upper versus lower tertile $= 2.15$; $p < 0.05$.

IV. EXPERIMENTAL STUDIES

A. Children

Our group has also had one recent opportunity to do a controlled experiment in high school students on dietary sodium, sodium metabolism, and blood pressure. This involved 64 high school students at the Seventh Day Adventist Broadview Academy in LaFox, Illinois, where the high degree of health consciousness of students, faculty, and staff and the boarding school cafeteria arrangements made it possible to control sodium intake closely over a 24-day period. The habitual lacto-ovo-vegetarian diet at the Academy contained a daily average of about 216 mEq of sodium, and the experiment involved randomly assigning half of the 67 students to this usual diet. For the other half, careful planning of recipes and menus was done to reduce average daily sodium intake about 70%, to 72 mEq. The findings of the study are displayed in Tables VIII and IX.

Though systolic blood pressure decreased slightly from baseline for the experimental group and rose slightly for the control group, the mean difference in

TABLE VIII

Broadview Academy Dietary Study: Systolic Blood Pressure

Group	n	Baseline		Final		Change	
		Mean	SD	Mean	SD	Mean	SD
Experimental	30	110.3[a]	12.0	109.0	11.8	−1.3	11.1
Control	34	108.2	10.0	109.3	10.6	+1.1	8.7

[a] mm Hg.

TABLE IX

Broadview Academy Dietary Study: Red Blood Cell Sodium Concentration

Group	n	Baseline		Final		Change	
		Mean	SD	Mean	SD	Mean	SD
Experimental	14	7.85[a]	1.10	7.43	0.96	−0.43[b]	0.87
Control	10	8.33	2.09	8.62	1.95	+0.29	0.98

[a] mEq/liter RBC.
[b] $p < 0.05$.

change between the two groups—2.4 mm Hg—was not significant, given the small sample size. Possibly the reduction in sodium intake (verified by chemical analysis of representative meal homogenates) for the experimental group compared to the control group, was not low enough to have had a significant effect on blood pressure, or the duration may have been too short. The limitations of the academic calendar at the Academy restricted the time available for the experimental period to 24 days, and precluded use of a crossover design in this study.

The data in Table IX show that RBC [Na] was significantly reduced in the group on the lower sodium diet, compared both with values for this same group at baseline and values for the control group. This findings, in addition to those reported earlier, showing a significant negative relationship between RBC [Na] and urinary sodium excretion, as well as a significant relationship between Li efflux and systolic blood pressure for the subgroup of Chicago school children, suggests complex interrelationships among sodium intake, sodium metabolism, and blood pressure which need further investigation.

B. Adults

1. Long-Term Control of Hypertension by Dietary Means

The interrelationship between dietary factors and blood pressure are currently being investigated in a randomized controlled trial in hypertensive individuals as part of a cooperative effort with a second center in Minneapolis. Most of these adult men and women originally had mean diastolic pressures in the range 90–104 mm Hg, and their blood pressures were controlled by pharmacologic treatment over the previous 5–6 years as part of the national cooperative Hypertension Detection and Follow-up Program (HDFP) (Hypertension Detection and Follow-up Program Cooperative Group, 1979a,b). The major goal of this trial is to assess ability to maintain satisfactory blood pressure levels through modification of overweight and excessive sodium consumption without the use of antihypertensive medication.

The volunteers are being randomized into one of three groups. Group I is receiving nutritional–hygienic intervention with discontinuation of pharmacologic treatment. For those in this group whose blood pressures cannot be completely controlled by dietary means, the use of less medication (step or degree) than that in the entry regimen is to be tried. Those in Group II are discontinuing pharmacologic treatment with no other intervention to determine if long-term blood pressure control by pharmacologic means has made it possible to discontinue or reduce drug treatment without nutritional–hygienic intervention. Those in Group III are continuing pharmacologic treatment with no other intervention.

Data on the initial participants of Group I in the preliminary stages of the trial are displayed in Table X. Comparable weight losses and sodium reductions have been achieved by the two centers. No data are available at this time as to the effect on blood pressure of these weight and sodium changes after removal from medication.

2. Primary Prevention of Hypertension by Nutritional–Hygienic Means

Though great progress has been made in recent years in detection, treatment, and control of hypertension in the U.S. population, pharmacologic means of dealing with the high blood pressure problem must be recognized as a limited interim approach to this mass disease. Primary prevention is the key long-term strategy.

Though current understanding of the etiology and pathogenesis of this disease

TABLE X

Two-Month Intervention Results: Hypertension Control Program

Center	Baseline invitation visit	2-Month visit	Change
Minneapolis Center ($n = 14$)			
Weight (lb)	172.6	165.6	−6.9
Relative weight	123.8	118.9	−4.9
Urinary Na (mg/day)	5974	3755	−2219
Systolic BP (mm Hg)	122.8	118.6	−4.1
Diastolic BP (mm Hg)	79.4	78.4	−0.9
Chicago Center ($n = 8$)			
Weight	181.0	172.5	−8.5
Relative weight	124.1	118.6	−5.5
Urinary Na	5636	3751	−1885
Systolic BP	116.5	114.6	−1.9
Diastolic BP	77.6	76.5	−1.1

is still limited, substantial evidence is available on risk factors for hypertensive disease, e.g., overweight, high sodium intake, rapid heart rate, and high-normal blood pressure level (Stamler, 1979, Stamler *et al.*, 1975). This information makes possible both identification of hypertension-prone individuals and institution of preventive measures. Previous experience of our group in the Chicago Coronary Prevention Evaluation Program indicated that moderate weight reduction with a diet low in saturated fat and cholesterol, plus moderate rhythmic exercise to improve cardiopulmonary fitness, was effective in reducing high-normal blood pressures (average diastolic readings 80–89 mm Hg) and in preventing long-term rise in blood pressure for middle-aged coronary-prone men (Table XI) (Stamler *et al.*, 1980). Regression analysis indicated that weight loss in particular was significantly related to blood pressure fall (Table XII) (Stamler *et al.*, 1980). Sodium consumption was not systematically studied in this earlier trial, but it is reasonable to suggest that the dietary recommendations probably resulted in moderate reduction in sodium intake (Stamler, 1978).

On the basis of these findings by our group and extensive data available from the work of others, indicating the possibility of achieving the primary prevention of hypertension by safe nutritional–hygienic means, a 5-year randomized controlled trial has been undertaken to test ability of nonpharmacologic intervention to influence blood pressure in individuals age 30–44 assessed to be hypertension-prone. With the support of Chicago companies, 200 persons are

TABLE XI

Mean Change in the Six Variables of Cohort of 70 Nondropouts Never Receiving Antihypertensive Medication[a]

Year	Δ Weight (lb)	Δ Relative weight	Δ Pulse rate (beats/ min)	Δ Systolic BP (mm Hg)	Δ Diastolic BP (mm Hg)	Δ Serum cholesterol (mg/ dliter)
0	192.4	127.5	77.7	130.3	83.0	258.5
1	180.8[b]	119.8[b]	74.9[c]	123.0[b]	78.6[b]	243.2[b]
2	180.2[b]	119.3[b]	74.5[c]	123.0[b]	78.4[b]	237.8[b]
3	181.3[b]	120.2[b]	73.8[b]	123.1[b]	78.8[b]	241.8[b]
4	183.5[b]	121.6[b]	74.0[b]	124.2[b]	80.2[b]	243.7[b]
5	183.4[b]	121.5[b]	74.1[b]	123.8[b]	79.5[b]	244.4[b]
1–5	181.8[b]	120.5[b]	74.3[b]	123.4[b]	79.1[b]	240.4[b]
Change 1–5	−10.5	−7.1	−3.4	−6.8	−3.9	−18.1
% Change 1–5	−5.5	−5.6	−4.4	−5.2	−4.7	−7.0

[a] Last baseline diastolic blood pressure (BP) was 80–89 mm Hg; relative weight, 115 or greater.
[b] $p \leq 0.001$.
[c] $p \leq 0.01$.

TABLE XII

Relationship between Percent Change in Weight, Pulse Rate, and Blood Pressure (BP) for Years 1-5[a]

Statistic	70 Men with last baseline relative weight ≥ 115		24 Men with last baseline relative weight 115-123		46 Men with last baseline relative weight ≥ 124	
	% Δ Systolic BP	% Δ Diastolic BP	% Δ Systolic BP	% Δ Diastolic BP	% Δ Systolic BP	% Δ Diastolic BP
Simple r, % Δ BP and % Δ weight	0.325[b]	0.459[c]	0.314	0.368[d]	0.323[d]	0.522[c]
Partial r, % Δ BP and % Δ weight[e]	0.309[b]	0.449[c]	0.318	0.381[d]	0.306[d]	0.519[c]
Simple r, % Δ BP and % Δ pulse rate	0.247[d]	0.179	−0.018	−0.080	0.383[b]	0.353[b]
Partial r, % Δ BP and % Δ pulse rate[f]	0.225[d]	0.146	−0.057	−0.132	0.370[b]	0.348[b]

[a] Cohort of 70 nondropouts with last baseline diastolic BP 80-89 mm Hg and relative weight 115 or greater and its subgroup, correlation analyses.

[b] $p \leq 0.01$.

[c] $p \leq 0.001$.

[d] $p \leq 0.05$.

[e] Controlled for percent change in pulse rate.

[f] Controlled for percent change in weight.

TABLE XIII

Change in Weight and Relative Weight of 30 Intervention Participants in Primary Prevention of Hypertension Program

Variable	Baseline	6 Months	Change
Weight (lb)	184.0	176.8	−7.2 lb[a]
Relative weight	119.0	114.3	−4.7

[a] Number who lost $\geq$ 10 lb = 9; number who lost $\geq$ 5 lb = 16.

being identified with sustained high normal diastolic blood pressure (80–89 mm Hg). Those whose pressures are at the lower end of this range (80–84 mm Hg) must also have a rapid heart rate and/or a weight 10–49% above desirable weight. One-half of the eligible persons are being randomly assigned to the intervention group in which each individual receives individualized diet and exercise prescriptions. The intervention goals consist of at least a 10-lb weight loss, a reduction in daily sodium intake to no more than 75 mEq (1760 mg Na), a reduction in alcohol intake to no more than two drinks/day, and institution of a regular program of frequent aerobic exercise. Emphasis is placed on frequent contact with the interventionists to reinforce progress and on inclusion of a family member in planning lifestyle changes.

Tables XIII and XIV give results in regard to 6-month changes in weight and sodium intake achieved by the initial entrants into the Intervention Group. Comparison with changes in the control group is not possible until 1 year, since data are collected from persons in this group only at annual intervals. The mean decrease in weight from baseline was 7.2 lb (4.7%). Reduction in urinary sodium excretion for 21 participants who collected 6-month urine samples was 33.1%.

Experience of the study to date indicates that changing aspects of lifestyle, particularly habitual ingestion of excess calories and sodium, and low level of activity, is a complex process requiring sustained and intensive motivation and education, constant reinforcement, and sensitivity to individual problems. Clearly, with these approaches, many people are willing to make changes they deem beneficial to their own health and the health of their families.

In summary, the recent experiences of our research group reinforce the long-

TABLE XIV

Change in Average Daily Urinary Sodium Excretion of 21 Intervention Participants in Primary Prevention of Hypertension Program

Baseline (mg Na)	6 Months (mg Na)	% Change
4918	3290	−33.1

standing judgment that dietary sodium and sodium metabolism are of central importance in the etiology and pathogenesis of the mass public health problem of hypertension, and hence in its control and prevention.

ACKNOWLEDGMENTS

The authors acknowledge the contributions of the many individuals whose efforts helped to make these investigations possible: Francesco del Greco, M.D. and the excellent technical support received from the laboratory of the Clinical Research Center, Northwestern University Medical School; David Ostrow, M.D., Ph.D. and Steven Sparks, Veterans Administration Lakeside Medical Center; the staff of the Primary Prevention of Hypertension Program and the Hypertension Control Program; and Reuben Berman, M.D., Richard Grimm, M.D., and Patricia Elmer, M.S., R.D. as co-investigators of the Hypertension Control Program, Minneapolis Center, Minneapolis, Minnesota.

The authors are grateful for the cooperation of the students, staff, and teachers of the Chicago community schools and the Broadview Academy, La Fox, Illinois, and to Yolita Leonas, William Miller, Irma Robinson, Michael J. Steinhauer, and Jean Thiry for their valuable assistance. Appreciation is also expressed to the following colleagues and publishers for permission to cite from published works: L. B. Page, M.D., K. Liu, Ph.D., and R. Cooper, M.D., American Heart Association, American Medical Association, and the School of Hygiene and Public Health of The Johns Hopkins University.

Grant support: This work was supported by grants from the National, Heart, Lung, and Blood Institute, National Institutes of Health (HL21823-03, HL24999, HL23468), the Research Career Development Award for Kiang Liu, Ph.D. (HL00577), and postdoctoral training in cardiovascular epidemiology, nutrition, and biostatistics for Arline McDonald Allen, Ph.D. (HL07113-05).

REFERENCES

Chapman, C. B., and Gibbons, T. B. (1950). The diet and hypertension—A review. *Medicine (Baltimore)* **29**, 29-69.

Childe, V. G. (1951). "Man Makes Himself." New American Library, New York.

Cooper, R., Soltero, I., Liu, K., Berkson, D., Levinson, S., and Stamler, J. (1980). The association between urinary sodium excretion and blood pressure in children. *Circulation* **62**, 97-104.

Dahl, L. K., and Love, R. A. (1954). Evidence for a relationship between sodium intake and human essential hypertension. *Arch. Intern. Med.* **94**, 525-531.

Freis, E. D. (1976). Salt, volume and the prevention of hypertension. *Circulation* **53**, 589-595.

Hypertension Detection and Follow-up Program Cooperative Group (1979a). Five years findings of the Hypertension Detection and Follow-up Program. I. Reduction in mortality of persons with high blood pressure, including mild hypertension. *JAMA, J. Am. Med. Assoc.* **242**, 2562-2571.

Hypertension Detection and Follow-up Program Cooperative Group (1979b). Five year findings of the Hypertension Detection and Follow-up Program. II. Mortality by race-sex and age. *JAMA, J. Am. Med. Assoc.* **242**, 2572-2577.

Leakey, R. E., and Lewin, R. (1977). "Origins," pp. 120–177. Dutton, New York.

Leakey, R. E., and Lewin, R. (1979). "People of the Lake. Mankind and Its Beginnings," pp. 90–114. Avon Books, New York.

Liu, K., Cooper, R., McKeever, J., McKeever, P., Byington, R., Soltero, I. Stamler, R., Gosch,

F., Stevens, E., and Stamler, J. (1979a). Assessment of the association between habitual salt intake and high blood pressure: Methodological problems. *Am. J. Epidemiol.* **110**, 219–226.

Liu, K., Dyer, A. R., Cooper, R. S., Stamler, R., and Stamler, J. (1979b). Can overnight urine replace 24-hour urine collection to assess salt intake? *Hypertension* **1**, 529–536.

Liu, K., Cooper, R., Soltero, I., and Stamler, J. (1979c). Variability in 24-hour urine sodium excretion in children. *Hypertension* **1**, 631–636.

Meneely, G. R., and Battarbee, H. D. (1976). Sodium and potassium. *Nutr. Rev.* **34**, 225–235.

Meneely, G. R., and Dahl, L. K. (1961). Electrolytes in hypertension: The effects of sodium chloride. *Med. Clin. North Am.* **45**, 271–283.

Multhauf, R. P. (1978). ''Neptune's Gift—A History of Common Salt.'' Johns Hopkins Univ. Press, Baltimore, Maryland.

Page, L. B. (1976). Epidemiological evidence on the etiology of human hypertension and its possible prevention. *Am. Heart J.* **91**, 527–534.

Page, L. B., Damon, A., and Moellering, R. C. (1974). Antecedents of cardiovascular disease in six Solomon Islands societies. *Circulation* **49**, 1132–1146.

Stamler, J. (1978). Improving life styles to control the coronary epidemic. *Nutr., Diet. Sport [Proc. Int. Conf.], 1976* pp. 5–48.

Stamler, J. (1979). Hypertension: Aspects of risk. *In* ''Hypertension Update: Cardiovascular Risk Factors and Consequences of Hypertension'' (J. C. Hunt, T. Cooper, E. D. Frohlich, R. W. Gifford, Jr., N. M. Kaplan, J. H. Laragh, M. H. Maxwell and C. G. Strong, eds.), pp. 22–37. Health Learning Systems Inc., Bloomfield, New Jersey.

Stamler, J., Katz, L. N., Pick, R., and Rodbard, S. (1955). Dietary and hormonal factors in experimental atherogenesis and blood pressure regulation. *Recent Prog. Horm. Res.* **11**, 401–452.

Stamler, J., Berkson, D. M., Dyer, A., Lepper, M. H., Lindberg, H. A., Paul, O., McKean, H., Rhomberg, P., Schoenberger, J. A., Shekelle, R. B., and Stamler, R. (1975). Relationship of multiple variables to blood pressure—Findings from four Chicago epidemiologic studies. *In* ''Epidemiology and Control of Hypertension'' (O. Paul, ed.), pp. 307–356. Stratton Intercontinental Med. Book Corp., New York.

Stamler, J., Farinaro, E., Mojonnier, L. M., Hall, Y., Moss, D., and Stamler, R. (1980). Prevention and control of hypertension by nutritional-hygienic means. *JAMA, J. Am. Med. Assoc.* **243**, 1819–1823.

Swartz, M. J., and Jordan, D. K. (1976). ''Anthropology. Perspective on Humanity,'' pp. 372–391. Wiley, New York.

Tannahill, R. (1973). ''Food in History.'' Stein & Day, New York.

Trevisan, M., Ostrow, D., Cooper, R., Liu, K., Sparks, S., and Stamler, J. (1982). Methodological assessment of assays for red cell sodium concentration and sodium-dependent lithium efflux. (In press.)

Wilson, C. A. (1974). ''Food and Drink in Britain.'' Harper (Barnes Noble Imprint Div.), New York.

6

The Effect of Dietary Sodium in Infancy on Blood Pressure and Related Factors

CHARLES F. WHITTEN AND ROBERT A. STEWART

I. INTRODUCTION

Our studies on the role of salt in infant nutrition were initiated in the late 1960s with the objective of determining whether the levels of salt in commercial baby foods influenced blood pressure and/or other factors related to blood pressure of infants.

The first approach was to carry out sodium and potassium balance studies with infants 5–9 months old. A total of 33 infants were fed for 12–18 days using

THE ROLE OF SALT IN
CARDIOVASCULAR HYPERTENSION

TABLE I

Effect of Dietary Sodium Level on Sodium Retention during 21-Day Balance Study

Factor	Unit	Low	Medium	High
Sodium intake	mEq/day	20.8	47.8	79.3
Urinary Na excretion	mEq/day	16.0	39.1	59.7
Stool Na excretion	mEq/day	1.7	2.2	3.1
Sweat Na loss (corrected)	mEq/day	2.5	3.4	3.7
Estimated retention	mEq/day	-0.4	1.4	10.4
Estimated growth requirement	mEq/day	1.0	1.2	1.0
Extracellular fluid volume (day 12, 3 infants per group)	% Body wt	31.2	31.8	30.8
Urinary aldosterone	μg/day	2.93	2.37	1.11
Urinary 17-ketogenic steroids	mg%/day	1.19	1.02	1.15
Weight gain	g/12 days	159 ± 80	183 ± 139	151 ± 154
Initial serum Na	mEq/liter	137.5	136.5	136.6
Change in serum Na (day 12)	mEq/liter	$+0.6$	$+0.2$	-0.5

dietary intakes of 2.3, 6.4, and 10.4 mEq Na/kg/day. Sodium balances, calculated from sodium ingested and sodium excreted in urine, stool, and sweat, showed an average retention of 0.4, 1.0, and 10.4 mEq Na/day on the three diets. Infants on the low, medium, and high sodium diets were not statistically different with respect to weight gain, serum sodium concentration, basal metabolic rate, or ECF volume. They were significantly different with respect to urinary excretion of aldosterone and sodium as well as sodium and potassium losses in sweat (Table I). The high retention of sodium on the high sodium diet could not be explained by delay in sodium diuresis, inaccuracies in sweat losses, errors in balance collections, growth requirements, Na retention in the ECF compartment, or Na deposition in bone.

Because of the enigmatic results of these balance studies, long-term feeding studies with a thorough examination of blood pressure relationships was undertaken.

The procedure and results of these studies have been reported (Whitten and Stewart, 1980). Our purpose here will be to review these findings and present some additional data on the interrelationships of dietary sodium, extracellular fluid (ECF), urine volume, sodium excretion, and blood pressure.

II. PROCEDURE

Two groups of black male infants were fed identical foods with and without added salt for 5 months, starting at 3 months of age. These diets, as consumed

TABLE II

Effect of Dietary Sodium in Infancy on Blood Pressure, Extracellular Fluid Volume, Exchangeable Chloride, and Urinary Excretions

	1 Month					5 Months					8 Years				
	Low salt		p^a	High salt		Low salt		p^a	High salt		Low salt		p^a	High salt	
	Mean	SD		Mean	SD	Mean	SD		Mean	SD	Mean	SD		Mean	SD
Sodium intake															
mEq Na/100 kcal/day	1.91	0.13	0.001	7.09	0.54	1.96	0.16	0.05	10.37	0.40	Uncontrolled				
mEq Na/100 kcal/day	1.85	0.47	0.001	6.53	1.23	1.71	0.37	0.001	9.55	3.03	Uncontrolled				
mEq Na/day	12.8	3.7	0.001	46.1	8.7	15.1	3.2	0.001	81.1	18.8	Uncontrolled				
Percentile in 1969	6th	—	—	97.5th		7th		—	99th						
Percentile in 1977[b]	30th	—	—	98.3rd		30th		—	99.5th						
Blood pressure															
Diastolic	49	5	0.6	50	5	48	5	0.5	49	5	75	5	0.6	76	5
Systolic	97	21	0.5	102	16	88	5	0.4	90	1	103	5	1.0	103	6
ECF (% change in ECF)	37.8	2.8	0.6	38.6	3.8	37.2	2.5	0.02	39.5	2.0	—			—	
(% change in ECF)				2.1%					6.2						
Exchangeable chloride	40.8	3.8	1.0	40.8	2.8	39.9	2.7	0.02	42.4	2.1	—			—	
(% change in Cl)	0%			6.3					6.3						
Urinary excretion															
Volume (ml/72 hr)	1101	228	0.50	1212	408	1124	310	0.90	1106	395	1345	668		1810	731
Na (mEq/day)	7.6	2.2	0.001	51.6	11.0	11.3	3.2	0.001	54.8	9.4	3.20	0.84	0.14	2.75	1.03
K (mEq/day)	11.6	2.6	0.001	18.1	3.4	13.1	2.1	0.001	17.2	2.8	—			—	
Na/K (mEq/day)	0.66	0.15	0.001	2.9	0.5	0.86	0.2	0.001	3.18	0.3	—			—	
Aldosterone (mEq/day)	5.25	1.9	0.001	2.16	1.08	6.1	2.9	0.001	2.37	1.15	—			—	

[a] Values less than 0.05 indicate a significant difference between low and high salt groups.

[b] No salt.

during the third to fifth month of feeding, provided 1.9 and 10.4 mEq Na/100 kcal/day or a total of 15.1 and 81.1 mEq Na/day (Table II).

After 1, 3, and 5 months of feeding at home, the infants were admitted to the Clinical Research Center of the Children's Hospital of Michigan for 3 days to obtain blood pressure, growth, blood composition, body compartment, and urinary excretion measurements.

During their eighth year of age, 23 subjects were located. Growth and blood pressure measurements were taken over a 3-day period and urinary sodium was determined to gain an indication of salt usage.

III. RESULTS

A. Effect on Blood Pressure

From 27 to 123 BP measurements were taken during the evaluation periods and wide variations in both systolic and diastolic pressure were noted in the measurements of a given individual. The means and standard deviation were calculated for each individual and for the dietary groups. These group means are shown in Table II. There is no significant difference in either the systolic or diastolic pressure between the groups after feeding 1 month or 5 months or after 8 years on uncontrolled diets.

B. Effect on ECF

After one month of feeding, there was no significant difference in the ECF or exchangeable chloride between the two groups. However, with continued feeding the ECF of most (seven of ten) infants on the low salt diet tended to go down while the ECF of most (six of nine) infants on the high salt diet tended to go up. This resulted in a significant difference in the extracellular fluid volume of the two groups after 5 months of feeding.

Although the changes in exchangeable chloride did not parallel the changes in ECF, they were similar so that the high salt group also had a significantly higher exchangeable chloride than the low salt group. The ECF increase amounted to 6.2% and the p value was 0.02 (Table II). This finding is similar to the results of Tobian's (1975) experiments with rats fed 0.3% NaCl, 8% NaCl, and 8% NaCl plus thiazide. The low salt diet as well as the thiazide treatment resulted in a 4.6% difference in ECF ($p < 0.03$). The group fed 8% salt, however, had a significantly increased blood pressure compared to the thiazide-treated and the low salt-treated groups ($p < 0.0001$). As was seen in Table II, salt feeding at the 99th percentile did not result in increased blood pressure but it was noted that within the high salt group, there was a significant ($p < 0.05$) positive correlation

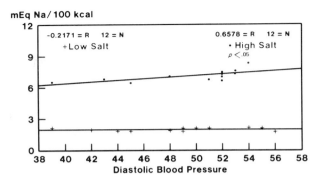

Fig. 1. Diastolic blood pressure versus sodium intake in mEq Na/100 kcal intake, 4 month infants.

$(r = 0.66)$ of diastolic blood pressure with sodium intake calculated as mEq Na/ 100 kcal/day (Fig. 1). This relationship was seen only after 1 month and disappeared after 5 months of feeding. Significant correlations with either systolic or diastolic pressure and sodium intake were not found in either feeding group when sodium intake was calculated as mEq Na per kg of body weight per day or as mEq Na per day.

To study the relationship further, blood pressure was plotted against ECF for all the infants in each feeding group; regression lines and correlation coefficients were also calculated. The regression lines are practically flat and the correlation coefficients show no significant relationship between ECF and blood pressure (Figs. 2 and 3).

C. Effect on Urine Volume and Na Excretion

To maintain homeostasis of ECF, kidneys must excrete increased levels of water and salt. Tobian (1975) has shown that in "post salt" hypertensive rats, kidney infusion pressure must be raised to obtain normal urine volume and sodium output. Normotensive kidneys will handle this increased load at normal blood pressure. An examination of our blood pressure–urine volume data indicates that after 1 month of feeding, lower urine volumes are associated with higher blood pressure. After 5 months of feeding, there was no significant correlation of blood pressure, with urine volume (Figs. 4, 5, 6, and 7).

Further study of the sodium excretion and the urinary sodium/potassium ratio failed to show any significant correlations with blood pressure. The urinary Na/K ratio of infants on the high sodium diet was 3.0–3.5 which suggests that the potassium level of the diet was high enough to exert a protective effect against hypertension.

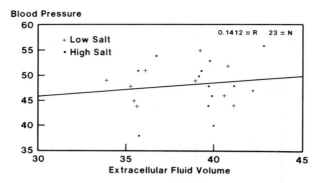

Fig. 2.   Extracellular fluid volume versus diastolic blood pressure at 8 months, all infants.

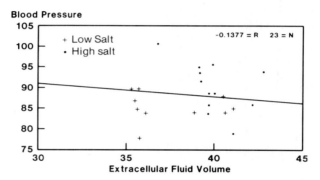

Fig. 3.   Extracellular fluid volume versus systolic blood pressure at 8 months, all infants.

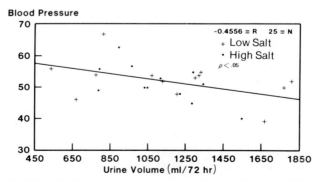

Fig. 4.   Diastolic blood pressure versus urine volume at 4 months, all infants.

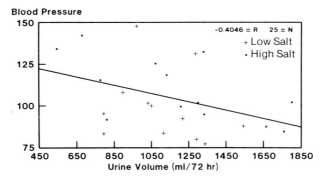

Fig. 5. Systolic blood pressure versus urine volume at 4 months, all infants.

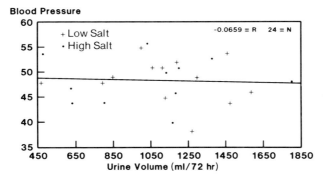

Fig. 6. Diastolic blood pressure versus urine volume at 8 months, all infants.

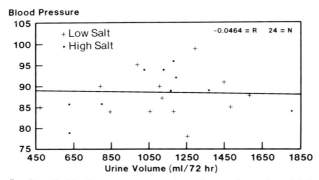

Fig. 7. Systolic blood pressure versus urine volume at 8 months, all infants.

D. Effect of Weight

The positive correlation of blood pressure with weight described by Lauer *et al.* (1976) has been confirmed in these studies. Figure 8 shows the systolic blood pressure versus weight after 5 months of feeding. The correlation ($r = 0.59$) was statistically significant ($p < 0.01$).

Correlation of diastolic and systolic BPs with weight after 1 month and 5 months of feeding the test diets was also noted. This correlation also carried over to the 8-year-old children. Table III lists these correlation coefficients which summarize the relationships noted between blood pressure, ECF, urinary excretion, sodium intake, and weight.

Other measures of obesity such as skinfold measurements, excessive weight gain, and Quetelet Index were also correlated with increased blood pressure, particularly at 8 years of age, but these correlates are not listed here.

IV. SUMMARY

We have concluded from these studies that commercially salted baby foods at the 1969 level, namely 0.75% added NaCl, did not cause an increase in blood pressure of black male infants during a 5-month feeding test. Nor did this diet influence blood pressure or preference for salt in later childhood (8 years). The high salt diet did result in a significantly expanded ECF (6%) but this was not correlated with increased blood pressure, sodium excretion, urine volume, or body weight.

The diet without added salt provided ample sodium for growth, obligatory sodium losses, and maintenance of normal serum sodium and chloride levels.

Blood pressure of these test infants at 8 years of age was not correlated with either early salt feeding or salt intake as indicated by Na excretion or the mother's

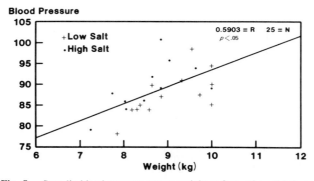

Fig. 8.   Systolic blood pressure versus weight at 8 months, all infants.

TABLE III

Correlates of Blood Pressure after 1 and 5 Months of Feeding Salted and Unsalted Baby Foods

	ECF		Urine volume		Na excretion		Na/K excretion		Body weight		Na intake (mEq Na/100 kcal)		mEq Na/day		Weight	
	Sys.	Dia.	Sys.	Dia.	Sys.	Dia.	Sys.	Dia.	Sys.	Dia.	Sys.	Dia.	Sys.	Dia.	Sys.	Dia.
1 Month																
Low salt group	0.35	0.58	−0.21	−0.63[a]	0.24	−0.31	0.55	−0.10	0.57	0.39	−0.1	−0.22	−0.12	0.14	0.57	0.39
High salt group	−0.15	−0.22	−0.64[a]	−0.43	0.36	0.05	−0.15	0.24	0.26	0.55	−0.22	0.66[a]	−0.09	0.15	0.26	0.55
All infants	0.13	0.18	−0.40[a]	−0.46[a]	0.05	0.04	0.35	0.09	0.39	0.47[a]	0.10	0.16	−0.12	0.13	0.39	0.47[a]
5 Months																
Low salt group	−0.23	0.30	0.09	−0.17	0.05	0.04	0.34	0.39	0.67[a]	0.23	0.22	0.61	−0.34	−0.33	0.67[a]	0.23
High salt group	−0.48	−0.11	−0.11	0.03	0.43	0.13	0.44	0.47	0.64[a]	0.48	0.4	0.53	0.40	0.07	0.64[a]	0.48
All infants	−0.13	0.14	−0.05	−0.07	0.29	0.12	0.08	0.18	0.59[a]	0.35	0.20	−0.17	0.05	−0.05	0.59[a]	0.35
8 Years																
Low salt group	—	—	−0.19	−0.21	0.27	0.19	—	—	0.77[b]	0.56	—	—	—	—	0.77[b]	0.56
High salt group	—	—	−0.30	0.05	0.21	0.25	—	—	0.39	0.48	—	—	—	—	0.32	0.48
All subjects	—	—	−0.27	0.09	0.23	0.21	—	—	0.55[b]	0.45[a]	—	—	—	—	0.57[b]	0.45[a]

[a] p = 0.05.
[b] p = 0.01.

perception of salt preference and usage. Blood pressure was correlated with weight and skinfold thickness and Quetelet Index at 8 years of age.

REFERENCES

Lauer, R. M., Filer, L. J., Reiter, M. A., and Clarke, W. R. (1976). Blood pressure, salt preference, salt threshold and relative weight. *Am. J. Dis. Child.* **130,** 493–497.

Tobian, L. (1975). Current status of salt in hypertension. *In* "Epidemiology and Control of Hypertension" (P. Oglesby, ed.), pp. 131–143. Year Book Med. Publ., Chicago, Illinois.

Whitten, C. F., and Stewart, R. A. (1980). The effect of dietary sodium in infancy on blood pressure and related factors. *Acta Paediatr. Scand., Suppl.* **279,** 3–17.

7

Blood Pressure and Sodium Intake in the First Two Years of Life

JOSEPH SCHACHTER, LEWIS H. KULLER, AND
CAROL PERFETTI

I. INTRODUCTION

In a previous report of a prospective study of infants, among infants at 6 months of age, a positive association was found between sodium intake and blood pressure (BP) (Schachter *et al.*, 1979). This report presents the results of re-examining this cohort at 15 and at 24 months to determine whether this sodium intake–BP relationship persists.

THE ROLE OF SALT IN
CARDIOVASCULAR HYPERTENSION

II. MATERIALS AND METHODS

A. Subjects

A group of 392 healthy, full-term (37–42 weeks gestation), appropriate weight (above the 10th percentile in birth weight for gestational age) infants, stratified by ethnic group (black or white) and socioeconomic status (Green, 1970) (high or low) was selected. Adequate blood pressure (BP) measurements were obtained on 340 newborns. At 6 months of age 318 infants were re-examined; 277 infants were again re-examined at 15 months and 232 infants at 24 months.

B. Procedure

Examinations at 15 and 24 months of age were carried out in the home by research assistants who previously had visited the families at the 6-month examination. At 15 months attempt was made to obtain BP measurements while the infant was sleeping during a nap, as had been done at 6 months of age. At the 24-month examination attempt was made to obtain waking BP measurements on all infants, as very few of them napped with regularity.

BP measurements were obtained with a Roche Arteriosonde 1010. Comparison of BP measurement by the Arteriosonde with intra-arterial BP measurement in infants and children indicates a degree of validity approximately the same as that of sphygmomanometer measurement in adults for SBP, and somewhat less for DBP (Hochberg and Saltzman, 1971; Zahed et al., 1971; Black et al., 1972; Poppers, 1973; Whyte et al., 1975; Reder et al., 1978). A cuff was selected in which bladder length exceeded 75% of the biceps circumference (Blumenthal et al., 1977). The bladder width conformed reasonably to the additional recommendation that bladder width be 40% of arm circumference (Geddes and Whistler, 1978).

C. Results

Effects of Attrition

The effects of attrition of subjects during the course of the study was examined. A total of 108 of the original 340 infants was lost to the study by 24 months of age. Those lost from the study either because they refused to continue, they moved away, or they could not be located did not differ from those infants who remained in the study in any of the following characteristics: socioeconomic score, mother's age or weight, the infant's gestational age, birthweight or length at birth and infant's sex ratio, or the newborn's SBP or DBP or heart rate.

Among those lost from the study because they could not be located, a higher proportion were black than among those who remained in the study.

In addition, those infants examined at 6 months were compared with those infants not examined at 6 months, separately among the whites and blacks, with regard to the following newborn characteristics: gestational age, birth weight, SBP, DBP, and heart rate. There were no significant differences. Similarly, those infants examined at 15 months were compared with those infants not examined at 15 months, separately among the whites and blacks, with regard to the following characteristics at 6 months of age: weight, height, SBP, DBP, and heart rate. Again, there were no significant differences.

Finally, the effects of attrition were assessed by comparing the mean of a particular variable at each of the four ages examined for each of the following groups of infants: (1) all of the infants with data at each age; (2) infants with data at all four ages; (3) infants missing data only at 6 months; (4) infants missing data only at 15 months; and (5) infants missing data only at 24 months. There were no significant differences between the means of these five groups for SBP, DBP, heart rate, infant weight, or infant height.

There is no evidence that the attrition of subjects has biased the results of either cardiovascular or physical examinations.

III. BLOOD PRESSURE IN RELATION TO AGE, SEX, AND ETHNIC GROUP

At 15 months of age average BP during sleep in 276 infants was 89/49 mm Hg; at 24 months of age average BP during waking in 230 infants was 97/55 mm Hg. BP at 2 or 2.5 years as reported by other investigators is presented in Table I. With the exception of Berenson's Infrasonde measurements, which were made with a much wider bladder than was used with the other instruments, mean SBP ranged from 94 to 99 mm Hg. Again, with the exception of the Infrasonde measurements, mean DBP ranged from 55 to 63 mm Hg. The average for all the studies (excepting the Infrasonde measurements) weighted by the number of subjects was 97 mm Hg SBP and 59 mm Hg DBP.

BP as a function of ethnic group and age from newborn to 24 months is presented in Table II. Differences in average BP between white infants and black infants are small, 2.5 mm Hg or less. SBP is lower among black infants at 15 and 24 months; DBP is higher among black newborns. BP did not vary significantly as a function of socioeconomic class or sex. Health of the infant on either the day of the visit or the week preceding the visit did not affect either SBP or DBP for either white infants or black infants.

TABLE I

Comparison of Blood Pressure Measurements

Investigator	Age (years)	n	Bladder size (cm)	Instrument	No. measurements	Blood pressure (mmHg)	
						Systolic	Diastolic
Allen-Williams (1945)	2–3	89	6.0 × —	Sphygmomanometer	2	96	62
Jesse and Blumenthal (1977)	2	97		Sphygmomanometer	2	99	63
Berenson et al. (1978)	2.8	101	5.8 × 17.8	Sphygmomanometer	3	98	62
			7.0 × 21.6				
Berenson et al. (1978)	2.8	101	13.0 × 23.5	Infrasonde	3	87	49
Berenson et al. (1978)	2.8	101	9.5 × 21.6	Arteriosonde	3	94	60
Schachter et al. (1982)	2	203	5.5 × 13.0	Arteriosonde	6	97	55

TABLE II

Blood Pressure as a Function of Ethnic Group and Age

	Systolic				Diastolic			
	White	Black	Δ	p	White	Black	Δ	p
Newborn	75.0	76.4	−1.4	n.s.	50.1	51.9	−1.8	.047
6 months	86.9	86.0	0.9	n.s.	48.3	48.0	0.3	n.s.
15 months	88.8	86.3	2.5	.011	49.8	48.6	1.2	n.s.
24 months	97.4	95.3	2.1	.043	54.6	54.5	0.1	n.s.

IV. BLOOD PRESSURE–NUTRITION RELATIONSHIP

Nutritional data were derived from 3-day food records which were obtained for 126 15-month-old and 96 24-month-old infants. A comparison of our caloric intake results by age and ethnic group with those of other investigators is presented in Table III. Protein intake results are compared with those of other investigators in Table IV.

Caloric intake failed to correlate with either SBP or DBP at 6, 15, or 24 months. Protein intake (with a single exception) also failed to correlate with SBP or DBP. Caloric intake at 6 months correlated positively with caloric intake at 15 months ($p < 0.004$) which, in turn, correlated with caloric intake at 24 months ($p < 0.001$).

Caloric intake correlated with sodium intake at each age, the highest correlation occurring at 24 months (0.74, $p < 0.001$). Protein intake also correlated with sodium intake at each age; the correlation at 24 months was 0.60 ($p < 0.001$).

V. BLOOD PRESSURE–ELECTROLYTE INTAKE RELATIONSHIP

Sodium and potassium intakes were estimated from 3-day food records. In 29 infants at 15 months of age sodium intake estimated from food records averaged 20% less than spectrophotometric measurement of sodium in food portions equivalent to what the infant had eaten.

In a separate study of the validity of the estimates of sodium and potassium intakes of nine adults from daily food records, the estimate of sodium intake from 3-day food records averaged 11% lower than measurement of sodium excretion in three 24-hr urines; the estimate of sodium intake from food portions averaged less than 2% higher than urinary sodium excretion. Individual differences, however,

TABLE III

Comparison of Caloric Intake by Age and Ethnic Group

Investigator	Age (months)	Year	Number	Average calories	Calories per kg
White infants					
Stearns et al. (1958)[a]	12	1930–1958	194	1094	
Eagles and Steele (1975)[a]	12	1965–1966	93	1255	
Brown and Ho (1972)[b]	12	1966–1971	145	1186	
Crawford et al. (1978)	12	1969–1970	284	947	95
Hanes I (National Center, 1979)	12	1971–1974	400	1288	114
Reuda-Williamson and Rose (1962)[a]	12–15	1959–1960	67	1080	106[c]
Guthrie (1963)	12–15	1963	12	1026	
Beal (1970)	15	1953–1967	45	1073	101
Schachter et al.	15	1978	91	1148	108
Fryer et al. (1971)	12–18	1965	279	1282	
Owen et al. (1974)	12–23	1968–1970	635[d]	1083[c]	
Ten State (National Center, 1972)	12–23	1968–1970	316	1429	
Widdowson (1947)[a]	12–24	1935–1939	43	1153	101
Burke et al. (1959)[a]	12–24	1959	125	1280	
Eagles and Steele (1975)[a]	12–24	1967–1966	810	1405	
Fryer et al. (1971)	18–24	1965	218	1394	
Stearns et al. (1958)[a]	24	1930–1958	152	1219	
Beal (1970)	24	1953–1967	45	1252	
Schachter et al.	24	1978	76	1221	95
Black infants					
Crawford et al. (1978)	12	1969–1970	58	942	
Hanes I (National Center, 1979)	12	1971–1974	145	1182	105
Schachter et al.	15	1978	35	1069	99
Ten State (National Center, 1972)	12–23	1968–1970	277	1233	
Schachter et al.	24	1978	20	1210	95

[a] Ethnicity not specified; probably 80–90% white.

[b] Hawaiian population, one-third white.

[c] 50th percentile.

[d] 80% white.

were large between both the 3-day food records and the food portion analysis in comparison to urinary sodium excretion (Schachter et al., 1980). The estimate of potassium intake from food records deviated from the average urinary excretion by less than 8%. Differences for individuals between 3-day estimates of potassium intake from either food record or food portion analysis and of urinary excretion showed a smaller variance than for sodium, although a considerable number of differences exceeded 10% and 3 out of 18 differences exceeded 25%.

TABLE IV

Comparison of Protein Intake by Age and Ethnic Group

Investigator	Age (months)	Year	Number	Average protein (g)	Protein per kg
White infants					
Stearns et al. (1958)[a]	12	1930–1958	194	43	
Brown and Ho (1972)[b]	12	1966–1971	145	47	
Crawford et al. (1978)	12	1969–1970	284	45	4.5
Hanes I (National Center, 1979)	12	1971–1974	400	52	4.5
Reuda-Williamson and Rose (1962)[a]	12–15	1959–1960	67	45	4.4
Guthrie (1963)	12–16	1963	12	44	
Fryer et al. (1971)	12–18	1965	279	56	
Schachter et al.	15	1978	91	48	4.5
Owen et al. (1974)[c]	12–23	1968–1970	635	46[d]	
Widdowson (1947)[a]	12–24	1935–1939	43	38	3.3
Eagles and Steele (1975)[a]	12–24	1965–1966	810	56	
Fryer et al. (1971)	18–24	1965	218	56	
Stearns et al. (1958)[a]	24	1930–1958	152	48	
Schachter et al.	24	1978	76	46	3.6
Black infants					
Crawford et al. (1978)	12	1969–1970	57	40	
Hanes I (National Center, 1979)	12	1971–1974	145	47	4.3
Schachter et al.	15	1978	35	42	3.9
Schachter et al.	24	1978	20	46	3.7

[a] Ethnicity not specified; probably 80–90% white.

[b] Hawaiian population, one-third white.

[c] 80% white.

[d] 50th percentile.

Estimates of sodium intake from our food record analyses are presented by age and ethnic group in Table V. Our value for white infants 15 months of age of 6.3 mEq sodium/kg/day corresponds closely to the value of 6.5 mEq/kg/day for infants 14 months of age from a report by Puyau and Hampton (1966, Fig. 1). Analysis of variance of logarithmically transformed sodium intake per kilogram indicated no change from 15 to 24 months.

Analyses of variance of the effects of ethnic group and socioeconomic class on both sodium intake and potassium intake were calculated for 6, 15, and 24 months of age. For sodium intake the only significant effects were at 15 months; sodium intake was higher among whites ($p < 0.027$) and among low socioeconomic class infants ($p < 0.022$). For potassium intake the effect of ethnic group was significant only at 6 months; white infants had a higher potassium intake. High socioeconomic class infants had a higher potassium at 6 months ($p < 0.032$) and 15 months ($p < 0.029$). At 24 months neither ethnic

TABLE V

Sodium Intake by Age and Ethnic Group

Age (months)	n	mEq/day	mEq/kg/day
White infants			
6	114	24	3.1
15	91	67	6.3
24	76	74	5.8
Black infants			
6	39	21	2.6
15	35	55	5.1
24	20	69	5.4

group nor socioeconomic class had any significant effect on either sodium intake or potassium intake.

The analysis of the association between sodium intake and blood pressure in the infant was calculated for infants at 15 and at 24 months, as it had been for 153 infants at 6 months (Schachter *et al.*, 1979). Among white infants 15 months of age, whose mother's mean blood pressure was above the median for this population, there was no association between infant sodium intake and infant BP. At 24 months of age, results of the same analysis were also negative. Results remained negative when infants were selected on the basis either of the father's mean BP above the median or the parents' combined mean BP above the median. These results were uniformly negative, although a considerable number of the infants were the same ones who at 6 months of age had exhibited a positive association between infant sodium intake and BP. Several different BPs of the parents were used, such as SBP rather than the mean BP. Regardless of the BP chosen, results remained consistently negative.

In order to determine whether the association between sodium intake and BP at 6 months of age among white infants whose parent's mean BP was above the median had any persistent effect, the subsequent identification of the one-third of these infants with the highest salt intake as well as the one-third with the lowest salt intake allowed a comparison of their BPs. There was no difference between these two groups at either 15 or 24 months of age with respect to SBP, weight, or height. There was little relationship between salt intake at 6 months and salt intake either at 15 or 24 months of age.

Several other approaches to this analysis were utilized. Since our study of intake and excretion of sodium indicated that estimates of sodium intake from dietary data were reasonably valid for groups of nine or larger (Schachter *et al.*, 1980), we examined sodium intake and BP in groups of ten. Again, no relationship was found between infant sodium intake and BP.

TABLE VI

Average Systolic Blood Pressure in mm Hg at 24 Months of Age as a Function of Levels of Potassium and of Sodium Intake

| Sodium intake | Potassium intake | | | | | |
| | Low | | | High | | |
	n	Mean	SD	n	Mean	SD
High	14	99.3	9.2	35	97.4	7.0
Low	31	96.3	6.3	12	97.9	7.7

Next, infants were selected not on the basis of having a parent whose BP was above the median for this population, but on the basis of having at least one parent who reported a history of hypertension. Among these offspring of a hypertensive parent, infant sodium intake failed to correlate with BP.

In order to determine whether high potassium intake might have protected against a pressure-elevating effect of high sodium intake, infants were selected who were either above or below the median for potassium intake and for sodium intake at each age. Among low-potassium-intake infants, mean BP levels were not significantly higher among the high-sodium groups at 6, 15, or 24 months of age. Table VI presents mean BPs for infants above and below the median in potassium intake (2.9 mEq/kg or 38 mEq/day) and in sodium intake (5.1 mEq/kg or 66 mEq/day) at 24 months of age. Among low-potassium-intake infants, high-sodium-intake infants averaged 3.0 mm Hg higher than low-sodium-intake infants, though this difference was not statistically significant.

Finally, on the assumption that sodium intake might be correlated among family members, mean BP for each parent of an infant whose sodium intake was above the median was compared with the mean BP for each parent of an infant whose sodium intake was below the median. There were no significant differences in the mean BP of mothers or fathers as a function of the level of sodium intake of the infant.

VI. DISCUSSION

The most intriguing finding in our earlier report was that among white infants whose parents' BP was above the median there was a positive association between sodium intake and infant BP at 6 months of age (Schachter *et al.*, 1979). The present report fails to replicate this association in infants at 15 and at 24 months of age.

Numerous factors may account for this failure of replication in older infants. There is no evidence to suggest any greater errors in measurement of either BP or sodium intake at 15 or 24 months of age than there was at 6 months of age. BP at 15 months was measured during nonrapid-eye-movement sleep as it had been at 6 months; only the measurements at 24 months which were in the waking state were characterized by greater intraindividual variability. Average BP at 24 months agreed reasonably well with the findings of other investigators. Tracking correlations from 6 to 15 months and from 15 to 24 months were similar to those reported by other investigators and suggest that measurement errors did not exceed those in other studies. With regard to sodium intake, there is close agreement with one other study of 15-month-old infants. Further, caloric intake and protein intake, which correlated closely with sodium intake, and which were derived from the same food records as the estimates of sodium intake, showed reasonable agreement with the averages reported by numerous investigators at both 15 and 24 months of age. There is, therefore, no indication of greater errors of measurement of either BP or salt intake at 15 and 24 months than there had been at 6 months when the association was found.

The possibility remains that interindividual errors in assessment of sodium intake may be substantially greater in the older ages when the infants are on more variable diets and that this may vitiate the association of sodium intake with infant BP. This seems unlikely since forming the infants into groups of 10 also failed to provide substantiation, and a separate study indicated that average sodium intake estimated from food records for groups of this size are reasonably accurate (Schachter *et al.*, 1980).

Selection of infants on the basis of a parent with hypertension, rather than on the basis of the parent's BP being above or below the median, also failed to provide evidence of a sodium intake–BP relationship in infants. This fails to provide support for the report that normotensive adults with a first degree relative who was hypertensive exhibited significant correlations between sodium excretion and BP (Pietinen *et al.*, 1979). The significant association in the latter study cannot be attributed to any wider range of sodium values. In the latter, sodium excretion ranged from 60 to 370 mEq/day; the maximum is 6.2 times the minimum. In our data from infants 6 months of age the maximal sodium value was also 6.2 times the minimum when a significant association was found. At 15 months of age, when no significant association was observed, the maximal sodium value was 10.8 times the minimal value; at 24 months of age the maximal sodium value was 5.7 times the minimal value.

Another hypothesis was considered to try to account for finding a sodium intake–BP relationship at 6 months, but not at 15 or 24 months: Was the ratio of the sodium load to the infant's capacity to excrete sodium substantially greater at 6 months than at the later ages? The ability to excrete a sodium load increases linearly through the first year of life (Aperia *et al.*, 1975). Aperia *et al.* (1979)

have shown that in infants averaging 2.5 months of age (assuming an average weight of 5.0 kg), maximal sodium excretion in response to sodium load averaged 15 mEq/day. Aperia's earlier works (Aperia *et al.*, 1975) had shown that maximal sodium excretion at 6 months was 2.1 times as great as that at 2.5 months. Therefore, maximal sodium excretion in response to sodium load at 6 months of age is approximately 32 mEq/day; in our cohort average sodium intake for white infants at 6 months of age was 24 mEq/day (Table V). Extrapolating similarly from Aperia's data (Aperia *et al.*, 1975) maximal sodium excretion in response to sodium load at 15 months of age is approximately 77 mEq/day; in our cohort average sodium intake for white infants at 15 months of age was 67 mEq/day. The relationship of maximal excretory capacity to sodium intake at 15 months seems quite similar to that at 6 months of age. Whitten and Stewart (1980) report higher levels of sodium excretion among infants who were fed a diet containing 68 mEq of sodium per day. Average urinary excretion of sodium was 52 mEq/day at 4 months and 55 mEq/day at 8 months. These levels would not provide any support for the hypothesis that the ratio of sodium load to sodium excretory capacity may be greater at 6 than at 15 months.

The higher levels of sodium excretion reported by Whitten and Stewart (1980) may reflect an effect on sodium excretion of a high sodium intake. Aperia *et al.* (1979) reported that placing infants 2–3 months of age on a diet with the sodium intake increased to approximately 12 mEq/day for 1 week increased the infants' capacity to excrete a sodium load; in one group of infants the capacity to excrete a sodium load was doubled. Aperia *et al.* (1979) suggested, "It might therefore be an advantage to increase the daily sodium intake stepwise during the first months of life provided that infants are healthy, show no signs of renal disease and have a negative family history of hypertension."

It is appropriate to mention also that the sodium intake–BP relationship at 6 months of age may have been a chance finding that happened to conform to our expectation.

Our results indicated that those infants who showed a salt intake–BP relationship and who had a high salt intake at age 6 months did not show any persistent effects. That is, their BPs were no higher at 15 or 24 months of age. These results are consistent with those of Whitten and Stewart (1980).

The failure to observe the sodium intake–BP relationship in infants at 15 and 24 months of age may have been a function of the protective action of potassium (Parfrey *et al.*, 1981). However, the sodium/potassium ratio failed to correlate with BP. In addition, selecting infants with below the median intake in potassium failed to show a BP effect among high-sodium-intake infants. Among 24-month-old infants, however, there was some tendency toward a higher BP among high-sodium-intake infants. Perhaps with a larger population, where it would be possible to examine more levels of electrolyte intake than just high or low sodium or potassium, the degree to which relatively high levels of potassium may protect against a BP-elevating effect of relatively high sodium intake could more clearly be elucidated.

VII. SUMMARY

In a prior report, measurements of BP and estimates of sodium intake from food records among 153 infants at 6 months of age failed to show any significant association. However, at this 6-month age, among white infants whose parent's BP was above the median for this population, there was a positive association between the infant's BP and the infant's sodium intake. The present report provides results of subsequent examinations of this cohort. Measurements of BP and estimates of sodium intake were obtained from 126 infants at 15 months and 96 infants at 24 months of age. The association between the infant's BP and the infant's sodium intake, among white infants whose parents' BP was above the median, could not be replicated either at 15 or at 24 months of age. There was no evidence that this failure of replication was due to the ratio of the sodium load to the infant's capacity to excrete sodium having been substantially greater at 6 months than at the later ages. The positive association between the infant's BP and the infant's sodium intake at 6 months of age may have been a chance finding that happened to conform to our expectation. The failure to observe the BP–sodium intake relationship among the older infants may have been a function of the protective action of potassium since among 24-month-old infants there was some tendency toward a higher BP among low-potassium- and high-sodium-intake infants.

REFERENCES

Allen-Williams, G. M. (1945). Pulse-rate and blood pressure in infancy and early childhood. *Arch. Dis. Childhood* **20,** 125–128.

Aperia, A, Broberger, O, Thodenius, K., and Zetterström, R. (1975). Development of renal control of salt and fluid homeostasis during the first year of life. *Acta Paediatr. Scand.* **64,** 393–398.

Aperia, A, Broberger, O, Herin, K., Thodenius, K., and Zetterström, R. (1979). Renal sodium excretory capacity in infants under different dietary conditions. *Acta Paediatr. Scand.* **68,** 351–355.

Beal, V. A. (1970). Nutritional intake. *In* "Human Growth and Development" (R. W. McCammon, eds.), p. 63. Thomas, Springfield, Illinois.

Berenson, G. S., Foster, T. A., Frank, G. C., Frerichs, R. R., Srinivasan, S. R., Voors, A. W., and Webber, L. S. (1978). Cardiovascular disease risk factor variables at the preschool age—The Bogalusa Heart Study. *Circulation* **57,** 603–612.

Black, I. F. S., Kotrapu, N., and Massie, H. (1972). Application of Doppler ultrasound to blood pressure measurement in small infants. *J. Pediatr.* **81,** 932–935.

Blumenthal, S., Epps, R. P., Havenrich, R., Lauer, R. M., Lieberman, E., Mirkin, B., Mitchell, S.

C., Naito, V. B., O'Hare, D., Smith, W. M., Tarazi, R. C., and Upson, D. (1977). Report of the task force on blood pressure control in children. *Pediatrics* **59**, Suppl., 797–820.

Brown, M. L., and Ho, C. H. (1972). Infant and childhood feeding practices among low-income families in urban Hawaii. DHEW Publ. (HSA) (U.S.) **HSA75-5605**, 91–92.

Burke, B. S., Reed, R. B., van den Berg, A. S., and Stuart, H. C. (1959). Caloric and protein intakes of children between 1 and 18 years of age. *Pediatrics* **24**, 922–940.

Crawford, P. B., Hankin, J. H., and Huenemann, R. L. (1978). Environmental factors associated with preschool obesity. III. Dietary intakes, eating patterns and anthropometric measurements. *J. Am. Diet. Assoc.* **72**, 589–596.

Eagles, J. A. and Steele, P. D. (1975). Food and nutrient intake of children from birth to four years of age. DHEW Publ. (HSA) (U.S.) **HSA75-5605**, 19–25.

Fryer, B. A., Lamkin, G. H., Vivian, V. M., Eppright, E. S., and Foy, H. M. (1971). Diets of preschool children in the North Central Region. *J. Am. Diet. Assoc.* **59**, 228–232.

Geddes, L. A. and Whistler, S. J. (1978). The error in indirect blood pressure measurement with the incorrect size of cuff. *Am. Heart J.* **96**, 4–8.

Green, L. W. (1970). Manual for scoring socioeconomic status for research on health behavior. *Public Health Rep.* **85**, 815–827.

Guthrie, H. A. (1963). Nutritional intake of infants. *J. Am. Diet. Assoc.* **43**, 120–124.

Hochberg, H. M. and Saltzman, M. B. (1971). Accuracy of an ultrasound blood pressure instrument in neonates, infants and children. *Curr. Ther. Res.* **13**, 482–488.

Jessee, M. J. and Blumenthal, S. (1977). Report of the task force on blood pressure control in children. *Pediatrics* **59**, 819, 820, Appendix 1 and 2.

National Center for Health Statistics (1972). "Ten-State Nutrition Survey 1968–1970. V. Dietary," DHEW Publ. No. (HMSM) 72-8133. Health Serv. Ment. Health Admin., Center for Disease Control, Atlanta, Georgia.

National Center for Health Statistics (1979). "Caloric and Selected Nutrient Values for Persons 1–74 Years of Age: First Health and Nutrition Examination Survey United States, 1971–1974," Vital and Health Statistics, Ser. II, No. 209, DHEW Publ. No. (PHS) 79-1657. Office of Health Research, Statistics and Technology. US Govt. Printing Office, Washington, D.C.

Owen, G. M., Kram, K. M., Garry, P. J., Lowe, J. E., and Lubin, A. H. (1974). A study of nutritional status of preschool children in the United States, 1968–70. *Pediatrics* **53**, 597–646.

Parfrey, P. S., Vanderberg, M. J., Wright, P., Holly, J. M. P., Goodwin, F. J., Evans, S. J. W., and Ledingham, J. M. (1981). Blood pressure and hormonal changes following alteration in dietary sodium and potassium in mild essential hypertension. *Lancet* **1**, 113–117.

Pietinen, P. I., Wong, O., and Altschul, A. M. (1979). Electrolyte output, blood pressure, and family history of hypertension. *Am. J. Clin. Nutr.* **32**, 997–1005.

Poppers, P. I. (1973). Controlled evaluation of ultrasonic measurement of systolic and diastolic blood pressure in pediatric patients. *Anaesthesiology* **38**, 187–191.

Puyau, F. A. and Hampton, L. P. (1966). Infant feeding practices, 1966. *Am. J. Dis. Child.* **3**, 370–373.

Reder, R. F., Dimich, I., Cohen, M. L., and Steinfeld, L. (1978). Evaluating indirect blood pressure techniques: A comparison of three systems in infants and children. *Pediatrics* **62**, 326–330.

Rueda-Williamson, R. and Rose, H. E. (1962). Growth and nutrition of infants. *Pediatrics* **30**, 639–653.

Schachter, J., Kuller, L. H., Perkins, J. M., and Radin, M. E. (1979). Infant blood pressure and heart rate: Relation to ethnic group (black or white), nutrition and electrolyte intake. *Am. J. Epidemiol.* **110**, 205–218.

Schachter, J., Harper, P., Radin, M., Caggiula, A. W., McDonald, R. H., and Diven, W. F. (1980). Comparison of sodium and potassium intake from food ingested with sodium and potassium urinary excretion. *Hypertension* **2**, 695–699.

Schachter, J., Kuller, L. H., Perfetti, C. (1982). Blood pressure during the first two years of life. *Am. J. Epidemiol.* In press.

Stearns, G., Newman, K. J., McKinley, J. B., and Jeans, P. C. (1958). The protein requirements of children from one to ten years of age. *Ann. N.Y. Acad. Sci.* **69,** 857–868.

Whitten, C. F. and Stewart, R. A. (1980). The effect of dietary sodium in infancy on blood pressure and related factors. Studies of infants fed salted and unsalted diets for five months at eight months and eight years of age. *Acta Paediatr. Scand., Suppl.* **279,** 3–17.

Whyte, R. K., Elseed, A. M., Fraser, C. B., Shinebourne, E. A., and de Swiet, M. (1975). Assessment of Doppler ultrasound to measure systolic and diastolic blood pressures in infants and young children. *Arch. Dis. Child.* **50,** 542–544.

Widdowson, E. M. (1947). A study of individual children's diets. *Med. Res. Counc. (G.B.), Spec. Rep. Ser.* **SRS-257.**

Zahed, B., Sadove, M. S., Hatano, S., and Wu, H. H. (1971). Ultrasound versus Korotkoff blood pressure techniques. *Anesth. Analg. (Cleveland)* **50,** 699–704.

8

The Control of Sodium Chloride Intake by Normotensive and Hypertensive Rats

MELVIN J. FREGLY

103

THE ROLE OF SALT IN
CARDIOVASCULAR HYPERTENSION

I. INTRODUCTION

The regulation of both food and water intakes by animals is well known. Food intake is normally adjusted to energy expenditure (Adolph, 1943) and water intake is related both to food intake and to water loss (Cizek, 1959; Cizek and Nocenti, 1965; Wolf, 1958). Less well studied is the possibility that animals may control their sodium intake.

Regulation of the sodium concentration of plasma and/or the sodium content of the body involves two main processes: the control of sodium intake and the control of sodium loss. A great deal of information is available regarding the physiological control of sodium loss from the body and the hemodynamic, hormonal, and other factors that influence it (Davis, 1976; Oparil, 1976). Physiologists, particularly, have concentrated their efforts in this area. Much less solid information is available regarding control of sodium intake. In fact, it is unknown in most species whether sodium intake is controlled or whether it is fickle and independent of control. There is, however, evidence in sheep and rabbits that sodium intake may be as closely controlled as sodium output (Denton, 1969; Denton and Nelson, 1980).

Early experiments of Richter (1936) called attention to the role of the adrenal gland in the control of the intake of NaCl solution by rats. When choice was offered between water and a NaCl solution to drink, adrenalectomized rats ingested the NaCl solution predominately and survived.

Others noted that rats rendered hypertensive by bilateral encapsulation of their kidneys with latex envelopes manifested a relative aversion to NaCl solutions under the same conditions as used by Richter (1936) earlier to study adrenalectomized rats (Abrams *et al.*, 1949; Fregly, 1955, 1961). Since the responses of both adrenalectomized and renal hypertensive rats seemed appropriate to the experimental situation, an objective was to study further the relative aversion to NaCl solutions reported in renal hypertensive rats. In addition, the preference (taste) threshold for detection of NaCl was studied as was the time course for development of the aversion. Additional studies were performed to determine whether normotensive rats could control their intake of NaCl and whether hypertension altered regulatory ability.

II. METHODS

A. Experiment 1: Time Course of the Development of Hypertension, NaCl Aversion, and Polydipsia in Renal Hypertensive Rats

Thirty-two male rats of the Sprague–Dawley strain weighing 250–280 g were used. They were maintained on Purina Laboratory Chow and tap water *ad libitum* in a temperature controlled (26° ± 1°C) room illuminated from 7 A.M. to 7 P.M.

Control measurements were made on all rats during the first 2 weeks of the experiment. During this time, daily intakes of food (ground Purina Laboratory Chow) and fluids (distilled water and 0.15 M NaCl solution) were measured, as was body weight. Food was provided in spill-proof containers as described by Fregly (1960) while fluid containers were infant nursing bottles with cast aluminum spouts as described by Lazarow (1954). Systolic blood pressure of each rat was measured weekly by means of the microphonic manometer technique of Friedman and Freed (1949) as modified by Fregly (1963). All rats were unanesthetized when blood pressure was measured.

Upon completion of the 2-week control period, both kidneys of half of the rats were encapsulated with latex envelopes following anesthesia with pentobarbital (Abrams and Sobin, 1947; Fregly, 1966). One week was allowed for postoperative recovery after which daily measurements of body weight and intakes of food and fluids, and weekly measurements of systolic blood pressure, were resumed for 9 weeks and at 2- or 3-week intervals thereafter. Between measurements, the rats were given the same food and fluids as during the periods of observation.

B. Experiment 2: Effect of Renal Hypertension on the Preference Threshold of Rats for Sodium Chloride

Ten male Sprague–Dawley rats were used. Bilateral renal encapsulations were performed on half of the rats at age 11 weeks, while the remaining rats were used as control. The experiment began 20 weeks after renal encapsulation when all operated rats had a significantly elevated systolic blood pressure which was at least 35 mm Hg above the highest single blood pressure in the control group. At this time the rats weighed 410–440 g. During the period prior to the initiation of this study, the rats were maintained under conditions identical to those described in Experiment 1.

During the study, daily measurements of individual food and fluid intakes, as well as body weight, were made. Systolic blood pressure of each rat was measured once weekly by the microphonic manometer technique of Friedman and Freed (1949) but without anesthesia and as modified by Fregly (1963). The food and fluid containers were the same as those described in Experiment 1.

Two separate drinking fluids were available to the rats at all times. One bottle always contained distilled water and will be designated as reference solution while the second bottle contained a NaCl solution designated as the test solution. The concentration of the test solution was changed every fourth day (with the single exception of period 1 lasting 8 days). Each of the following concentrations of test (NaCl) solution was given in the order stated: 0.00 (distilled water); 0.0005, 0.001, 0.002, 0.004, 0.008, 0.016, 0.024, 0.032, 0.045, 0.060, 0.075,

0.090, 0.105, and 0.00 M. Sixty-four days (15 test periods) were required to complete the experiment. Additional details of the experimental procedure have been described elsewhere (Fregly, 1955).

C. Experiment 3: Effect of Sodium Content of Diet on Spontaneous Intake of Sodium Chloride Solutions by Normotensive Rats

The first study used 15 male rats of the Sprague–Dawley (Holtzman) strain while the last two studies each used 10 different male rats of the same strain. The rats were caged individually in all studies and were maintained under conditions identical to those described in Experiment 1. Each rat was given choice between distilled water and a NaCl solution to drink. The food was a commercially available (U.S. Biochemicals Corp., Cleveland, Ohio) sodium-deficient diet into which 2, 4, and 6% by weight of NaCl (345, 690, and 1026 mEq NaCl/kg of food) was thoroughly mixed. The rats were given each diet for 5 days. The three studies differed only in that the concentration of the NaCl solution offered to the rats was 0.15 M in part 1, 0.20 M in part 2, and 0.25 M in part 3. Food and fluid intakes as well as body weights were measured daily. Other details of the experimental procedure have been described previously (Fregly *et al.*, 1965).

D. Experiment 4: Effect of Sodium Content of Diet on Spontaneous Intake of Sodium Chloride Solution by Normotensive and Hypertensive Rats

Ten male Sprague–Dawley (Holtzman) rats were used. Five rats had their kidneys bilaterally encapsulated with latex envelopes 10 weeks prior to the experiment. The remaining five rats were used as controls. Each rat was kept in an individual cage and allowed to choose between distilled water and 0.15 M NaCl solution to drink. The food given was a commercially available sodium-deficient diet (U.S. Biochemicals Corp., Cleveland, Ohio) supplemented in chronological sequence with 100, 250, 500, 750, 1000, and 100 mEq NaCl/kg food. Each ration was given for 5 days; the experiment lasted 30 days. Body weight and intakes of water, 0.15 M NaCl solution, and food by each rat were measured daily. Additional details of this experiment have been described elsewhere (Fregly, 1961).

III. RESULTS

A. Experiment 1

Following renal encapsulation with latex envelopes, water intake of the operated group increased above that of the control group and remained elevated for the duration of the 29-week experiment (Fig. 1A). Intake of 0.15 M NaCl solution, on the other hand, decreased and remained below that of the control group for the duration of the experiment (Fig. 1B). Food intakes of the two groups were similar throughout the experiment (Fig. 1C). The ratio of NaCl intake to total fluid ingested by the hypertensive group decreased by the seventh week after operation and remained below that of the control group throughout the experiment (Fig. 2A). Body weights of the two groups were similar throughout the experiment (Fig. 2B) while systolic blood pressure of the operated group was elevated above the level of the control group within 2 weeks after operation (Fig. 2C). Hypertension affected survival of the rats. Half of the hypertensive group was dead by 23 weeks after operation while all normotensive controls survived (Fig. 2D).

Table I compares the times during the experiment at which significant changes

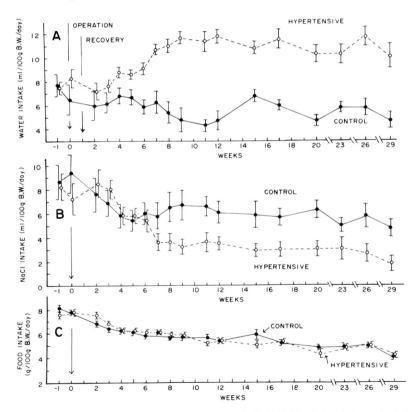

Fig. 1. This figure depicts the intakes of water (A), 0.15 M NaCl solution (B), and food (C) by normotensive control (closed circle) and hypertensive (open circle) rats during the course of Experiment 1. Kidneys of the hypertensive group were bilaterally encapsulated at 0. One standard error is set off at each mean.

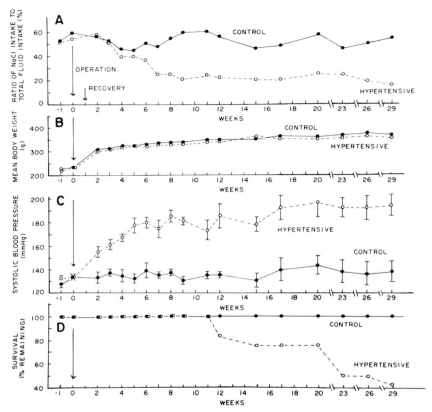

Fig. 2. This depicts the ratio of NaCl intake to total fluid intake (A), mean body weight (B), systolic blood pressure (C), and percent survival (D) of normotensive control (closed circle) and hypertensive (open circle) rats during the course of Experiment 1. One standard error is set off at each mean in panel C.

first occurred for four of the measured variables. Thus, the first significant elevation of blood pressure above the level of the control group occurred during the second week after renal encapsulation. As shown in Fig. 2C, blood pressures were maximally elevated by 6 weeks after operation. Water intake first increased significantly by 4 weeks after operation (Table I) and reached maximal levels by 8–10 weeks after renal encapsulation (Fig. 1A). Intake of 0.15 *M* NaCl solution showed a first significant decrease ($p = 0.03$) during the eighth week of the experiment (Table I) and reached minimal values within a week or two thereafter (Fig. 1B). Excepting only the second and third weeks after operation, food intakes of both groups were similar throughout the experiment (Table I).

Thus, the chronological sequence of events occurring after induction of renal hypertension by this technique is an elevation of blood pressure, an increase in

TABLE I

Comparison[a] of Hypertensive and Control Rats

Week	Blood pressure	Water intake	0.15 M NaCl intake	Food intake
Preoperation				
1	0.16	0.74	0.80	0.69
2	1.00	0.22	0.29	0.81
Postoperation				
1	Recovery	—	—	—
2	<0.01	0.39	0.32	<0.01
3	<0.01	0.14	0.42	0.02
4	<0.01	<0.01	0.98	0.70
5	<0.01	<0.01	0.73	0.35
6	<0.01	<0.01	0.68	0.23
7	<0.01	<0.01	0.07	0.73
8	<0.01	<0.01	0.03	0.21
9	<0.01	<0.01	<0.01	0.89
11	<0.01	<0.01	0.02	0.70
12	<0.01	<0.01	0.02	0.67
15	<0.01	<0.01	0.01	0.06
17	0.11	<0.01	<0.01	0.65
20	<0.01	<0.01	<0.01	0.52
23	0.04	<0.01	0.10	0.73
26	0.13	<0.01	0.02	1.00
29	<0.01	<0.01	<0.01	0.77

[a] Probability values.

water intake, and a reduction in intake of NaCl solution. The hypertensive rats in this study developed an absolute aversion to NaCl solution in that less was ingested by them than by the normotensive control group. At least 8 weeks elapsed after the operation before the aversion manifested itself. Since the rats had a choice between water and 0.15 M NaCl solution to drink throughout the 29-week experiment, the relationship between them and systolic blood pressure was determined. These are shown in Fig. 3. Since the variability of blood pressure and water intake of control rats was relatively small throughout the experiment, the mean systolic blood pressure and the mean water intake are shown as a single dot on the figure. The mean water intake by hypertensive rats during each week of the experiment is also shown. It appeared to be related linearly and directly to systolic blood pressure. On the other hand, the intake of 0.15 M NaCl solution was related inversely to systolic blood pressure. The ratio of intake of NaCl solution to intake of total fluid (water plus NaCl solution) was also related inversely to systolic blood pressure. Thus, intakes of water and 0.15 M NaCl solution and the ratio of NaCl intake to total fluid intake are variables that are functions of systolic blood pressure (Fig. 3).

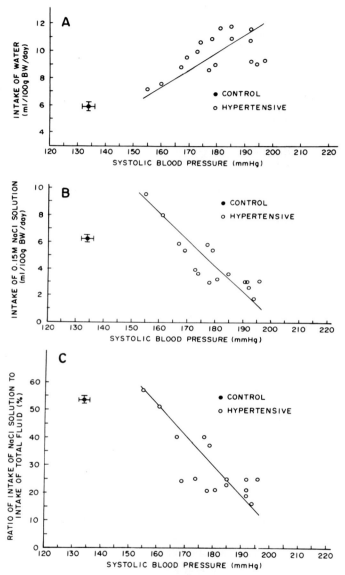

Fig. 3. The relationships between intakes of water (A), 0.15 *M* NaCl solution (B), and the ratio of NaCl intake to total fluid intake (C) and systolic blood pressure are shown here. Control data for the entire experiment are shown as the single dot at the left of each figure. The open circles represent the mean of each weekly measurement during the experiment and the corresponding weekly systolic blood pressure for the hypertensive group.

Since water and NaCl intakes were related to blood pressure, their relationship to each other was determined by regression analysis using the average weekly intakes of water and NaCl solution for each group throughout the experiment (Fig. 4). The results suggest that the two variables are inversely related to each other and that the relationship for the hypertensive group differs from the control group in intercept but not slope. The surprising aspect of this relationship is the negative slope. Thus, as intake of 0.15 M NaCl solution increased, water intake decreased for both groups. The significance of this relationship is not clear at present but probably cannot be accounted for by differences in food intake or by postulating a ceiling on total fluid intake. With respect to the latter, the total fluid intake increases as the intake of NaCl solution increases. If a ceiling on fluid intake were being controlled, it would be expected that the intakes of NaCl solution plus water would add to a reasonably constant value. This does not appear to be the case (Fig. 4). The significance of this relationship remains to be uncovered.

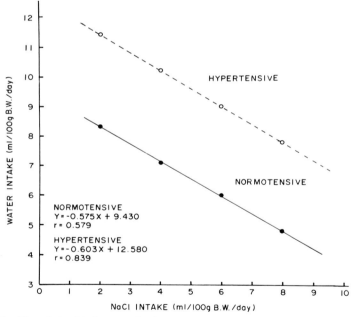

Fig. 4. The relationship between simultaneous intakes of water and 0.15 M NaCl solution by normotensive (closed circle) and hypertensive (open circle) rats in Experiment 1 is shown. A regression analysis of the mean weekly intakes of water and 0.15 M NaCl solution throughout the experiment was made. The equations derived for each group, with their correlation coefficients, are shown in the figure. The lines were derived from the equations.

B. Experiment 2

The objectives of this experiment were to determine whether hypertensive rats could detect NaCl in the same concentrations as normotensive rats and whether the aversion for NaCl solution was present at all concentrations above their detection threshold.

Figure 5 shows an inverse relationship between intakes of water and NaCl solution by control rats. When intakes of distilled water decreased, intake of NaCl solution increased simultaneously. This inverse relationship between intakes of water and NaCl solution is, in general, also true for hypertensive rats (Fig. 6).

Food intakes of both groups of rats were stable and similar throughout the experiment. The mean body weights of the two groups remained relatively con-

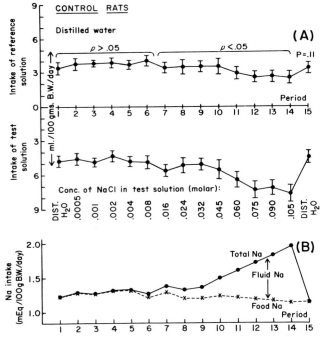

Fig. 5.   Fluid intakes of control rats in Experiment 2 are shown in A. Simultaneous intakes of distilled water (above the zero line) and NaCl solution (below the zero line) are shown for each period. One standard error is set off at each mean. Periods are arranged in chronological sequence and each period consists of 4 days with the exception of period 1 comprising 8 days. Probability values indicate significance of the difference between simultaneous volumes taken from the distilled water and salt bottles during each period. Panel B shows the total sodium intake partitioned into its food and fluid components for each period.

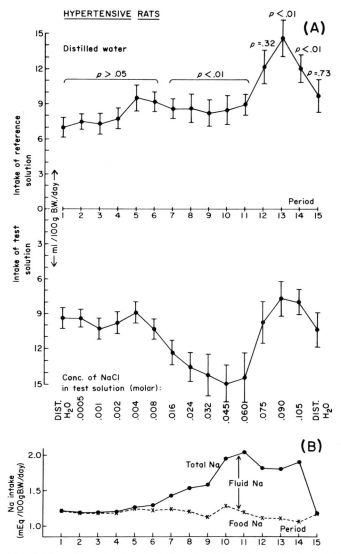

Fig. 6. Fluid intakes of hypertensive rats in Experiment 2 are shown. See legend of Fig. 5 for explanation.

stant throughout the experiment. Systolic blood pressures of the hypertensive rats (160–200 mm Hg) were significantly ($p < 0.01$) higher than those of controls (100–130 mm Hg) throughout the experiment.

The criterion of preference threshold used was similar to that of Richter (1939); namely, the concentration of test solution at and above which the simultaneous volumes taken from test and reference bottles differed significantly ($p < 0.05$) from each other. Figure 5A shows the simultaneous volume intakes of both reference (above the zero line) and test (below the zero line) solutions for each 4 day period throughout the experiment. The first significant difference between the two fluid intakes by control rats occurred during the period when the rats were given a choice between water and 0.016 M NaCl solution to drink. Therefore, the preference threshold concentration for NaCl solution lies between 0.008 and 0.016 M. The control animals ingested more NaCl solution than water at all concentrations of NaCl solution above the threshold value.

Using the same criterion of preference threshold, Fig. 6A indicates that hypertensive rats have a similar threshold to that of control rats (0.008–0.016 M). In addition to the similar thresholds, hypertensive rats also ingested more NaCl solution than water but only when the concentrations of the test solution ranged from 0.016 to 0.060 M (Fig. 6A). At concentrations above 0.075 M, a NaCl aversion (relative to water) occurred (periods 13 and 14).

During the periods in which the low concentrations of test solution (0.0005–0.008 M) were offered to both groups, the sodium ingested with the food constituted almost all of the total sodium intake (Figs. 5B and 6B). Consequently, the amount of sodium ingested remained relatively constant. When preference threshold was reached, total sodium intakes of both groups of rats rose above the level of the sodium ingested with the food (Figs. 5B and 6B). These figures show that when maximal sodium intake was achieved, sodium ingested by way of fluid contributed approximately half of the total sodium ingested. The maximal level of total sodium intake attained by each group was about 2.0 mEq/100 g of body wt/day and was achieved by hypertensive rats when 0.045 M NaCl solution was provided as the test solution. Control rats achieved the same level only when 0.105 M NaCl solution was given.

The preference thresholds observed here agree with those reported by Richter (1939) and Bare (1949) for normotensive rats by a similar criterion and technique. Patton and Ruch (1944) suggested calculating preference threshold by another method which has the advantage of eliminating the large difference in total fluid intakes between the control and hypertensive groups. This uses a ratio of the volume of NaCl solution ingested to the total fluid intake for comparison. A plot of this ratio versus the concentration of the test solution offered is shown in Fig. 7. By this method, as in the previous one, the preference thresholds of both groups of rats are the same. Preference thresholds for each group may be found in Fig. 7 by connecting the first and last points on the abscissa (distilled

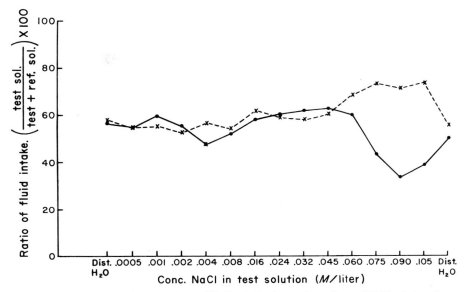

Fig. 7. Ratio of fluid intake (volume of NaCl solution ingested to volume of NaCl solution plus water ingested) is plotted against the concentration of NaCl solution offered as choice with distilled water. Preference thresholds of normal (×) and hypertensive (closed circles) rats lie between 0.008 and 0.016 M. (From Fregly, 1959; used by permission.)

water points). In the cases of both the control and hypertensive groups, the first concentration at which the points lie consistently above the line is 0.016 M. Hence, preference threshold is between 0.008 and 0.016 M for both groups. In addition, the hypertensive rats appeared to have an aversion threshold for NaCl solution. By this technique, it appears to be between 0.060 and 0.075 M.

C. Experiment 3

When graded levels of NaCl were added to the diet and choice was allowed between distilled water and NaCl solution to drink, normotensive rats appeared to ingest approximately the same amount of either 0.15, 0.20, or 0.25 M NaCl solution without regard to the concentration of NaCl in the food (Fig. 8). In all three studies, food intake remained relatively constant while water intake increased with increases in the dietary content of NaCl.

When the intake of NaCl solution is considered separately, it appears that decreasing volumes of NaCl solution were ingested as the concentration of NaCl solution increased (Fig. 9).

The amount of sodium ingested (mEq/100 g body wt/day) by way of fluid and food at each dietary concentration of NaCl is shown in Fig. 10. The amount of

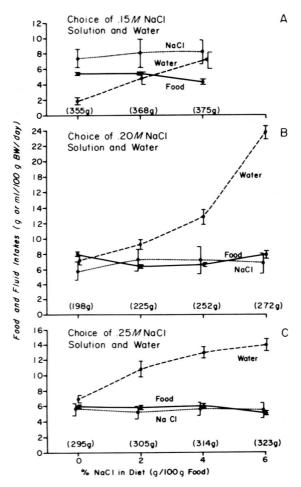

Fig. 8. This figure shows the means of daily intakes of water, NaCl solution, and food when the diet was supplemented with NaCl. Fluid choice was between distilled water and 0.15 *M* NaCl solution in Part 1 of the experiment (A); water and 0.20 *M* NaCl solution in Part 2 (B), and water and 0.25 *M* NaCl solution in Part 3 (C). One standard error is set off at each mean. Mean body weights of the groups during each period are shown in parenthesis. (From Fregly *et al.*, 1965; used by permission.)

sodium ingested by way of fluid was approximately the same for all concentrations of NaCl solution offered and for all concentrations of NaCl in the diet. Sodium intake by way of food increased in a nearly linear fashion as NaCl content of the diet increased. These results suggest that the amount of food ingested was not greatly influenced by the NaCl added to the diet, at least up to levels of 6%.

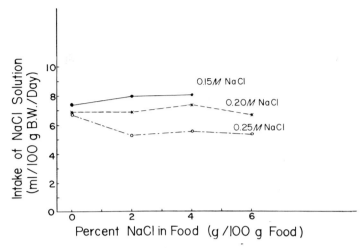

Fig. 9. This figure shows the volumes of each concentration of NaCl solution ingested when the diet was supplemented with 2, 4, and 6% NaCl. Intakes are the same as in Fig. 8 but are shown together to illustrate that the volume ingested decreased as the concentration of NaCl solution increased. (From Fregly *et al.*, 1965; used by permission.)

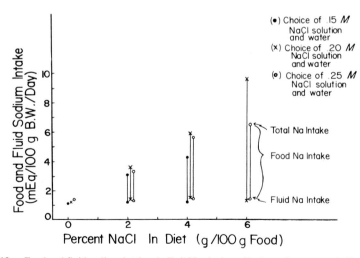

Fig. 10. Food and fluid sodium intakes (mEq/100 g body wt/day) are shown at each dietary level of NaCl. The amount of sodium ingested with drinking fluid is shown by the symbols in the lower part of the figure. The different symbols represent the three different NaCl concentrations given in fluid. The amount of sodium ingested with food is indicated by the solid line between any two points. Total sodium ingested is the sum of fluid and food sodium intakes. (From Fregly *et al.*, 1965; used by permission.)

Figure 11 reveals that total fluid intake is related to total sodium intake. Total fluid intake is the sum of the water and NaCl solution ingested, and total sodium ingested is the sum of food and fluid sodium. This line, drawn by eye, suggests that about 2.2 ml of total fluid are ingested for each mEq of sodium ingested.

D. Experiment 4

This experiment was similar to that of Experiment 3. Hypertensive and nor-motensive rats were given a choice between water and 0.15 M NaCl solution while the concentration of NaCl in their diet was changed. The objective was to determine whether a change in dietary NaCl concentration influenced their intake of NaCl solution.

Water intake of control rats (Fig. 12A, column with parallel lines) varied from 5 to 9 ml/100 g/day, while that of hypertensive rats varied from 12 to 16 ml/100 g/day (Fig. 12F). Intake of NaCl solution (stippled portions of Fig. 12A and F) by control rats was more variable than that of hypertensive rats. The latter consumed approximately 5 ml/100 g/day regardless of the NaCl content of the diet. Control rats consumed from 6 to 9 ml/100 g/day. Total fluid intakes (NaCl solution plus water) tended to increase as the NaCl content of the food increased. The sum of the heights of each column (stippled plus parallel lines) at a given concentration of sodium in food is the total fluid intake (Fig. 12A and F). Food intakes of the two groups (Fig. 12B and G) were nearly identical. Food intake

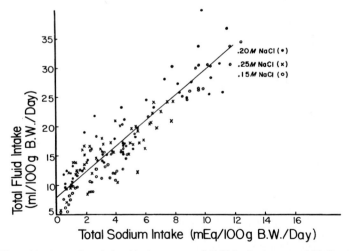

Fig. 11. This shows the relationship between total fluid intake (water and NaCl solution) and total sodium intake during the three experiments illustrated in Fig. 8. Symbols for each experiment are shown in the figure. Each point represents the daily intake of an individual rat. (From Fregly *et al.*, 1975; used by permission.)

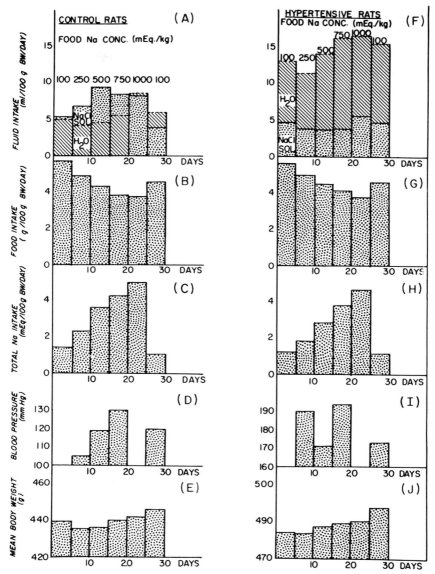

Fig. 12. This shows the results of measurements made on control (left side of figure) and hypertensive (right side of figure) rats. Fluid, food, and total sodium intakes are shown for control rats in A, B, and C, respectively, and for hypertensive rats in F, G, and H, respectively. Systolic blood pressures of control rats are shown in D and for hypertensive rats in I. Mean body weights of the two groups are shown in E and J, respectively. (From Fregly, 1961; used by permission.)

tended to decrease as NaCl content of the diet increased. Total sodium intake (both food and fluid, Fig. 12C and H) of hypertensive rats was less than that of control rats at any period during the experiment. This reflects the absolute NaCl aversion of these rats. Blood pressures (Fig. 12D and I) of the two groups were significantly different at any period during the experiment. The blood pressure of control rats tended to rise as NaCl content of the diet increased. Mean systolic blood pressure rose from 105 mm Hg when food contained 250 mEq/kg to 130 mm Hg when food contained 1000 mEq/kg. This was a significant ($p < 0.01$) rise in blood pressure. Hypertensive rats failed to show any effect of increasing NaCl content of the diet on their blood pressure (Fig. 12I). Mean body weight of both groups increased during the course of the experiment (Fig. 12E and J).

The sodium intakes by way of food and fluid are shown separately for control and hypertensive rats at each level of dietary sodium used (Fig. 13). The amount of sodium ingested with food was the same for both groups of rats and was related linearly to sodium content of the diet. Hence, daily food intake was approximately constant in spite of increasing amounts of sodium in the diet. This demonstrates the results observed earlier by Adolph (1947) that the rat eats for calories primarily. In contrast to the linear increase of sodium intake with food, fluid sodium intake remained relatively constant for both groups of rats. Fluid sodium intake of control rats increased when food content of NaCl was increased

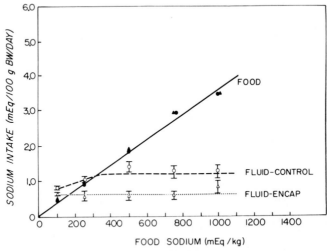

Figure 13. Sodium intakes (mEq/100 g body wt/day) in food and fluid are shown for five normotensive control (circle) and five hypertensive rats (triangle) given food containing the sodium contents shown on the abscissa of the figure and choice between distilled water and 0.15 *M* NaCl solution to drink. One standard error is set off at each mean. (From Fregly, 1961; used by permission.)

from 100 to 500 mEq/kg but remained constant thereafter. Fluid sodium intakes of control rats were significantly ($p < 0.01$) greater than those of hypertensive rats when 250, 500, and 750 mEq Na/kg food were given. The results suggested that both control and hypertensive rats may regulate their voluntary intake of sodium and that the physiological factor (or factors) involved in this regulation senses NaCl in solution only. Sodium chloride in food appears not to be sensed. If it were, one might expect a large intake of dietary NaCl to decrease voluntary NaCl intake as salt solution. The level of NaCl ingested voluntarily (in fluid) by the control rats is nearly the same as the minimal sodium intake required for normal growth as cited by McCoy (1942).

IV. DISCUSSION

When hypertension is induced in rats by encapsulation of their kidneys with latex envelopes, a sequence of events occurs which includes an elevation of blood pressure within 2 weeks, an increased water intake within 4 weeks, and a reduction in the spontaneous intake of 0.15 M NaCl solution within 8 weeks. The systolic blood pressure reached maximal levels by 8 weeks after renal encapsulation.

Manifestation of the "aversion" to NaCl solution is dependent on at least several factors. The first is the time after renal encapsulation at which the measurement is made. Prior to maximal elevation of blood pressure, the aversion is relative to the total fluid ingested. The hypertensive rats may ingest the same volume of NaCl solution voluntarily as that ingested by normotensive rats. However, when considered in relation to the total volume of fluid ingested, the ratio is significantly less than that of controls.

Manifestation of the "aversion" is also dependent on the concentration of the NaCl solution offered to the rats. Hypotonic concentrations (0.016 to 0.060 M) may be ingested in excess of water offered simultaneously by rats tested at a sufficient period of time after renal encapsulation for blood pressure to be maximal.

Earlier studies have also shown that age of the rat at the time of renal encapsulation is a factor (Fregly, 1955). Rats that were 20 weeks old (360 g) at the time of renal encapsulation developed a relative NaCl aversion less consistently than those whose kidneys were encapsulated at 10 weeks of age (250 g). Reasons for this difference are not apparent.

Other studies showed that renal hypertensive rats manifest an aversion for lithium chloride and reject it in favor of water offered simultaneously at concentrations one-half lower (0.008 M) than that at which it was rejected by control rats (0.016 M) (Fregly, 1959). Lithium chloride appears to be the only inorganic salt with taste characteristics that are similar to NaCl.

It is particularly interesting that renal hypertensive rats had the same preference threshold for detecting the difference between water and a NaCl solution offered simultaneously (Figs. 2 and 3). Hence, the aversion occurred independently of a change in preference threshold. This is opposite to the relationship between the appetite for NaCl solution and preference threshold. To date, experimental conditions manifesting an appetite for NaCl solution in rats have been accompanied by a reduction in preference threshold (Fregly, 1967, 1969; Fregly and Newsome, 1974; Fregly and Waters, 1965; Herxheimer and Woodbury, 1960; Richter, 1939; Thrasher and Fregly, 1980). By analogy, it might be expected that renal hypertensive rats should have a preference threshold higher than that of normotensive rats. No explanation can be advanced for this difference.

Hypertension in rats is not always accompanied by an aversion to NaCl solution although it has been reported in at least one other type, the Dahl genetically hypertensive strain (Wolf *et al.*, 1965). In contrast, the spontaneously hypertensive rat, derived from the Okamoto–Aoki strain, has an appetite (Catalanotto *et al.*, 1972; McConnell and Henkin, 1973; Fregly, 1975) and a reduced preference threshold for NaCl solution (Fregly, 1975).

When the food was salt loaded and rats were offered choice between water and NaCl solution to drink, water intake increased in proportion to the amount of salt ingested, but intake of NaCl solution remained independent of salt load in food and continued at the level observed when the food was salt deficient. The selective constancy of intake of NaCl solution, in spite of increases in water intake, is taken to suggest, but not prove, that rats "regulate" their intake of NaCl and that "regulation" apparently occurs by way of NaCl in solution rather than by way of NaCl in food. The ingestion of NaCl with food can be considered obligatory since the rat is known to eat primarily for calories (Adolph, 1947). If salt intake is regulated, it seems therefore unlikely that it could be regulated by way of food. It is clear, however, that food-choice studies need to be conducted to determine with what accuracy rats can both regulate their NaCl intake and detect differences in NaCl concentration of food.

Other results also suggest that regulation of NaCl intake exists and occurs by way of NaCl in solution. For example, increasing the concentration of the NaCl solution offered to rats whose food is salt loaded results in a proportional decrease in volume intake of NaCl solution. It seems that the amount of sodium (1.3–1.5 mEq/100 g body wt per day) ingested by way of salt solution is approximately that required for normal growth and reproduction in young rats (McCoy, 1942).

In earlier studies normotensive rats also maintained a constant intake of sodium when food was sodium deficient and choice was offered between two NaCl solutions of different concentration as their sole source of sodium (Fregly, 1961). One of the salt solutions (reference) was always 0.15 M while the other (test) solution varied in concentration every fourth day. When the concentration of the test solution changed, the rats varied the volumes of fluid ingested from each bottle, but maintained a very constant sodium intake (1.2 mEq/100 g body wt per day) over the range of concentrations of test solution from 0.004 to 0.150 M. The results again suggest that rats can regulate their NaCl intake.

The apparent failure of the normotensive rats used in these studies to detect the NaCl added to the food seems puzzling. However, the amount of food-borne NaCl that goes into solution in the saliva will be related to the amount of time the food spends in the mouth of the rat. The fundamental equation on which the theory of taste stimulation of Beidler (1954–1955) is based relates the magnitude of neural response to the concentration of the applied chemical stimulus. If food is swallowed by the rat before its content of NaCl goes into solution in saliva, it is conceivable that the salt content of the food might not be detected.

Hypertensive rats also appear to "regulate" their intake of NaCl when graded levels of NaCl are added to food and choice is offered between water and 0.15 M NaCl solution to drink. Regulation, however, was at a lower level than that observed in normotensive rats. Hypertensive rats also appeared to disregard the sodium content of their diet and appeared to regulate intake by means of sodium chloride solution.

In earlier studies in which there was choice of drinking fluids between a bottle that always contained 0.15 M NaCl solution (reference bottle) and a second bottle in which the concentration of NaCl was varied every fourth day (test bottle), hypertensive rats were less able than control rats to maintain a constant intake of sodium (Fregly, 1961). It is possible that this experimental paradigm may uncover a regulatory defect in hypertensive rats more readily than loading of food with NaCl and allowing choice between water and NaCl solution to drink. It is clear that additional studies will be required to understand this.

Denton and Sabine (1961) reported that sheep containing a unilateral parotid fistula, which results in continuous loss of alkaline saliva, spontaneously ingested greater quantities of $NaHCO_3$ (420 mEq/liter) than of either NaCl (420 mEq/liter) or KCl (140 mEq/liter) offered simultaneously during 24-hr periods. When such sheep were made sodium deficient for 23 hr and allowed choice between water and $NaHCO_3$ solution for only 1 hr, roughly 50% of the sodium deficit was ingested during the first 5 min. The animals generally returned to sodium balance by the end of the hour. When the concentration of the $NaHCO_3$ appetite was increased, the volume ingested was reduced proportionately to maintain a relatively constant sodium intake and sodium balance. The $NaHCO_3$ appetite was induced experimentally by sodium depletion but not by water depletion (Beilharz et al., 1962). Other evidence also suggests that the mechanisms regulating thirst are separate from those regulating $NaHCO_3$ intake. When a sheep that was both water- and sodium-depleted was offered water, it drank 3.32 liters in 72 sec. When water was offered 1 min after the end of the drinking session, none was ingested, indicating satiation. $NaHCO_3$ was then offered and the sheep immediately drank 1.25 liters in 27 sec. Appetite appeared to be unrelated either to reduction in plasma volume or to change in plasma sodium concentration (Beilharz and Kay, 1963).

Falk and Herman (1961) have put forth experimental evidence that depletion of body sodium by intraperitoneal dialysis with 5% glucose solution stimulates

NaCl appetite of rats. Such animals were shown to prefer 33% NaCl solution to water after dialysis but not before it. This suggests that regulation of salt intake is adjusted to body sodium content. Falk has pointed out elsewhere, however, that while this may explain the salt appetite under this specific condition, it does not explain salt appetites under certain other conditions, e.g., the increased NaCl intake when rats are given choice between a hypotonic NaCl solution and water (Falk, 1961). Epstein and Stellar (1955) conclude from their studies that salt preferences of both normal and adrenalectomized rats are under multifactor control. The most important factor is also visualized by them as the level of salt in the internal environment, while taste stimulation and gastric factors also contribute. The studies presented here neither confirm nor refute the notions of these investigators. The maintenance of a relatively constant salt intake in spite of dietary supplementation with NaCl cannot at present be attributed to depletion of body sodium. However, the increase in spontaneous intake of NaCl solution after 5 days on a salt-deficient diet, which was observed earlier in this laboratory (Fregly *et al.*, 1965), seems to point toward the possibility that relative sodium depletion may influence NaCl intake under these conditions.

It is clear from the results of these studies that much more experimental work will be required to understand the mechanism concerned with the regulation of sodium intake by both normotensive and hypertensive rats.

V. SUMMARY

Induction of hypertension by bilateral encapsulation of the kidneys with latex envelopes in rats given choice between distilled water and 0.15 M NaCl solution to drink is accompanied in chronological sequence by an elevation of blood pressure, an increase in water intake, and an aversion to NaCl solution. The latter occurs when blood pressure is maximally elevated and suggests that its occurrence is secondary to that of some other aspect of the processes involved in the development of renal hypertension. Certain characteristics of the intake of NaCl solution by hypertensive rats have been observed. Thus, an appetite for NaCl solution may actually occur when choice of drinking fluids is offered between hypotonic concentrations (0.016–0.060 M) of NaCl solution and water to drink. The aversion appears to occur at concentrations of NaCl solution exceeding 0.075 M. Further, the preference ("taste") threshold for NaCl is unaffected by hypertension, implying the receptor sensitivity is unchanged. A mechanism to account for the aversion under these conditions remains for further experimentation.

The possibility that rats may control their intake of sodium was also studied. The results suggest that both normotensive and hypertensive rats may control their intakes of NaCl, but only by way of NaCl in solution. In terms of control of sodium intake, the sodium ingested with food appeared to be undetected. However, in terms of its effect on fluid balance, the increasing amounts of sodium chloride ingested with food called forth a specific increase in water intake. In this experimental situation the rats clearly differentiated between the need for ingestion of water and NaCl solution. The mechanism accounting for this ability to differentiate remains speculative.

The results of these studies, as well as those of others using different animal species, suggest the need for more information in these areas.

ACKNOWLEDGMENT

This research was supported by grant HL 14526-09 from the National Heart, Lung, and Blood Institute.

REFERENCES

Abrams, M., and Sobin, S. (1947). Latex rubber capsule for producing hypertension by perinephritis. *Proc. Soc. Exp. Biol. Med.* **64,** 412–416.

Abrams, M., DeFriez, A. I. C., Tosteson, D. C., and Landis, E. M. (1949). Self-selection of salt solutions and water by normal and hypertensive rats. *Am. J. Physiol.* **156,** 283–247.

Adolph, E. F. (1943). "Physiological Regulations," p. 17. Jacques Cattell Press, Lancaster, Pennsylvania.

Adolph, E. F. (1947). Urges to eat and drink in rats. *Am. J. Physiol.* **151,** 110–125.

Bare, J. K. (1949). The specific hunger for sodium chloride in normal and adrenalectomized rats. *J. Comp. Physiol. Psychol.* **42,** 242–253.

Beidler, L. M. (1954–1955). A theory of taste stimulation. *J. Gen. Physiol.* **38,** 133–139.

Beilharz, S., and Kay, R. N. B. (1963). The effects of ruminal and plasma sodium concentrations on the sodium appetite of sheep. *J. Physiol. (London)* **165,** 468–483.

Beilharz, S., Denton, D. A., and Sabine, J. B. (1962). The effect of concurrent deficiency of water on sodium appetite of sheep. *J. Physiol. (London)* **163,** 378–390.

Catalanotto, F., Schechter, P. J., and Henkin, R. I. (1972). Preference for NaCl in the spontaneously hypertensive rat. *Life Sci.* **11,** 557–564.

Cizek, L. J. (1959). Long-term observations on relationship between food and water ingestion in the dog. *Am. J. Physiol.* **197,** 342–346.

Cizek, L. J., and Nocenti, M. R. (1965). Relationship between water and food ingestion in the rat. *Am. J. Physiol.* **208,** 615–620.

Davis, J. O., and Freeman, R. H. (1976). Mechanisms regulating renin release. *Physiol. Rev.* **56,** 1–56.

Denton, D. A. (1969). Salt appetite. *Nutr. Abstr. Rev.* **39,** 1043–1049.

Denton, D. A., and Nelson, J. F. (1980). The influence of reproductive processes on salt appetite. *In* "Biological and Behavioral Aspects of Salt Intake" (M. R. Kare, M. J. Fregly, and R. A. Bernard, eds.), pp. 229–246. Academic Press, New York.

Denton, D. A., and Sabine, J. R. (1961). The selective appetite for Na$^+$ shown by Na$^+$ deficient sheep. *J. Physiol. (London)* **157,** 97–116.

Epstein, A. N., and Stellar, E. (1955). The control of salt preferences in the adrenalectomized rat. *J. Comp. Physiol. Psychol.* **48,** 167–172.

Falk, J. L. (1961). Behavioral regulation of water-electrolyte balance. *In* "Nebraska Symposium on Motivation" (M. R. Jones, ed.), pp. 1–33. Univ. of Nebraska Press, Lincoln.

Falk, J. L., and Herman, T. S. (1961). Specific appetite for NaCl without postingestional repletion. *J. Comp. Physiol. Psychol.* **54,** 405–408.

Fregly, M. J. (1955). Hypertension, polydipsia and sodium chloride averson in rats; time course and relation to age. *Am. J. Physiol.* **182**, 139–144.

Fregly, M. J. (1959). Specificity of sodium chloride aversion of hypertensive rats. *Am. J. Physiol.* **196**, 1326–1332.

Fregly, M. J. (1960). A simple and accurate feeding device for rats. *J. Appl. Physiol.* **15**, 539.

Fregly, M. J. (1961). Regulation of sodium chloride intake by normotensive and hypertensive rats. *Am. J. Cardiol.* **8**, 870–879.

Fregly, M. J. (1963). Factors affecting indirect determination of systolic blood pressure of rats. *J. Lab. Clin. Med.* **62**, 223–230.

Fregly, M. J. (1966). The thyroid gland and experimental hypertension. *Arch. Biol. Med. Exp.* **3**, 148–177.

Fregly, M. J. (1967). Effect of hydrochlorothiazide on preference threshold of rats for NaCl solutions. *Proc. Soc. Exp. Biol. Med.* **125**, 1079–1084.

Fregly, M. J. (1969). Preference threshold and appetite for NaCl solution as affected by propylthiouracil and desoxycorticosterone acetate in rats. *In* "Olfaction and Taste" (C. Pfaffmann, ed.), pp. 554–561. Rockefeller Univ. Press, New York.

Fregly, M. J. (1975). NaCl intake and preference threshold of spontaneously hypertensive rats. *Proc. Soc. Exp. Biol. Med.* **149**, 915–920.

Fregly, M. J., and Newsome, D. G. (1974). Oral contraceptive-induced salt appetite in rats. *In* "Oral Contraceptives and High Blood Pressure" (M. J. Fregly and M. S. Fregly, eds.), pp. 141–158. Dolphin Press, Gainesville, Florida.

Fregly, M. J., and Waters, I. W. (1965). Effect of propylthiouracil on preference threshold of rats for NaCl solutions. *Proc. Soc. Exp. Biol. Med.* **120**, 637–640.

Fregly, M. J., Harper, J. M., Jr., and Radford, E. P., Jr. (1965). Regulation of sodium chloride intake by rats. *Am. J. Physiol.* **209**, 287–292.

Friedman, M., and Freed, S. C. (1949). Microphonic manometer for indirect determination of systolic blood pressure in the rat. *Proc. Soc. Exp. Biol. Med.* **70**, 670–672.

Herxheimer, A., and Woodbury, D. M. (1960). The Effect of desoxycorticosterone on salt and sucrose taste thresholds and drinking behavior in rats. *J. Physiol. (London)* **151**, 253–260.

Lazarow, A. (1954). Methods for the quantitative measurement of water intake. *Methods Med. Res.* **6**, 225–229.

McConnell, S. D., and Henkin, R. I. (1973). NaCl preference in spontaneously hypertensive rats: Age and blood pressure effects. *Am. J. Physiol.* **225**, 624–627.

McCoy, R. H. (1942). Dietary requirements of the rat. *In* "The Rat in Laboratory Investigation" (J. Q. Griffith and E. J. Farris, eds.), p. 70. Lippincott, Philadelphia, Pennsylvania.

Oparil, S. (1976). "Renin, 1976," pp. 25–38. Eden Press, Montreal.

Patton, H. D., and Ruch, T. C. (1944). Preference thresholds for quinine hydrochloride in chimpanzee, monkey and rat. *J. Comp. Psychol.* **37**, 35–49.

Richter, C. P. (1936). Increased salt appetite in adrenalectomized rats. *Am. J. Physiol.* **115**, 155–161.

Richter, C. P. (1939). Salt taste threshold of normal and adrenalectomized rats. *Endocrinology* **24**, 367–371.

Thrasher, T. N., and Fregly, M. J. (1980). Factors affecting salivary sodium concentration, NaCl intake and preference threshold and their interrelationship. *In* "Biological and Behavioral Aspects of Salt Intake" (M. R. Kare, M. J. Fregly, and R. A. Bernard, eds.), pp. 145–164. Academic Press, New York.

Wolf, A. V. (1958). "Thirst," p. 32. Thomas, Springfield, Illinois.

Wolf, G., Dahl, L. K., and Miller, N. E. (1965). Voluntary sodium chloride intake of two strains of rats with opposite genetic susceptibility to experimental hypertension. *Proc. Soc. Exp. Biol. Med.* **120**, 301–305.

9

Central Effects of Angiotensin II on Hypertension and Sodium Intake

M. IAN PHILLIPS

I. INTRODUCTION

The idea that sodium plays an important role in high blood pressure is based on our understanding of sodium in fluid balance, studies on rat models of hypertension, and clinical correlations between sodium diet and the incidence of hypertension. For example, among the Eskimos where salt in the diet is low on the average, there is also a low incidence of hypertension. Among the Northern Japanese where salt intake is over 200 mEq/liter per day the incidence of hypertension is extremely high. Among rats, the Dahl strain has one type that becomes

127

THE ROLE OF SALT IN
CARDIOVASCULAR HYPERTENSION

hypertensive when fed a high sodium diet, the salt-sensitive strain, and another type that does not develop hypertension even when the sodium in the diet is raised to large concentrations (Dahl, 1967). In fluid balance sodium has a pivotal role in drawing water to the extracellular space. Since sodium does not passively diffuse into the intracellular space, the content outside the cell is maintained at a higher level than the content inside the cell. This imbalance retains water in the extracellular space and contributes to the volume and pressure of blood in vessels.

In addition to these three pieces of evidence that sodium is involved in blood pressure, it is known from classical studies of Richter (1936) that sodium appetite can be altered by the hormonal balance in the body. Adrenalectomized rats develop high sodium intake feeding and drinking patterns, which, if sodium is available, compensate for the loss of sodium through the kidneys when aldosterone is not present. There can be at least three physiological mechanisms where one can study the effects of sodium on blood pressure. One is the intake which involves the brain. The second is the cardiovascular system on which sodium exerts an influence. The third is the kidney which controls the output of sodium. Clearly, the role of the kidney is of prime importance in controlling the amounts of sodium retained in the body but the tendency to eat more salt and its control by hormones and the brain cannot be overlooked as a factor. In this chapter some experiments are described which have implicated a role of angiotensin II in sodium intake and hypertension via an effect on the brain.

II. CENTRAL EFFECTS OF ANGIOTENSIN II ON SODIUM INTAKE

It is well known that angiotensin II (A II) in the plasma reaches the adrenal glands and stimulates the release of aldosterone. Aldosterone acts to conserve sodium by inhibition of urinary sodium excretion. Absence of aldosterone or very low levels lead to an increase in sodium appetite, so we may consider aldosterone to be the hormone for sodium control. Angiotensin may be considered the hormone of water balance. To achieve water balance, it is necessary to have both water conservation, sodium retention, and water replenishment. Angiotensin achieves these different effects by inducing thirst to replace water loss, by releasing vasopressin to enhance water retention and releasing aldosterone to favor sodium retention (Fig. 1). The effects of angiotensin on thirst and vasopressin release are by far better seen when angiotensin is injected into the brain ventricles than when it is injected into the peripheral blood vasculature. It has proved difficult to release vasopressin by infusions of angiotensin in the blood but large quantities are consistently released when angiotensin is injected into the brain. Similarly, much lower doses of angiotensin are required to produce thirst

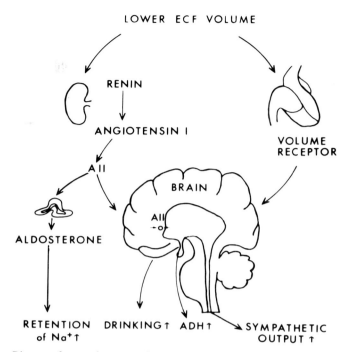

Fig. 1. Diagram of events that occur when extracellular fluid (ECF) volume is reduced resulting in retention of sodium, drinking, vasopressin, and sympathetic output all being increased, partly by volume receptor and partly by the renin–angiotensin system, both acting on the brain.

when A II is injected into the brain than when it is injected into the periphery. It has been our experence that to achieve either vasopressin release or drinking by peripheral A II infusions one must carefully manipulate the physiological conditions whereas central injections of A II produce effects almost regardless of the animals' physiological state. In one experiment, for example, the animals were waterloaded for a bioassay of vasopressin release and these animals drank to A II i.v.t. even though they were overhydrated (Hoffman *et al.*, 1977).

Sodium intake to A II injections centrally was first reported by Buggy and Fisher (1974). In their study, rats were given a two bottle choice test with one bottle containing water and the other 1.8% saline. In 32 rats, A II i.v.t. produced an average intake of 9.6 ml of water and 6.8 ml of 1.8% saline. This was in contrast to control injections of carbachol. Fifteen animals treated with carbachol ingested an average of 9.5 ml of water but only 0.5 ml of 1.8% saline. These tests were made during a 1-hr period. The results were repeated in our laboratory (Buggy *et al.*, 1979). There was a distinct difference between carbachol and NaCl injections, which produced no sodium intake and angiotensin injections,

which produced increasing amounts of sodium ingestion with increasing dose
(Fig. 2). When rats were made sodium deficient by a diet low in sodium,
angiotensin injections into the brain increased the intake of 2.7% sodium chloride
(Buggy and Fisher, 1974). These results were curiously ignored on the grounds
that the doses used were very high and it was not until 4 years later that Fitzsimons published results using a lower dose which confirmed the findings (Fitzsimons, 1980). A II was infused by osmotic minipumps for up to 1 week causing
increasing amounts of 2.7% saline to be ingested (Fig. 3). The effect was so
dramatic that the makers of the osmotic pumps jauntily offered a prize for what
the limit of sodium intake would be.

According to another report, 1 μg of A II infused per hour over 4 days led to

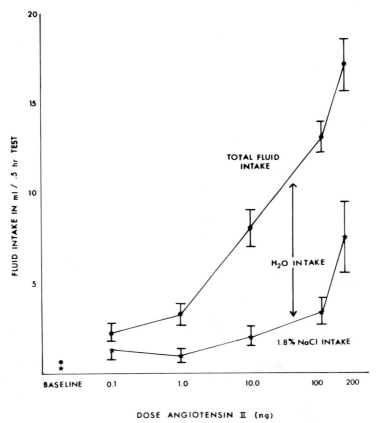

Fig. 2. The effect of increasing doses of angiotensin II on sodium chloride intake and water
intake. The rats tested had two bottles available, one containing water and the other saline (see Buggy
et al., 1979).

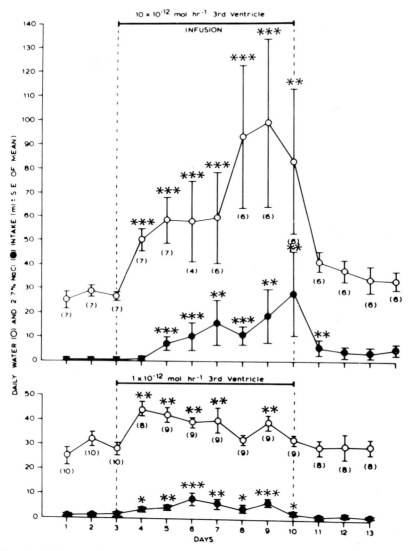

Fig. 3. Daily water intake and 2.7% NaCl over 7 days of continuous infusion with 2 doses of angiotensin into the third ventricle by osmotic pumping. (From Fitzsimons, 1980; reprinted with permission.)

intakes of over 100 ml per day of 3% saline (Epstein, 1978). When one considers rats would not normally drink 1 ml of such a high concentration of sodium chloride, this effect of A II is even more impressive than its effect on water intake. So far, however, the mechanism for this phenomenon has not been elucidated. One possibility is that the angiotensin infused into the brain is leaking into the periphery and stimulating the adrenal glands. Fregly and Waters (1966) have shown that high levels of aldosterone, which could be released by A II, increased sodium chloride intake. It was found that in adrenalectomized rats, sodium appetite had a V-shaped dose response relationship with increasing amounts of deoxycorticosterone acetate (DOCA). The intake of 0.15 M NaCl solution was high at very low doses and became progressively less until a dose of 100 μg/100 g body wt/day. Increasing the amount of DOCA increased the amount of NaCl ingested by the adrenalectomized rats. However, it is unlikely that this is the mechanism of the angiotensin effects for the following reasons: First, the levels of sodium intake in response to A II given i.v.t. are vastly higher than the sodium intake of adrenalectomized DOCA-treated rats. Also, the angiotensin-treated rats were ingesting 3% saline solutions, which are aversive to untreated rats, whereas the adrenalectomized rats were drinking physiological saline, which a significant number of any given group of rats prefer over water.

Second, infusions of an angiotensin antagonist, Saralasin, given systemically do not inhibit the effects of A II i.v.t. whereas the effects of A II i.v. are antagonized. Unless a very high dose of Saralasin is given which can cause a pressor response by its agonistic action, Saralasin does not enter into the brain at the same sites as A II i.v.t. has its effects. In an earlier study, Hoffman and Phillips (1976b) thought that the antagonism between a high dose of Saralasin (70 μg/ml i.v.) with angiotensin II i.v.t. (100 ng/ml) did show that sufficient doses could reach the receptor sites for A II. Others have also postulated this (Johnson and Schwob, 1975). A different interpretation is that when high levels of Saralasin are given, they cause a sudden acute hypertension which is sufficient to open the blood–brain barrier (Johansson, 1979). Therefore, our earlier results may be interpreted as resulting from a change in the hemodynamics of the blood–brain barrier allowing abnormal access of Saralasin to A II receptor sites. Within physiological ranges, injections of peptides into the brain do not leak into the periphery and injections of peptides into the peripheral vasculature do not gain access to the brain. This is illustrated when one injects bradykinin into the brain where it causes a pressor response, but when it is injected i.v. it causes a depressor response. Finally, infusions of A II systemically do not produce the dramatic increase in sodium intake seen with i.v.t. injections (Fitzsimons, 1980).

Another possibility for the phenomenon of sodium ingestion to angiotensin in the brain is that A II modulates the sensation of taste for sodium chloride. After adrenalectomy, the taste threshold for sodium chloride is altered encouraging rats to seek or accept higher levels of sodium than they would normally tolerate. This possibility of the effect of A II has not been tested but is more complex than the effect of adrenalectomy. For adrenalectomized rats, there is an ever-present need to ingest more sodium since they are unable to control the loss of sodium by urinary excretion. With the A II phenomenon there is no regulatory factor involved and the volumes ingested are greater than would be expected if the animals simply could not taste the concentration of sodium in the solutions. It would seem that the compulsive drinking of concentrated sodium chloride results from a direct action of angiotensin on neurocircuits in the brain which control sodium taste.

III. BRAIN CIRCUITS AND ANGIOTENSIN II

The brain circuitry for the effects of angiotensin has been under intensive investigation for the last few years. It was shown that angiotensin had its action via the brain ventricle system. Johnson and Epstein (1975) demonstrated that in order for angiotensin to be effective in the brain, it had to reach the brain ventricle. Angiotensin is injected via metal cannuli implanted into the brain. Although the tips of these cannuli can be localized in certain parts of the brain, the trajectory of the path of the cannula is commonly through the ventricular system. This allowed A II to leak back up the cannuli into the ventricular system. Proof of this was given by using radioactively labeled A II and also by the lack of effect when cannuli were specifically aimed at brain sites without traversing the ventricles. Among the possible sites within the ventricular system where A II might act are the circumventricular organs which are dotted around the third and fourth ventricle. By injecting angiotensin into different parts of the ventricular system, Hoffman and Phillips (1976a) showed that the effective area for angiotensin was in the anterior third ventricle and not in the fourth ventricle. This dismissed the role of the area postrema as a site of angiotensin action in the rat brain. In the dog brain, however, there is still considerable evidence that the area postrema is an important site of A II action (Ferrario, 1972). In the anterior third ventricle of the rat, there are two prominent circumventricular organs that appear to play a crucial role in the central actions of angiotensin II. These are the subfornical organ (SFO) and the organum vasculosum lamina terminalis (OVLT). There is now considerable evidence for both organs containing receptors for A II. When the SFO is lesioned, A II given systemically is without effect in producing drinking and less effective in producing a pressor response (Mangiapane and Simpson, 1980). It has been claimed that lesioning the SFO abolished the intraventricular effects of A II, but a series of studies using a ventricular plugging technique indicated that another site within the third ventricle was more efficacious for A II i.v.t. When the SFO was lesioned electrically, a certain amount of debris built up in the narrow channel between the lateral ventricle and the third ventricle. It was hypothesized that such an obstruction could prevent A II injected into the lateral ventricle from reaching receptor sites within the third ventricle (Buggy *et al.*, 1975). Two tests of this hypothesis were made and proved we were correct. The plugging experiments in which a cream plug was placed in the ventricle were designed to simulate ventricular obstruction. Hoffman and Phillips (1976a) demonstrated that a ventricular plug in all parts of the ventricular system except over the OVLT did not prevent the action of angiotensin II, but when access to the OVLT was blocked by a plug, none of the responses to A II could be elicited by intraventricular injection, even though the A II could reach the surface of the SFO. A II given i.v., however, was still effective (Buggy and Fisher, 1975). It was also shown that after SFO lesions A II was still effective if injected into the third ventricle on the caudal side of the lesion site thereby voiding the obstructive block of necrotic tissue. The difference between the SFO and OVLT was in the response to i.v.t. A II. In all other respects, however, there was evidence that both organs are sensitive to A II. Both the SFO and OVLT have receptor binding sites for A II. In normal rats the SFO had higher binding levels than the OVLT but in spontaneously hypertensive rats the binding for A II increased over 120% whereas there was no change in the SFO (Stamler *et al.*, 1980). In order for an area to contain receptors one must show not only binding but also a biological response. In both the OVLT and the SFO, there is evidence of a biological response when A II is applied directly to the tissue. This comes from studies on microiontophoresis (Phillips and Felix, 1976; Knowles and Phillips, 1980; Felix and Phillips, 1979). In studies on anesthetized cat, rat, and unanesthetized rat brain slices, angiotensin II was shown to produce a marked excitation of cells within the SFO and OVLT. These excitatory responses were specifically inhibited by the specific antagonist for A II, Saralasin. Some of the cells identified were also sensitive to acetylcholine; other cells were exclusively sensitive to A II. Having established that there are receptors for A II in the circumventricular organs, the next step has been to trace the neural connections from these structures. In two studies, the techniques of horseradish peroxidase tracing and radioactive labeled tracing have been used. Horseradish peroxidase injected discretely into the OVLT has revealed connections to cell bodies in the SFO (Camacho and Phillips, 1981). Injections of labeled amines into the SFO demonstrated terminal fields in the OVLT (Miselis *et al.*, 1979). Both organs have connections to the preoptic area and possibly the supraoptic nucleus. It is probable, however, that the connections to the supraoptic nucleus from these organs are not direct but involve another synapse before arriving at the supraoptic. Other areas connected to the OVLT include the hippocampus, septum, and sites as far away as the locus ceruleus and dorsal vagal motor nucleus. Which of these connections are involved in the effects of A II has still to be established. The effects that A II produces on vasopressin release, sympathetic activation, and water and sodium drinking require a widespread involvement of various brain sites. For example, the connection to the hippocampus from the OVLT was at first surprising. When one considers, however, that drinking behavior must involve a component of memory in seeking out the source of water even within the small confines of a cage for our experimental subjects, a memory function in the hippocampus would not be inappropriate. Finally, there have been several investigations on the pharmacology of A II-induced effects. Recently, we separated the blood pressure response from the drinking response pharmacologically (Camacho and Phillips, 1980). Phentolamine, an α-adrenergic blocking agent, inhibits the A II pressor effect substantially without significant effects on the drinking response. Sumners *et al.* (1979) have shown that dopamine blockers significantly inhibit the drinking response to A II. Thus, we are beginning to see a separation of the neurocircuits involved in the various responses to A II. So far no separation of sodium drinking versus water drinking has been attempted.

IV. SODIUM INTAKE AND ANGIOTENSIN II RECEPTORS

The OVLT is contained within the area labeled AV3V (anteroventral third ventricle periventricular tissue). Lesions of the AV3V have profound effects on body fluid homeostasis (Brody and Johnson, 1980). After such lesions, rats go through an acute phase and, if they survive, through a chronic change in their body fluid responses. In the acute phase, the animals are adipsic, they fail to produce the appropriate antidiuresis, and they are unresponsive to angiotensin II injected systemically or intraventricularly. To get animals through this adipsic stage, it is necessary to artificially hydrate some of them. Recovered AV3V lesioned animals are chronically hyperosmotic, hypernatremic, and have attenuated responses to A II including drinking, vasopressin release, and pressor activity. The rats also do not respond to intraventricular injections of hyperosmotic sodium chloride. Bealer and Johnson (1979) placed rats on a sodium deficient diet and allowed continuous access to 2% (w/v) sodium chloride solution and distilled water from water bottles mounted in the same cage. Preoperatively, there was no difference between the groups but after AV3V lesions, the sodium intake was significantly reduced. To find whether this reduction was due to an insensitivity to body sodium levels, another test of sodium intake was performed by giving an injection of formalin (1.5%, 2.5 ml), which is known to induce hyponatremia. To this stimulus, the animals were still responsive as shown by their increased sodium intake above the level of the untreated AV3V rats. It was concluded that ablation of the AV3V area results in decreased sodium intake but does not alter the sensitivity of rats to their sodium levels. One possible interpretation of these results is that by destroying the receptors to angiotensin in the brain, more A II is produced in the periphery and this leads to hyperaldosteronism and increased sodium retention. This would imply a feedback circuit between the renin-producing cells of the kidney and the levels of active angiotensin in the brain.

V. BRAIN RECEPTOR BINDING AND SODIUM

When A II is injected into the brain ventricles of normotensive, sodium-deplete rats, there is a significant difference in the blood pressure response compared to the same injections into sodium-replete rats (Mann *et al.*, 1980). At 100 ng A II i.v.t., blood pressure increases in sodium-replete rats was 16.3 ± 1.0 mm Hg but in sodium-deplete rats, the pressor effect was 12.2 ± 0.8 mm Hg ($p < 0.05$). Carbachol is also known to raise blood pressure (Hoffman and Phillips, 1977), but on a test of sodium-deplete versus -replete rats there was no difference in their response to this cholinergic agent. These data imply that the receptors in the brain for A II are altered by giving the rats a low sodium diet. It has earlier been suggested by Andersson (1977) that angiotensin requires sodium at the receptor level in order for it to have biological effects. Buggy *et al.* (1979), however, were not able to find an interaction between sodium injections and angiotensin injections which would support this view. Receptor binding studies in our laboratory on brain tissue of sodium replete rats did not reveal any alterations in the level of binding in the presence of high sodium or low sodium concentrations. One possibility for failure to find an interaction is that the effect of altering sodium levels in the brain may take time to manifest itself. In a study by Mann *et al.* (1980) rat brains were dissected to produce a block of midbrain tissue and the binding method of Bennett and Synder (1976) using [^{125}I]A II was applied. The homogenized tissue was centrifuged, buffered, and incubated with [^{125}I]A II. Bound and unbound hormones were separated by centrifugation or filtration at 4°C. Radioactivity of the pellets was counted and the amount bound to the tissue calculated by subtracting the nonspecific binding with unlabeled Ile^{5}A II from the total amount bound. The results are shown in Fig. 4 for rats on normal sodium diets and low sodium diets. The saturation curves indicate that with increasing concentrations of angiotensin II the low sodium rats have less binding than the sodium replete rats. A Scatchard analysis of these data revealed that sodium depleted rat brains have fewer binding sites for A II than sodium replete rat brains. The K_d calculated from the slope of the regression line changed from 0.16 to 0.24 nM. This study implied that lowering the sodium in the diet reduces the responsiveness to angiotensin in the brain because there are fewer binding sites for angiotensin to bind to in the sodium deplete state. An implication that may be drawn from this study is that by lowering sodium in the diet the central effects of angiotensin on hypertension can be reduced. The next question, therefore, is whether the central effects of angiotensin are involved in hypertension.

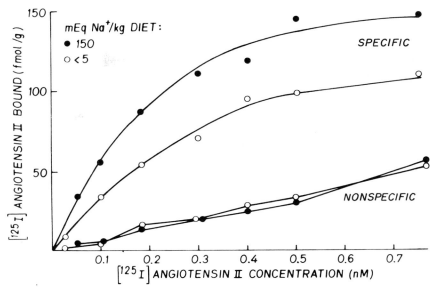

Fig. 4. Angiotensin binding in brain tissue from rats on normal sodium diets and low sodium diets. The saturation curves to increasing concentrations of angiotensin II indicate a lower saturation for rats given a low sodium diet. Scatchard analysis of these data revealed that the number of binding sites is reduced. (From Mann *et al.*, 1980; reprinted with permission.)

VI. CENTRAL BLOCKADE OF ANGIOTENSIN AND HYPERTENSION

There are several models of hypertension used for study which reflect on the three levels of sodium interaction outlined at the beginning of the chapter: the intake, the cardiovascular system, and the output (kidney). Many models require surgical manipulation of the kidneys either by clipping the renal arteries, removing a kidney, or combinations of both. Deoxycorticosterone is effective on the cardiovascular system when sodium is available. The development of high blood pressure with this treatment is accelerated when one kidney is removed. In addition to kidney function and increased sodium retention, there appears to be involvement of the brain in the genetically hypertensive rats of the spontaneous hypertensive strain (SHR). Higher levels of central angiotensin in the SHR or more activity at the receptor level is implied in experiments using a specific antagonist to A II, Saralasin acetate injected directly into the brain ventricle (Phillips *et al.*, 1977). This competitive antagonist for A II has also been tested in these other models of hypertension (Mann *et al.*, 1978). For the renal hypertensive rats, 1-clip, 1-kidney Goldblatt hypertensive rats were prepared and Saralasin infused i.v. or i.v.t. where blood pressure was recorded on chronic unanesthetized rats. No effect of the antagonist on blood pressure was seen by either route but in the 2-clip, 2-kidney hypertension, 20 µl given i.v.t. lowered mean arterial pressure by 0.1 mm Hg, a significant decrease in pressure. There was no significant effect of the drug by the i.v. route on blood pressure. In 1-clip, 2-kidney hypertension, 20 mg Saralasin i.v.t. lowered blood pressure by 12.1 mm Hg, again a significant fall in blood pressure. In this case, Saralasin also reduced blood pressure when given i.v. (Fig. 5). In the DOCA-salt treated rats with unilateral nephrectomy the i.v.t. administrated Saralasin resulted in a dose-dependent increase in mean arterial pressure (Fig. 6). At 40 mg the increase in blood pressure was 17.7 mm Hg. Finally, in the SHR rats, i.v.t. injections of the antagonist caused a fall in blood pressure in a dose-related fashion from 5 to 20 µg. Even after bilateral nephrectomy which by itself did not alter blood pressure, 20 µg of Saralasin given i.v.t. produced a significant lowering of blood pressure of 14 mm Hg (Fig. 7). Thus, the effects of Saralasin in the SHR could not be due to the peripheral action of the antagonist on the plasma renin angiotensin because bilateral nephrectomy abolished the circulating levels of plasma renin. Also, high levels of circulating Saralasin given i.v. failed to produce any lowering of blood pressure whereas central injections of Saralasin produced a distinctive dose-related lowering of the mean arterial pressure (Fig. 8).

There appears to be a central component in the 1-clip, 2-kidney hypertensive model, the 2-clip, 2-kidney model, and the SHR model. The increased respon-

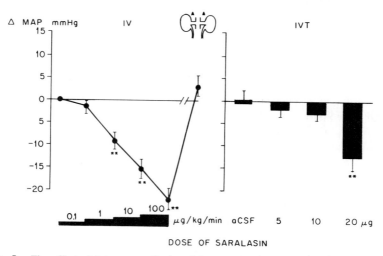

Fig. 5. The effect of intravenous (i.v.) and intraventricular (i.v.t.) Saralasin on the blood pressure of 1-clip, 2 kidney hypertensive rats. Blockage of angiotensin in this model produced a lowering of blood pressure.

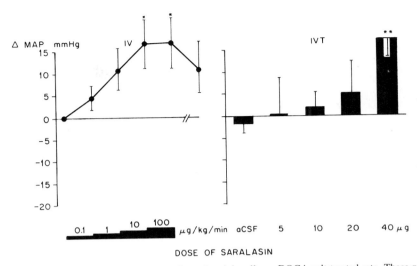

Fig. 6. The effect of Saralasin centrally and peripherally on DOCA-salt-treated rats. These rats have low circulating renin levels but it can be seen that the effects of Saralasin are to raise blood pressure rather than reduce it. The rise in blood pressure may reflect an alteration of the angiotensin II receptors in brain and tissue toward increased sensitivity, which increases the likelihood of the agonistic rather than the antagonistic actions of Saralasin.

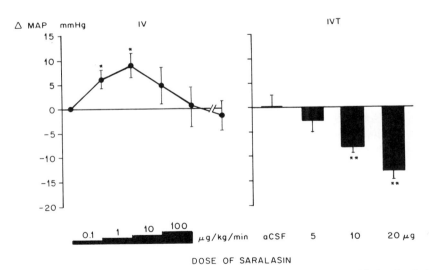

Fig. 7. The effect of Saralasin on spontaneously hypertensive rats. Note that while i.v. Saralasin tends to increase blood pressure, i.v.t. Saralasin significantly lowers blood pressure.

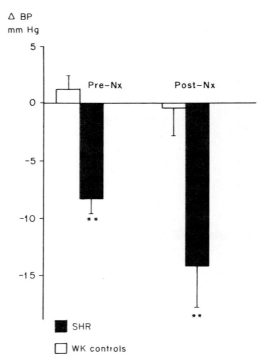

Fig. 8. The lowering of blood pressure effects by Saralasin i.v.t. in both nephrectomized and nonnephrectomized SHR rats.

siveness to Saralasin in DOCA-salt rats may indicate a change in the receptor binding sites for A II such that the antagonist acted as an agonist. If the high levels of sodium consumed by the DOCA-salt rats increased the number of binding sites for A II in the blood vessel walls and in the brain, Saralasin may have manifested its agonistic rather than its antagonistic effects. Thus, in each case in addition to peripheral effects on blood pressure in these models, it is possible that there is a brain component involving renin-angiotensin.

VII. CONCLUSION

In summary, the results imply that angiotensin, either from the periphery or from the brain directly, has an action in the brain which can produce hypertension. Active stimulation of central angiotensin receptors results in sodium retention and increased sodium intake. The role of the brain in sodium-dependent hypertension is relatively unexplored. There are data that indicate a central component, or at least a neural component, in the Dahl strain of rat. Salt-sensitive rats are more responsive to central injections of angiotensin II than salt-resistant rats. Furthermore, central sympathectomy by 6-OHDA reduces the blood pressure in salt-sensitive hypertensive Dahl rats (Westfall, Chapter 26, this volume). Although the early experiments of Dahl in transplanting kidneys clearly indicate a major role for the kidney in salt-sensitive hypertension (Dahl *et al.*, 1972), these experiments and the weight of the data above show that the brain may also play a part in sodium intake and high blood pressure. It would appear that the mediator in the brain of sodium ingestion is angiotensin II. The level of sodium in the brain can alter the state of blood pressure by an action on central angiotensin receptors.

It is clear that not all individuals are salt sensitive. Many people can eat salt without developing hypertension. The Dahl model of salt-sensitive rats indicates that genetic differences expressed hormonally occur in a number of individuals for whom salt in the diet is dangerous. In the genetically hypertensive rat we found an increased level of salt intake compared to controls (Fig. 9). Although this was not the cause of their hypertension, it could be a manifestation of their increased brain-angiotensin activity since angiotensin increases sodium intake and blood pressure. The data therefore hint at salt-sensitive individuals having an

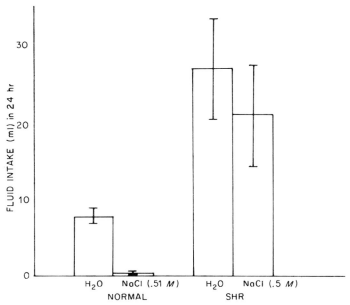

Fig. 9. The elevated sodium intake of spontaneously hypertensive rats given the choice of water and NaCl solution (0.51 *M*) compared to the response of the normotensive controls.

altered brain angiotensin system. This conclusion would have to be taken with a pinch of salt.

ACKNOWLEDGMENTS

I am very grateful to James Buggy, Hans Mann, and James Fitzsimons for permission to reprint their figures. Supported by grants from NIH and NSF.

REFERENCES

Andersson, B. (1977). Regulation of body fluids. *Annu. Rev. Physiol.* **39,** 185–200.

Bealer, S. L., and Johnson, A. K. (1979). Sodium consumption following lesions surrounding the anteroventral third ventricle. *Brain Res.* **4,** 287–290.

Bennett, J. P., Jr., and Snyder, S. H. (1976). Angiotensin II binding to mammalian brain membranes. *J. Biol. Chem.* **251,** 7423–7430.

Buggy, J., and Fisher, A. E. (1974). Evidence for a dual central role for angiotensin in water and sodium intake. *Nature (London)* **250,** 733–735.

Buggy, J., and Fisher, A. E. (1975). Water and sodium intake: Evidence for a dual central role for angiotensin. *Nature (London)* **250,** 733–735.

Buggy, J., Fisher, A. E., Hoffman, W. E., Johnson, A. K., and Phillips, M. I. (1975). Ventricular obstruction: Effect on drinking induced by intracranial injection of angiotensin. *Science* **190,** 72–74.

Buggy, J., Hoffman, W. E., Phillips, M. I., Fisher, A. E., and Johnson, A. K. (1979). Osmosensitivity of rat third ventricle and interactions with angiotensin. *Am. J. Physiol.* **236,** R75–R.82.

Camacho, A., and Phillips, M. I. (1980). Separation of drinking and pressor responses to central angiotensin by monoamines. *Am. J. Physiol.* **240,** R106–R113.

Camacho, A., and Phillips, M. I. (1981) Hypothalamic and extra-hypothalamic connections of the organum vasculosum of the lamina terminalis (OVLT). *Neurosci. Lett.* **25,** 201–204.

Dahl, L. K., Knudson, K. D., Heine, M., and Leitl, G. (1967). Effects of chronic excess salt ingestion. Genetic influence on the development of salt hypertension in parabiotic rats. Evidence for a humoral factor. *J. Exp. Med.* **126,** 687.

Epstein, A. N. (1978). Consensus, controversies, and curiosities. *Fed. Proc., Fed. Am. Soc. Exp. Biol.* **37,** 2711–2716.

Felix, D., and Phillips, M. I. (1979). Inhibitory effects of luteinizing hormone releasing hormone releasing hormone (LH-RH) on neurons in the organum vasculosum lamina terminalis (OVLT). *Brain Res.* **169,** 204–208.

Fitzsimons, J. T. (1980). Angiotensin and other peptides in the control of water and sodium intake. *Proc. R. Soc. London* **210,** 165–182.

Fregly, M. J., and Waters, I. W. (1966). Effect of mineralocorticoids on spontaneous sodium chloride appetite of adrenalectomized rats. *Physiol. Behav.* **1,** 65–74.

Hoffman, W. E., and Phillips, M. I. (1976a). The effect of subfornical organ lesions and ventricular blockade on drinking induced by angiotensin II. *Brain Res.* **108,** 59–73.

Hoffman, W. E., and Phillips, M. I. (1976b). Evidence for sar¹-ala⁸-angiotensin crossing the blood cerebrospinal fluid barrier to antagonize central effects of angiotensin II. *Brain Res.* **109,** 541–552.

Hoffman, W. E., and Phillips, M. I. (1976c). Regional study of cerebral ventricular sensitive sites to angiotensin II. *Brain Res.* **110**, 313–330.

Hoffman, W. E., and Phillips, M. I. (1977). Independent receptors for pressor and drinking responses to central injections of angiotensin II and carbachol. *Brain Res.* **124**, 305–315.

Hoffman, W. E., Phillips, M. I., Schmid, P. G., Falcon, J., and Weet, J. F. (1977). Antidiuretic hormone release and the pressor response to central angiotensin II and cholinergic stimulation. *Neuropharmacology* **16**, 463–472.

Johansson, B., Li, C. L., Olsson, Y., and Klatzo, I. (1970). The effect of acute arterial hypertension on the blood brain barrier to protein tracers. *Acta Neuropathol.* **16**, 117–124.

Johnson, A. K., and Epstein, A. N. (1975). The cerebral ventricles as the avenues for the dipsogenic action of intracranial angiotensin. *Brain Res.* **86**, 399–418.

Johnson, A. K., and Schwob, J. E. (1975). Cephalic angiotensin II receptor mediating drinking to systemic angiotensin II. *Pharmacol., Biochem. Behav.* **3**, 1076–1084.

Knowles, W. D., and Phillips, M. I. (1980). Angiotensin II responsive cells in the organum vasculosum lamina terminalis (OVLT) recorded in hypothalamic brain slices. *Brain Res.* **195**, 256–259.

Mangiapane, M. L., and Simpson, J. B. (1980). Subfornical organ lesions reduce the pressor effect of systemic angiotensin II. *Neuroendocrinology* **31**, 380–384.

Mann, J., Phillips, M. I., Dietz, R., Haebara, H., and Ganten, D. (1978). Effects of central and peripheral angiotensin blockade in hypertensive rats. *Am. J. Physiol.* **234**, H629–H637.

Mann, J. F. E., Schiffrin, E. L., Schiller, P. W., Rascher, W., Boucher, R., and Genest, J. (1980). Central actions and brain receptor binding of angiotensin II: Influence of sodium intake. *Hypertension* **2**, 437–443.

Miselis, R. R., Shapiro, R. B., and Hand, P. J. (1979). Subfornical organ efferents to neural systems for control of body water. *Science* **205**, 1022–1025.

Phillips, M. I., and Felix, D. (1976). Specific angiotensin II receptive neurons in the cat subfornical organ. *Brain Res.* **109**, 531–540.

Phillips, M. I., Mann, H., Dietz, R., and Ganten, D. (1977). Lowering of hypertension by central saralasin in the absence of plasma renin. *Nature (London)* **270**, 445–447.

Richter, C. P. (1936). Increased salt appetite in adrenalectomized rats. *Am. J. Physiol.* **115**, 115–161.

Sirett, N. E., McLean, A. S., Bray, J. J., and Hubbard, J. I. (1977). Distribution of angiotension II receptors in rat brain. *Brain Res.* **122**, 299–312.

Stamler, J. F., Raizada, M. K., Fellows, R. E., and Phillips, M. I. (1980). Increased specific binding of angiotensin II in the organum vasculosum of the laminae terminalis area of the spontaneously hypertensive ra brain. *Neurosci. Lett.* **17**, 173–177.

Sumners, C., Woodruff, C. N., Poat, J. A., and Munday, K. A. (1979). The effect of neuroleptic drugs on drinking induced by central administration of angiotensin or carbachol. *Psychopharmacology* **60**, 291–196.

10

Dietary Sodium and Salt Taste

MARY BERTINO, GARY K. BEAUCHAMP,
KARL ENGELMAN, AND MORLEY R. KARE

An adequate sodium intake is necessary for normal growth and survival. Balance of the sodium ion is crucial in maintenance of cellular osmolarity, neural activity, blood pressure, extracellular fluid volume, acid–base balance, and carbohydrate metabolism (Meneely and Battarbee, 1976). Mechanisms, some of which are behavioral, have evolved to conserve sodium and to stimulate its intake when sodium deficits occur. These behavioral mechanisms are dependent on a functioning sense of taste and have been the subject of much research.

Another aspect of behavioral sodium regulation, observed in many species, is that salt (NaCl) is often ingested in amounts considerably greater than are physiologically needed. In humans, this apparent supplemental intake is often attributed to an acquired appetite for the taste of salt. This aspect of sodium intake is not well understood and its origins, including whether or not it is indeed acquired, are not known.

In this chapter, we discuss relationships between the taste of salt and intake of sodium. First, we briefly review some of the literature on taste-mediated re-

145

THE ROLE OF SALT IN
CARDIOVASCULAR HYPERTENSION

sponses during actual sodium deficiency. The majority of our discussion, however, concerns dietary sodium and salt taste in humans who are not in a state of sodium deprivation. Parallels are drawn between sodium regulation in a sodium-deficient organism and in an organism ingesting supplemental sodium.

I. SODIUM DEFICIENCY AND THE TASTE OF SALT

Responses to the taste of salt vary with changes in sodium balance. In rats, sodium depletion results in increased intake in response to the taste of salt. For example, an adrenalectomized rat, an animal that is unable to efficiently retain sodium since the source of aldosterone has been removed, exhibits an increased salt appetite. Behavioral control of this increased sodium intake was studied in detail by Richter whose studies remain the classic work on the subject. Richter surgically removed the adrenal glands from rats and observed that they increased their intake of salt solutions, both of low and high concentration, and were thus able to survive if allowed to compensate behaviorally for the loss due to absence of the adrenals. This ability was dependent on a functioning sense of taste since many of the rats failed to increase adequately their sodium intake and died after sectioning the taste nerves (Richter, 1956).

Richter also observed that the lowest concentration of salt solution at which the rats showed a preference for salt, the preference threshold, was lower in an adrenalectomized rat. He hypothesized that the adrenalectomized rat was more sensitive to the taste of salt. Later work was unable to demonstrate changes in threshold sensitivity to salt in adrenalectomized rats, either through behavioral or electrophysiological techniques (see Contreras, 1978, for review). Behavioral studies demonstrated that although normal and adrenalectomized rats had the same detection threshold for sodium chloride, the adrenalectomized rats exhibited lower preference thresholds (Carr, 1953; Harriman and MacLeod, 1953; Morrison, 1974). Electrophysiological recordings of chorda tympani activity did not distinguish adrenalectomized rats from normal rats at the lowest concentration of salt that produced a change in electrical activity greater than water (Nachman and Pfaffmann, 1963; Pfaffmann and Bare, 1950).

Adrenalectomy has been one major manipulation used experimentally to produce sodium depletion in rats. Sodium depletion has also been produced by placing rats on very low sodium diets which, like adrenalectomy, result in an increased intake of NaCl solutions at both low and high concentrations (e.g., Richter, 1956). Recent work on sodium-deprived rats has provided insight into the source of the increased intake at suprathreshold concentrations of NaCl. Recordings made from the chorda tympani nerve, which carries impulses from the anterior two-thirds of the tongue, revealed differences in the way the nerve responds to stimulation with NaCl solutions. The sodium-depleted rat showed decreased responses to a range of NaCl solutions (0.03–3.0 M). This decreased response was specific only to NaCl solutions (responses to quinine, sucrose, and HCl were the same) and was most apparent at high concentrations. Although this lowered neural response was evident in whole fiber preparations, it was best shown in single fiber recordings. Of fiber types, NaCl-best fibers distinguished the sodium depleted from the sodium replete group. These recent electrophysiological data, along with the older behavioral work, suggest that the sodium depleted rat is *less* sensitive to the taste of salt in the suprathreshold range (Contreras and Frank, 1979).

Few experimental data are available on changes in taste during sodium deficiency in humans. The data that are available for humans suggest that taste responses to salt are influences by sodium balance. Patients with adrenal insufficiency may crave salt, presumably because aldosterone secretion and sodium retention are impaired. A particularly well-known case was reported by Wilkins and Richter (1940) in which a young boy died after he was placed on a hospital diet and denied his supplemental salt. Others have found lowered taste thresholds for salt in individuals with adrenal insufficiency (Digiesi, 1961). Hence, severe sodium depletion increases the attraction to salt. However, it is unknown whether a craving for salt accompanies a small reduction in sodium intake or whether the depletion must be severe.

II. CONSUMPTION BEYOND NEED

Another aspect of salt intake is that in many species it is consumed well beyond physiological need. In humans, the sodium requirement has been estimated to be 0.25 g/day whereas average consumption of NaCl in the United States is 6–18 g/day (Meneely and Battarbee, 1976). It is believed that much of this supplemental intake is due to enjoyment of the taste of salt in foods. This supplemental ingestion has been believed to be a consequence of habits learned during development (Dahl, 1958; Meneely and Battarbee, 1976) for at least two reasons. First, there is great cultural variation in intake with some peoples adding no salt in addition to that which occurs naturally in their foods and some consuming up to 26 g/day (Sasaki, 1962). The second reason the taste for salt is thought to be acquired is the *apparent* change in response to it during development from indifference or rejection to acceptance. The evidence for this developmental change is incomplete and conflicting.

The behavioral responses of newborn infants to stimulation by salt are not as easily interpretable as are their responses to stimulation by sucrose. When newborn infants' responses to sucrose were tested, it was evident that the sucrose solution was preferred to water. Sucrose stimulated anterior tongue movements associated with solution acceptance (Nowlis, 1973), altered heart rate (Ashmead *et al.*, 1980), lengthened sucking bursts (Crook, 1978), elicited facial expressions associated with pleasantness (Steiner, 1977), and stimulated intake (Desor *et al.*, 1973; Nisbett and Gurwitz, 1970). In contrast, responses of newborn infants to salt have not been as clear-cut. There is no evidence that salt solutions are preferred to plain water. In some newborn individuals, saline elicited posterior tongue movements not unlike those seen with quinine (bitter) stimulation (Nowlis, 1973). This may indicate rejection of saline. In contrast to sucrose, salt solutions also shortened sucking bursts relative to water (Crook, 1978). The consequence of these effects was unclear. Salt solutions were not ingested differenty from the diluent, either when the diluent was water or a weak (0.07 *M*) sucrose solution (Desor *et al.*, 1975).

   In summary, the response of the human newborn infant to salt is unclear; some methods indicate that salt solutions are unpleasant, others indicate indifference. There are no published data to indicate that they exhibit a preference for NaCl in the same way newborn infants show a preference for sucrose solutions. However, it still remains possible that if salt were tested in a medium other than water, newborn infants could manifest a preference. A full knowledge of newborn infants' responses to salt is not yet available.

   Little work exists on salt preference in children from a few days old to 2 years of age. By 2 years, children strongly reject salt solutions (Beauchamp and Maller, 1977). At 2 years, however, salt in some foods such as soup may increase the palatability and ingestion of that food (Beauchamp, 1981). The importance of the food medium in the taste test is shown in the results of the following experiment (G. K. Beauchamp and M. J. Moran, unpublished data). Two-year-old children were asked to sample two carrots, one from each of two distinctive bowls. One bowl contained carrot pieces that had been soaked overnight in tap water. The other bowl contained carrot pieces that had soaked overnight in a 0.34 *M* NaCl solution. After the child sampled a carrot from each bowl, he or she was told to take and eat as many carrots from either bowl as wished, for a 5-min period. The number of pieces taken from each bowl was recorded. Salty carrots were preferred to unsalty carrots (Fig. 1).

   Although the results of this experiment are clear, the interpretation is not. The simplest explanation for this preference for salty carrots is that the children liked the salty taste. An alternative explanation is that the salt masked or otherwise interacted with some flavor components in the carrots that the children found offensive. Mixing other taste substances with NaCl results in suppression of the taste of those substances (Bartoshuk, 1980). This hypothesis suggests that the children then may not be attracted to a salty taste per se, but to a carrot with fewer off or bad tastes. Some observations made during testing of the children tend to confirm, however, that the children were attracted to the salt taste. Many of the children were observed to chew the salty pieces and then spit them out, presumably after the salt and any other flavor had been extracted. Others would lick the

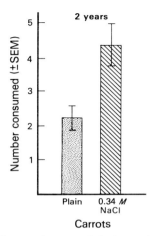

Fig. 1. Average number of carrot pieces sampled when soaked in plain water and in 0.34 M NaCl (n = 74).

salt water off the pieces and show no further interest once this was done. Older children (4–8 years old) preferred salted pretzels to unsalted pretzels (Beauchamp and Maller, 1977). Children then, do seem attracted to salt, but demonstration of this depends on the medium in which salt is tasted. When aqueous salt solutions were used, a salt preference did not emerge.

III. REDUCTION OF SODIUM INTAKE

Whether or not the salt preferences in childhood are present at birth, are the result of some physiological change, or the result of prior dietary experience with salt remains to be determined. Some evidence, although much of it anecdotal, does suggest that dietary experience influences the taste of salt in adults. A field study of the Siriono Indians of eastern Bolivia demonstrated this point. This group obtained most of their sodium from the meat they ate and did not add salt in preparation of food. When salt was first introduced to some individuals of the tribe they did not like the taste of it. By putting small quantities of salt in cooking, the Indians "soon developed craving for it" and it became a factor in establishing friendly relations with whites (Holmberg, 1950). Another account is from Stephannson (1946) who lived among Eskimos whose diet consisted of either boiled or frozen fish, their main source of sodium. He claimed that after a few months of this fare, he had acquired most of the tastes of the Eskimos and his craving for salt disappeared. Dahl (1958) reported that patients who initiate low sodium diets complained about the lack of taste for a few days but soon became accustomed to it and grew to like the reduction in salt. McCance (1936), on the other hand, reported a craving for salt when he went on an extremely low sodium diet to study physiological changes in sodium deprivation. In a rare experimental study, Yensen (1959) placed two individuals on a diet similar to McCance's for 7–8 days and monitored taste thresholds to all four taste qualities. He found large increases in sensitivity for NaCl with no changes in sensitivity to the other taste qualities (HCl, sucrose, quinine).

In these last two reports, sodium intake was below the suggested requirement and a deficiency may have been induced. The remaining anecdotal reports seem to indicate that as one remains on a low sodium diet, the taste of high concentrations of salt becomes more intense and less pleasant. This is contrary to the case in animal studies where induction of sodium deficiency results in behavioral and electrophysiological responses as if the high concentrations of salt were less intense and more pleasant.

There is a psychological mechanism that may offer an explanation for these anecdotal human observations and would work in direct opposition to the effect of deficiency on the taste of salt. Humans tend to judge sensory stimuli, including tastes, in terms of the contextual situation (Riskey et al., 1979). Ratings of the intensity and pleasantness of a particular taste can be changed by experimentally manipulating the context. For example, context can be manipulated by varying the frequency of presentation of various taste stimuli. If high concentrations of salt in soup are presented more frequently than low concentrations, a particular high concentration will be rated as tasting less intense and more pleasant. Restated, a given taste stimulus is judged as tasting more salty when presented in a context containing many low concentrations, less salty when placed in a context of many high concentrations of salt. These contexts also influence pleasantness ratings given to the stimuli (Riskey, 1980). If a low sodium diet is thought of as a context in which many taste stimuli of low concentration are presented frequently, it would be predicted that eventually the high concentrations of salt to which one was normally accustomed would begin to taste more salty and less pleasant.

In order to determine the effects of dietary sodium reduction on certain aspects of taste, three male students were placed on a low sodium diet containing 75 mEq sodium for 24 days and their taste responses were evaluated prior to, during, and following the experimental diet (Bertino et al., 1981). Compliance with the diet was monitored by unannounced 24-hr urine collections. Detection thresholds, that is, the smallest amount of either salt or of sucrose tasted in aqueous solution, were collected. We also measured the intensity and pleasantness of suprathreshold responses to salt in soup and sucrose in Kool-Aid. Subjects rated the saltiness and pleasantness of nine concentrations of salt in low sodium soup on nine-point rating scales. They also rated the sweetness and pleasantness of nine concentrations of sucrose in Kool-Aid. Taste responses to both salt and sucrose were measured to determine if the effects obtained were specific to the salt taste or were an effect on taste in general. Hedonic responses were also assessed through a preference task. At the end of a testing session, the nine concentrations were presented to the subject who was required to taste the samples and select the most pleasant tasting sample.

There was no effect of dietary manipulation on detection thresholds of sucrose in water or salt in water. Suprathreshold responses to NaCl in soup did change with the dietary manipulation. Soups with high concentrations of sodium (0.26–0.71 M) were rated by each subject as tasting less intense when they were on the low sodium diet when compared with the pre- and postdiet periods (Fig. 2). Most of these same soups were rated as tasting more pleasant when the subjects were on the low sodium diet. The preference task showed a comparable change. Each subject preferred a higher concentration during the low sodium diet. There were no systematic changes in intensity or pleasantness ratings of sucrose in Kool-Aid with the dietary manipulation. Urinary sodium excretion dropped with the low sodium diet to approximately one-third of the prediet level. All three subjects lost weight while they were on the diet ($\bar{X} = 4.21$ lb).

The taste effects of the low sodium diet were small but remarkably similar for each individual. Each subject rated the saltiness of the high NaCl concentrations as tasting less intense when on the diet and rated the same concentrations as tasting more salty when off the diet (Fig. 2). These results were surprising. Based on anecdotal reports, we had expected to see a decrease in the pleasantness of the

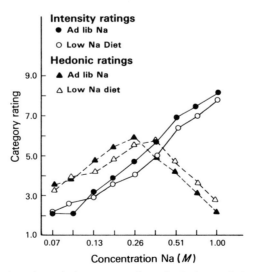

Fig. 2. Average intensity and pleasantness ratings of salted soup during *ad libitum* and low sodium intake ($n = 3$).

high concentrations of salt in soup and an increased pleasantness in the low concentrations. We observed the opposite. These data do, however, compare favorably with data obtained from rats placed in sodium deficit. When compared to sodium replete rats, sodium deprived rats respond to high concentrations of salt solutions as if they tasted less strong. This human experiment and the rat experiments of other researchers are methodologically quite different and different behaviors were measured. The rats were sodium deprived whereas the human subjects experienced only a reduced sodium intake. Caution must be exercised in drawing parallels between rat and human data.

Although these data do not match the anecdotal reports, this does not mean that the self-reports are necessarily in error. There may be a biphasic response to reduced sodium intake with salt initially becoming more pleasant. As time on the low sodium diet proceeds, perhaps a new level of sodium balance is reached and a new taste baseline is obtained by which salty tastes are now judged. The high concentrations of NaCl which at first had become more pleasant may fall in hedonic value and eventually become even less pleasant than they initially were. In recently completed research, taste effects of long-term, self-maintained, low sodium diets were examined. Individuals were tested with various concentrations of salt in water, soup, or crackers for 2 months prior to initiating the diet and, beginning 2 months after diet initiation, for 4 months. Analysis of the data indicated that a low sodium diet producing a 42% reduction in sodium excretion resulted in a decrease in the preferred concentration of salt in foods (soup and crackers). The taste changes occurred within 2–3 months of diet initiation.

Low sodium diets are often prescribed to hypertensive individuals for at least two reasons. High sodium intake can vitiate the effects of antihypertensive medication (Tobian, 1979), and low sodium diets alone can sometimes reduce high blood pressure (Meneely and Battarbee, 1976). The results of our first experiment suggest that in the initial stage of a low sodium diet, one source of difficulty in maintaining that diet may be an enhanced pleasantness of the taste of strong salt concentrations mediated by a reduced intensity of that taste. These effects were found in normotensive individuals. It is unknown if they would have been found and to what extent in hypertensive individuals. Hypertensive people may have altered taste responses to salt to begin with (e.g., Fallis, 1962). It is not known whether threshold differences are related to preference behavior. Some other studies have demonstrated greater sodium intake in hypertensive individuals (Langford et al., 1977; Schechter et al., 1973) with diuretics also increasing intake. These data may indicate an increased salt preference in hypertensive individuals. Compounded with this is the initial taste change demonstrated in our data, caused by reduction of sodium intake. This may give some indication of why difficulties ensue in initiation of a low sodium diet. However, the results of our recently completed study imply that if the individual is able to maintain a low sodium diet for 2–3 months, a lowered preference for salt in foods will develop.

IV. SUMMARY

At the deficiency end of the sodium intake spectrum, the involvement of taste in the control of intake, and taste responses to deficiency have been well studied. The role of taste in the control of supplemental intake is only beginning to be investigated. Initial findings indicate that there appear to be some similarities between the role of taste in supplemental intake and its role in need states. Superimposed on supplemental intake, however, is the influence of culture, with food availability and habits as well as sodium balance influencing the taste of salt. The role of taste in supplemental sodium intake may be even more complex than its role in response to sodium deficiency.

ACKNOWLEDGMENTS

This research was approved by the Committee on Studies Involving Human Beings of the University of Pennsylvania and the Clinical Research Advisory Committee at the Hospital of the University of Pennsylvania. Support for this research was provided by the USDA 59-32U4-0-3, the Clinical Research Center, and the NIH-5-M01-RR00040. We thank Marianne Moran for her assistance.

REFERENCES

Ashmead, D. H., Reilly, B. M., and Lipsitt, L. P. (1980). Neonates heart rate, sucking rhythm, and sucking amplitude as a function of the sweet taste. *J. Exp. Child Psychol.* **29,** 264–281.

Bartoshuk, L. M. (1980). Sensory analysis of the taste of NaCl. *In* "Biological and Behavioral Aspects of Salt Intake" (M. R. Kare, M. J. Fregly, and R. A. Bernard, eds.), pp. 83–98. Academic Press, New York.

Beauchamp, G. K. (1981). Ontogenesis of taste preference. *In* "Food, Nutrition and Evolution" (D. Walcher and N. Kretchmer, eds.). Masson, Paris.

Beauchamp, G. K., and Maller, O. (1977). The development of flavor preferences in humans: A review. *In* "The Chemical Senses and Nutrition" (M. R. Kare and O. Maller, eds.), pp. 291–311. Academic Press, New York.

Bertino, M., Beauchamp, G. K., Riskey, D. R., and Engelman, K. (1981). Taste perception in three individuals on a low sodium diet. *Appetite* **2,** 67–73.

Carr, W. J. (1953). The effect of adrenalectomy upon the NaCl taste threshold in the rat. *J. Comp. Physiol. Psychol.* **45,** 377–380.

Contreras, R. J. (1978). Salt taste and disease. *Am. J. Clin. Nutr.* **31,** 1088–1097.

Contreras, R. J., and Frank, M. (1979). Sodium deprivation alters neural responses to gustatory stimuli. *J. Gen. Physiol.* **73,** 569–594.

Crook, C. K. (1978). Taste perception in the newborn infant. *Infant Behav. Dev.* **1,** 52–69.

Dahl, L. K. (1958). Salt intake and salt need. *N. Engl. J. Med.* **258,** 1205–1208.

Desor, J. A., Maller, O., and Turner, R. (1973). Taste acceptance of sugars by human infants. *J. Comp. Physiol. Psychol.* **84,** 496–501.

Desor, J. A., Maller, O., and Andrews, K. (1975). Ingestive responses of human newborns to salty, sour and bitter stimuli. *J. Comp. Physiol. Psychol.* **89,** 966–970.

Digiesi, V. (1961). Le variazioni della sensibilita gustativa per il sapore salato nell'uomo in partico-
    lari situazioni fisiologiche e sperimentali ed in alcuni state morbosi. *Rass. Neurol. Veg.*
    15, 320-327.
Fallis, N., Lasagna, L., and Tetreault, L. (1962). Gustatory thresholds in patients with hypertension.
    Nature (London) **196,** 74-75.
Harriman, A. E., and MacLeod, R. B. (1953). Discriminative thresholds of salt for normal and
    adrenalectomized rats. *Am. J. Psychol.* **66,** 465-471.
Holmberg, A. R. (1950). "Nomads of the Long Bow: The Siriono of Eastern Bolivia." Inst. Soc.
    Anthropol. Publ. No. 10. Smithsonian Institution, Washington, D.C.
Langford, H., Watson, R. L., and Thomas, J. G. (1977). Salt intake and the treatment of hyperten-
    sion. *Am. Heart J.* **93,** 531-532.
McCance, R. A. (1936). Experimental sodium chloride deficiency in man. *Proc. R. Soc. London,*
    Ser. B **119,** 245-268.
Meneely, G. R., and Battarbee, H. D. (1976). Sodium and potassium. *In* "Present Knowledge in
    Nutrition" (D. M. Hegsted *et al.,* eds.), pp. 259-279. Nutr. Found., Inc., Washington, D.C.
Morrison, G. R. (1974). Taste thresholds, taste sensitivity and the effects of adrenalectomy in rats.
    Chem. Senses Flavour **1,** 77-78.
Nachman, M., and Pfaffmann, C. (1963). Gustatory nerve discharges in normal and sodium deficient
    rats. *J. Comp. Physiol. Psychol.* **56,** 1007-1011.
Nisbett, R. E., and Gurwitz, S. B. (1970). Weight, sex and the eating behavior of human newborn.
    J. Comp. Physiol. Psychol. **73,** 245-253.
Nowlis, G. (1973). Taste-elicited tongue movements in human newborn infants. *In* "Fourth Sym-
    posium on Oral Sensation and Perception: Development in the Fetus and Infant" (J. F. Bosma,
    ed.), pp. 292-303. US Govt. Printing Office, Washington, D.C.
Pfaffmann, C., and Bare, J. K. (1950). Gustatory nerve discharges in normal and adrenalectomized
    rats. *J. Comp. Physiol. Psychol.* **43,** 320-324.
Richter, C. P. (1956). Salt appetite in mammals: Its dependence on instinct and metabolism. *In*
    "L'Instinct dans le Comportement des Animaux et de l'Homme (M. Autuori, ed.), pp. 577-
    629. Masson, Paris.
Riskey, D. R. (1980). Effects of context and sensory adaptation in judgments of taste intensity and
    pleasantness. *Proc. Int. Symp. Olfaction Taste, 7th, 1980* pp. 385-388.
Riskey, D. R., Parducci, A., and Beauchamp, G. K. (1979). Effects of context in judgments of
    sweetness and pleasantness. *Percept. Psychophys.* **26,** 171-176.
Sasaki, N. (1962). High blood pressure and salt intake of the Japanese. *Jpn. Heart J.* **3,** 313-324.
Schechter, P. J., Horwitz, D., and Henkin, R. I. (1973). Sodium chloride preference in essential
    hypertension. *J. Am. Med. Assoc.* **225,** 1311-1315.
Steiner, J. E. (1977). Facial expressions of the neonate infant indicating the hedonics of food related
    chemical stimuli. *DHEW Publ. NIH (U.S.)* **(NIH) 77-1068,** 173-188.
Stephansson, V. (1946). "Not by Bread Alone." Macmillian, New York.
Tobian, L. (1979). The relationship of salt to hypertension. *Am. J. Clin. Nutr.* **32,** 2739-2748.
Wilkins, L., and Richter, C. P. (1940). A great craving for salt by a child with corticoadrenal
    insufficiency. *J. Am. Med. Assoc.* **114,** 866-868.
Yensen, R. (1959). Some factors affecting taste sensitivity in man. II. Depletion of body salt. *Q. J.*
    Exp. Psychol. **11,** 230-238.

11

The Interaction of Dietary Sodium and Potassium with the Adrenergic Nervous System and Peripheral Vasculature in Sodium-Induced Hypertension

HAROLD D. BATTARBEE, JOHN W. DAILEY,
AND GEORGE R. MENEELY

155

THE ROLE OF SALT IN
CARDIOVASCULAR HYPERTENSION

I. INTRODUCTION

Epidemiological studies of geographically or ethnically isolated populations consuming various quantities of sodium, intrapopulation studies of individuals consuming various amounts of salt, clinical information from normal and abnormal subjects treated with drugs such as diuretics and/or salt restriction or supplements, and studies of animal models offer compelling evidence of the association between dietary sodium and hypertension. Extensive reviews of the evidence for this effect of sodium have recently been conducted (Freis, 1976; Meneely and Battarbee, 1976; Battarbee and Meneely, 1978) and for the sake of brevity the readers are referred to these articles.

In contrast to the abundant literature relating sodium to hypertension, there is scant but mounting evidence that small increments in dietary potassium may have a modulating influence on the hypertensigenic effects of sodium excess. Early observations (Addison, 1928; Priddle, 1931; McQuarrie et al., 1936; Sasaki et al., 1959) showed increased dietary potassium can prevent hypertension or lower blood pressure in hypertensives. Epidemiological studies (Langford and Watson, 1975; Walker et al., 1979; Watson et al., 1980; Pietinen et al., 1979) suggest that a relative potassium deficit could aggravate the adverse effects of excessive salt intake on blood pressure. Parfrey et al. (1981a) very recently completed a study in which moderate amounts of dietary sodium were ingested by groups of normotensive and hypertensive subjects and their blood pressures monitored. Dramatic decreases in blood pressure were observed when hypertensives were given a dietary supplement of potassium and these decreases persisted for as long as the supplement was ingested. Upon discontinuance of the potassium supplement, blood pressures quickly rebounded to hypertensive levels.

Various models of experimental hypertension have borne out this hypothesized modulating role for potassium: the Dahl salt-sensitive rat (Dahl et al., 1972); spontaneously hypertensive rat (Louis et al., 1971); Sprague–Dawley rat (Meneely et al., 1957; Battarbee et al., 1979); and prenatal exposure to salt and kaliuretic diuretics (Grollman and Grollman, 1962). Recently, Battarbee et al. (1979) demonstrated that small increments in dietary potassium obtund the development of salt-induced hypertension and improve longevity while reducing the excretion of urinary catecholamines.

Studies of plasma catecholamines in essential hypertension are controversial. Results using newer, more sensitive, and specific techniques of measurement indicate that 25–75% of essential hypertensives manifest elevated norepinephrine (NE) values (Engleman *et al.*, 1970; DeQuattro and Chan, 1972; DeChamplain *et al.*, 1976; Miura *et al.*, 1978). Urinary excretion studies yield somewhat lesser percentages (DeQuattro, 1971; Hoeldtke, 1974; Januszewicz and Wocial, 1975). Attempts to correlate the degree of hypertension with indices of sympathetic nervous system activity have been largely fruitless. Some investigators using sympathetic blocking agents like hexamethonium (Louis *et al.*, 1973) or the α-agonist clonidine (Louis *et al.*, 1975) have found that decreases in blood pressure correlate well with plasma NE values. More recently, Weidmann *et al.* (1979) using debrisoquine found that essential hypertension may be maintained in part by inappropriate secretion of NE along with increased pressor sensitivity. In normotensives, very low levels of sodium ingestion result in greatly enhanced release of NE and epinephrine (E). As the sodium load is increased, plasma catecholamines suppress in a fashion that bears a very close resemblance to that of the renin–angiotensin–aldosterone axis (Murray *et al.*, 1978; Romoff *et al.*, 1978; Luft *et al.*, 1979). A recent study indicates that the plasma NE response to sodium loading may be biphasic—the level responding to increased sodium loading with suppression then a rebound to higher levels (Nichols *et al.*, 1980). Unfortunately, nearly all these studies were rather acute, short-term procedures. One study (Parfrey *et al.*, 1981a) was of a more chronic nature. In this study, essential hypertensive plasma NE values were higher than those of normotensives and suppressed upon sodium loading in a manner similar to normotensives. In a subsequent study of young normotensive adults whose parents were normotensive or hypertensive, this same group of investigators (Parfrey *et al.*, 1981b) suggested that all the objects of their study were sensitive to the pressor effects of sodium loading, but only those with a genetic predisposition to hypertension who are sensitive to the depressor effect of potassium proceed to develop hypertension if the intake of this electrolyte is inadequate. In addition, there was also evidence of enhanced sympathetic responsiveness to postural changes in those subjects with hypertensive parents.

With respect to sympathetic responsiveness, it has become obvious since the early work of Doyle and Black (1955) that vascular hyperreactivity is a regular feature of essential hypertension (Doyle and Fraser, 1961a; Mendlowitz, 1973; Sivertsson and Olander, 1968). A great deal of evidence has accumulated suggesting that structural redesign, as would be predicted from a simple increase in wall mass relative to luminal diameter (Folkow *et al.*, 1958, 1970; Folkow, 1971a; Sivertsson, 1970; Mulvany *et al.*, 1978), is an important contributor to this "apparent" hyperreactivity to pressor agonists.

Although the Swedish group was unable to demonstrate an altered threshold to pressor agonists in hypertension, other investigators have reported a decreased threshold and increased vascular reactivity that was additive to changes conferred by vessel wall geometry (Lais and Brody, 1975). Mendlowitz and Naftchi (1958) had much earlier demonstrated that more work was performed by vascular smooth muscle/unit of agonist injected in essential hypertensives, indicating a decreased threshold and found this hypersensitivity to be rapidly enhanced by aldosterone and salt in hypertensives, but not in normotensives (Mendlowitz et al., 1963). Furthermore, diuretics rapidly decreased both blood pressure and vascular responsiveness (Mendlowitz et al., 1960). Particularly suggestive are the studies of Doyle and Fraser (1961a) who demonstrated that the vascular bed of the hand was hyperresponsive in normotensive children of hypertensive parents. A recent report (Lais and Brody, 1978) indicates that there may be a specific hypersensitivity to norepinephrine and/or changes in geometry that precedes pressure changes in the anesthetized, spontaneously hypertensive rat model. Touw et al. (1980) report a specific hyperresponsiveness to NE in only certain vascular beds of young unanesthetized spontaneously hypertensive rats that is exclusive of changes in vascular geometry and argues against a nonspecific structural change that leads to increased vascular reactivity to all vasoconstrictor agonists.

Thus, there is compelling evidence that dietary sodium is an important factor in the genesis of essential hypertension. Many studies of the adrenergic nervous system, vascular geometry, and vascular sensitivity to agonists have been performed in individuals and animals that have *established* hypertension. Relatively few studies have been done during the transition period from normotension into arbitrary range described as hypertension. There is good reason to believe that the genesis of hypertension is intimately entwined with changes in sensitivity to agonists, changes in vascular geometry, and changes in the function of the sympathetic nervous system function, especially during the formative stages of the disorder. Superimposed on these interactions are the modulating effects of potassium. The present study was preliminary and was conducted to lend insight into many of these interactions and effects during the formative stages of sodium-induced hypertension.

II. METHODS

A. Animals and Diets

Male Sprague–Dawley derived rats were purchased from Holtzman Co. and, after a period of conditioning and observation, placed on special diets* consisting of Purina Lab Chow with the following total sodium and potassium content: 0.21 mEq Na/g and 0.23 mEq K/g (Control Diet); 0.91 mEq Na/g and 0.24 mEq K/g (High Na Diet); 0.98 mEq Na/g and 0.35 mEq K/g (High Na + K Diet).

*Bioserve, Inc., Frenchtown, New Jersey.

Deionized water and feed were provided *ad libitum*. Animal weights and systolic blood pressures (SBP) were measured twice weekly over a period of 1–4 weeks. Blood pressures were measured using the tail-cuff method and a programmed electrosphygmomanometer.[†]

B. Urinary Norepinephrine

Urinary norepinephrine (^{u}NE) levels were determined in a 24-hr urine sample by a modification (Battarbee *et al.*, 1979) of the semiautomated trihydroxyindole procedure of Viktora *et al.* (1968).

C. Vascular Resistance

Studies of vascular resistance in isolated perfused hindquarters were performed using the technique of Brody *et al.* (1963) as modified by Lais *et al.* (1974). In brief, rats were anesthetized with a dial–urethane solution and placed on a temperature controlled operating table. The abdominal aorta and nearby sympathetic nerve chains were exposed at approximately the level of the third lumbar vertebra through an abdominal midventral incision. Five mg/kg heparin (100 U/mg) were injected via the jugular vein. The blood from the proximal aorta above the level of the bifurcation was diverted through a cannula to a constant-flow pump that had been primed with blood from a treatment paired animal. The blood was then routed back to the abdominal aorta to perfuse the hindlimbs. At constant flow, changes in mean perfusion pressure reflect proportional changes in vascular resistance. Systemic pressure was monitored via a carotid cannula and perfusion pressure was measured via a T tube inserted into the perfusion tubing just proximal to the hindquarters. The pressure resulting from the resistance of the perfusion tubing was subtracted in the tabulation of perfusion pressure.

In general, the following protocol was used in evaluating each hindquarter preparation: (1) pressure–flow in innervated hindquarters, (2) pressure–flow in denervated hindquarters, (3) vasoconstrictor response to sympathetic nerve stimulation, (4) vasoconstrictor response to exogenous NE, and (5) vasodilator response to nitroprusside.

The contribution of neurogenic tone to hindquarters resistance was assessed by comparing vascular resistance before and after ganglionic blockade with hexamethonium chloride (12 mg/kg). Vascular resistance in the hindlimbs was evaluated at 3.0, 5.0, 7.0, and 10.0 ml/min $\cdot$ 500 g^{-1} body wt, and pressure–flow curves were constructed.

[†]Narco Biosystems, Houston, Texas.

Responses to direct sympathetic nerve stimulation were evaluated by stimulating the lumbar sympathetic nerve chains at L-3 with a supramaximal voltage (10 V, 3 msec) and a range of frequencies (1, 3, 10, 20, and 30 Hz) while measuring perfusion pressure at constant flow.

Responses to NE were obtained by the infusion of the agonist (norepinephrine bitartrate in 0.9% saline) into the perfusion tubing upstream from the hindlimbs at a rate calculated to deliver a known concentration of agonist to the hindquarters. Since Lais and Brody (1978) have demonstrated that the magnitude of the response elicited by pressor agonists is markedly affected by basal perfusion pressures, all basal perfusion flow rates were adjusted to yield a net pressure of 50 mm Hg. Dose–response curves were constructed from data obtained at 1, 3, 5, and 10 μg NE/ml.

To examine structural changes in the wall-to-lumen ratio in hindquarters vascular beds, maximal vasodilation was produced by administering sodium nitroprusside (45 μg) directly into the perfusion tubing, collecting pressure–flow data at 3, 5, 7, and 10 ml/min $\cdot$ 500 g^{-1}, and constructing pressure–flow curves.

Intrinsic vascular smooth muscle myogenic tone in the hindlimbs was assessed by comparing the differences between denervated pressure–flow curves and nitroprusside treated pressure–flow data.

Statistical comparisons were performed using least squares, best fit linear regression analysis, and analysis of variance. Values of $p < 0.05$ were regarded as statistically significant.

III. RESULTS

A. Effect of Diet on Systolic Blood Pressure

Figure 1 summarizes the effects of the various diets on SBP as a function of time on the diets. Perusal of the data at the end of the study suggested that there were two subgroups of animals within each of the high sodium fed groups: one whose SBP became only moderately elevated during the 4-week course of the study (SBP < 150 mm Hg) and a second that developed more severe hypertension (SBP $\geq$ 150 mm Hg). These subgroups were selected out, retrospectively, according to their SBP level and their data treated separately. At week 0, before the initiation of the dietary regimes, SBP of the various groups did not differ significantly, the mean SBP $\pm$ SEM being 120 $\pm$ 3 mm Hg ($n = 51$) for all groups combined. Initiation of the high sodium diets led to a significant increase in SBP in all groups within 1 week when compared to animals fed the control diet. The mean SBP was 123 $\pm$ 1 ($n = 11$), 141 $\pm$ 2 ($n = 10$, $p < 0.001$), 145 $\pm$ 3 ($n = 6$, $p < 0.001$), 141 $\pm$ 5 ($n = 7$, $p < 0.001$), and 146 $\pm$ 6 mm Hg ($n = 10$, $p < 0.001$) for the Control, High Na SBP < 150, High Na SBP $\geq$ 150, High Na + K SBP < 150, and High Na + K SBP $\geq$ 150 groups, respectively.

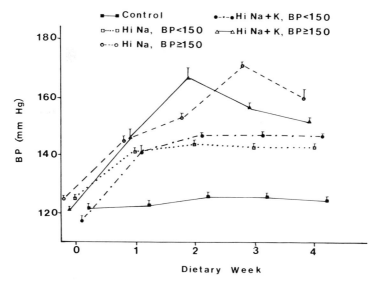

Fig. 1.   Systolic blood pressures (mean ± SEM) of rats fed diets varying in sodium and potassium content before and during the ingestion of the respective diets.

By the end of dietary week 2, the SBP of the moderately hypertensive animals from the High Na and High Na + K dietary groups had reached a plateau at approximately 145 mm Hg where they remained for the duration of the study. Animals that developed the more severe form of hypertension, however, had SBP that continued to increase. At the end of week 2 the High Na SBP ≥ 150 group's pressure had not risen significantly from week 1, but that of the High Na + K SBP ≥ 150 had continued to increase and reached its highest value (167 ± 7 mm Hg, $p < 0.01$). At dietary week 3, the High Na + K SBP ≥ 150 group's SBP had fallen to 157 ± 3 mm Hg whereas that of the High Na SBP ≥ 150 group had risen to its peak value of 171 ± mm Hg ($p < 0.01$). The pressures of both severely hypertensive groups declined by the end of dietary week 4 but remained significantly greater than that of the Control Diet Group ($p < 0.001$).

B. Effect of Diet on Body Weight

No significant differences were found among the various dietary groups at any given dietary week (see Table I).

C. Effect of Diet on Norepinephrine Excretion

During the course of the study, it was observed that the excretion of NE "tracked" with respect to time, i.e., values for animals that started off with high

TABLE I

Effect of Diets on Body Weight[a]

Group	Dietary week				
	0	1	2	3	4
Control	260 ± 15	298 ± 16	327 ± 15	350 ± 12	359 ± 9
High Na SBP < 150	268 ± 23	333 ± 20	346 ± 17	356 ± 18	370 ± 17
High Na SBP ≥ 150	241 ± 17	306 ± 15	341 ± 20	376 ± 17	375 ± 21
High Na + K SBP < 150	209 ± 26	286 ± 20	326 ± 14	355 ± 10	365 ± 12
High Na + K SBP ≥ 150	289 ± 17	334 ± 19	352 ± 18	373 ± 19	375 ± 18

[a] Animal body weights did not differ significantly among the various dietary groups at any given dietary week. Values are mean body weights in grams ± SEM.

^{U}NE values had a tendency to remain high for the duration of the study, and those that had intiially low ^{U}NE values remained low. Figure 2 depicts this tracking phenomenon in representative animals of the Control Diet Group. In order to take into account this tracking effect, the basal level of ^{U}NE at dietary week 0 was used to normalize each animal's ^{U}NE data for the subsequent dietary weeks, i.e., the ^{U}NE for each animal was expressed as percent of the dietary week 0 ^{U}NE values. Figure 3 illustrates changes in ^{U}NE for each of the dietary weeks. At the

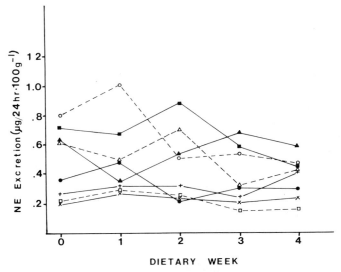

Fig. 2. Tracking of urinary NE excretion in animals from the Control Diet group. Each symbol represents data collected in the same animal over a period of 4 dietary weeks.

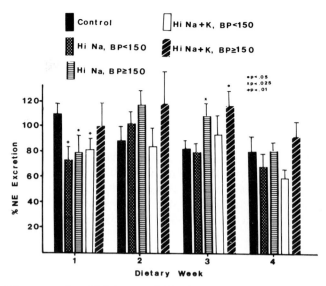

Fig. 3. Urinary excretion of NE (mean ± SEM) of animals fed control, high sodium, and high sodium plus potassium supplement over a period of 1 month. Data are expressed as percent excretion using dietary week 0 excretion rate of each animal as 100%.

end of dietary week 1, ^{U}NE was significantly suppressed in the High Na SBP < 150 ($-25 \pm 9\%$, $p < 0.01$), High Na SBP ≥ 150 ($-19 \pm 13\%$, $p < 0.05$), and the High Na + K SBP < 150 ($-17 \pm 8\%$, $p < 0.01$) groups when compared to the control value ($11 \pm 7\%$). The High Na + K SBP ≥ 150 group did not suppress significantly. By the end of dietary week 2, the ^{U}NE rates had returned to values insignificantly different from Control values, but the High Na SBP ≥ 150 and High Na + K SBP ≥ 150 groups reflected a tendency toward increased ^{U}NE. This tendency was significantly different from the Control Diet Group by the end of dietary week 3, the ^{U}NE values being $-14 \pm 6\%$, $14 \pm 9\%$ ($p < 0.025$), and $19 \pm 11\%$ ($p < 0.05$) for the Control, High Na SBP ≥ 150, and High Na + K SBP ≥ 150 groups, respectively. At the end of the dietary week 4 the ^{U}NE values for all groups were indistinguishable from the Control Diet Group's value.

D. Innervated and Denervated Pressure–Flow Curves

Neurogenic tone, assessed by taking the difference in perfusion pressure before and after sympathetic nervous system blockade with hexamethonium, was found to be significantly lower in the High Na SBP < 150 Group ($p < 0.01$) when compared to the Control Diet Group values at the end of dietary week 4. At this time the High Na SBP $\geq$ 150 group was found to have neurogenic tone that did not differ significantly from that of the Control Diet Group. There were no other significant differences in neurogenic tone among the various groups for dietary weeks 1 or 4. It was noted, however, that the innervated and denervated pressure–flow data for the High Na SBP $\geq$ 150 Group (dietary week 4) had a tendency to be lower than that of the Control Diet Group. The pressure for a given flow was reduced, but this did not differ in a manner considered statistically significantly ($p < 0.2$), perhaps because the number of animals in this particular group was small ($n = 5$). Innervated pressure–flow curves for the High Na + K SBP $\geq$ 150 and High Na + K SBP $<$ 150 Groups were superimposed on one another, as were the denervated pressure–flow curves; therefore, the data from these two groups were pooled to form a single High Na + K Group. Neurogenic tone in this pooled group did not vary significantly from that of the Control Diet Group at the end of either dietary week 1 or 4 (Figs. 4, 5, and 6).

E. Stimulus–Response Curves

At the end of the dietary week 4, the High Na SBP $<$ 150 group's vasoconstrictor responses to sympathetic nerve stimulation at L-3 were significantly attenuated when compared to that of the Control Diet Group ($p < 0.003$)(Fig. 7).

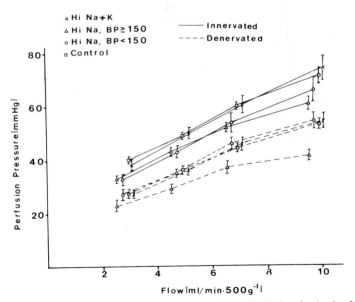

Fig. 4. Innervated–denervated pressure-flow curves of the hindlimbs of animals after 1 or 4 dietary weeks on the respective diets. Values are means ± SEM.

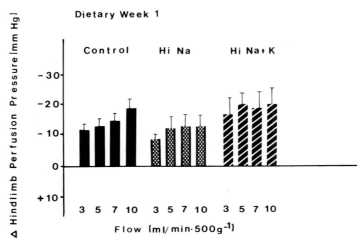

Fig. 5. Neurogenic tone calculated from the difference between innervated and denervated hindlimb pressure–flow curves for animals fed diets varying in sodium and potassium content for a period of 1 week. Values are mean change in perfusion pressure on denervation ± SE.

In contrast, the stimulus–response data of the High Na SBP ≥ 150 Group suggest a great enhancement of responsiveness when compared to controls, although the difference was significant only at the $p < 0.07$ level. Comparison of this group with the High Na SBP < 150 Group revealed a significant difference between the two groups ($p < 0.01$). Stimulus–response data for the two High Na

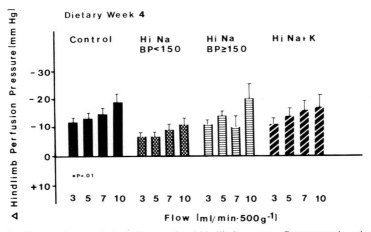

Fig. 6. Neurogenic tone derived from perfused hindlimb pressure–flow curves in animals fed diets varying in sodium and potassium content for a period of 4 weeks. Values are mean change upon denervation ± SEM.

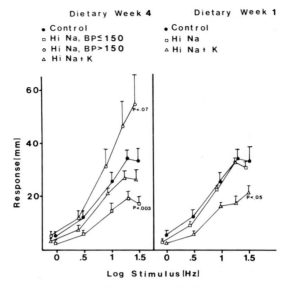

Fig. 7. Stimulus–response curves of the perfused rat hindlimb during sympathetic nerve stimulation at L-3 (10 V, 3 msec duration, monophasic). Animals were fed diets with various sodium and potassium contents for periods of 1 or 4 weeks. Values are means ± SEM.

+ K groups at dietary week 4 were again pooled to form a single group. Data from this pooled group did not differ significantly from that of the Control Diet Group. Stimulus–response data for the pooled High Na + K groups after dietary week 1 resembled very closely that of the High Na < 150 Group after dietary week 4, responsiveness being significantly depressed ($p < 0.05$) when compared to control data. The High Na Group at the end of dietary week 1 had no SBP values greater than 150 mm Hg, making it necessary to treat them as a single group. Their stimulus–response curves were indistinguishable from that of the Control Diet Group at this time.

F. Dose–Response Curves for Norepinephrine

Comparisons of the perfused hindlimb log dose–response data for NE revealed no significant differences in responsivess for the various dietary groups when compared to the Control Diet Group at dietary weeks 1 and 4 (Fig. 8).

G. Nitroprusside Vasodilated Pressure–Flow Curves

Evaluation of nitroprusside vasodilated perfused hindlimb data of the various dietary groups revealed no significant differences when compared to the Control Diet Group data (Table II). Determination of resistance vessel intrinsic myogenic

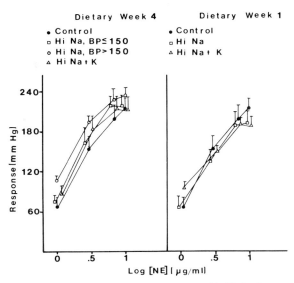

Fig. 8. Dose–response curves for NE in the perfused rat hindlimb after ganglionic blockade. Animals were fed diets with various sodium and potassium contents for periods of 1 to 4 weeks. Values are means ± SEM.

tone by taking the difference between denervated pressure and maximally vasodilated pressure at a given flow suggested a difference in myogenic tone in the High Na SBP < 150 Group when compared to Control Diet values, the intrinsic myogenic tone being reduced ($p < 0.05$)(Table III). Unfortunately, by the time the hindlimb preparation had reached this final stage, there had been some attrition, particularly in the High Na SBP ≥ 150 Group (dietary week 4) and the

TABLE II

Hindquarters Perfusion Pressures (mm Hg) during Maximal Vasodilation Produced by Nitroprusside

	Dietary week	n	Perfusion rate			
			3 ml/min	5 ml/min	7 ml/min	10 ml/min
Control	1,4	7	20 ± 2	26 ± 7	29 ± 3	36 ± 5
High Na, BP < 150	4	5	22 ± 2	30 ± 2	37 ± 4	43 ± 8
High Na, BP > 150	4	2	21 ± 1	27 ± 1	32 ± 1	38 ± 2
High Na + K	4	5	22 ± 5	29 ± 8	37 ± 8	43 ± 10
High Na	1	6	22 ± 1	29 ± 1	34 ± 2	39 ± 2
High Na + K	1	2	20 ± 4	30 ± 6	34 ± 6	37 ± 3

TABLE III

Hindquarter Intrinsic Myogenic Tone[a]

Group	Dietary week	n	Flow (ml/min · 500 g^{-1})			
			3	5	7	10
Control	1,4	7	5.1 ± 1.6	6.4 ± 2.6	11.4 ± 3.6	15.7 ± 4.2
High Na SBP < 150	4	5	2.5 ± 1.5	1.7 ± 2.5	5.2 ± 4	2.2 ± 9*
High Na SBP ≥ 150	4	2	Low	Low	Low	Low
High Na + K	4	5	11.7 ± 5.4	16.0 ± 6	13.0 ± 7.9	15.7 ± 9.1
High Na	1	6	7.8 ± 3.2	8.8 ± 2.9	9.0 ± 1.4	14.2 ± 3.1
High Na + K	1	2	Normal	Normal	Normal	Normal

[a] Intrinsic myogenic tone of resistance vessels of the perfused hindlimb was calculated from denervated pressure–flow and nitroprusside vasodilated pressure–flow curves. Values are mean perfusion pressure in mm Hg ± SEM. n Refers to the number of animals in each group. * indicates $p < 0.05$ when compared to the Control Diet Group.

High Na ± K Group (dietary week 1). Only a few animals in each of these two groups survived the nitroprusside vasodilation. Intrinsic myogenic tone in the High Na SBP ≥ 150 appeared low, whereas for the High Na + K Group (dietary week 1) it appeared normal or comparable to the values of the group given the Control Diet. Statistical analyses were not performed on these two groups due to the limited data obtained.

IV. DISCUSSION

Earlier studies conducted in the laboratory of the authors indicated that the Sprague–Dawley rat, when fed a moderately high sodium diet for 1 year, responded with a modest elevation in blood pressure and excreted more NE than did normotensive animals fed a control diet. The inclusion of a small dietary potassium supplement resulted in a reduction of the NE excretion rate to a value comparable to that of the control group and reduced the blood pressure to a level slightly greater than that of the control group. When normal cardiovascular reflexes were taken into account, the NE excretion rate in the hypertensive animals appeared inappropriately high for the level of blood pressure observed. The mechanisms of both the hypertensigenic effect of dietary sodium and the protective effect of potassium remained unknown. Recently, the effects of dietary sodium and potassium were reexamined during the early or formative stages of hypertension (Battarbee et al., 1980). Acute moderate sodium loading (1 week) suppressed catecholamine excretion at a time when blood pressure had already risen, much in the same manner as has been described for normotensive and hypertensive humans (Murray, 1978; Romoff *et al.*, 1978; Luft *et al.*, 1979; Parfrey *et al.*, 1981a, b). This suppression was promptly (2 weeks) followed by a return of catecholamine excretion rate to levels comparable to preload values, a level that appeared inappropriately high for the blood pressure observed. A small dietary potassium supplement had a modulating effect in that it prevented the suppression of catecholamine excretion despite the fact that blood pressure rose to a comparable level.

The present study was conducted as a further extension of the above acute study to gain insights into the mechanisms of the effects of dietary sodium and potassium on blood pressure during the transition from normotension into the range of blood pressure considered hypertensive. In order to address the matter of the "appropriateness" of changes in indices of function of the sympathetic nervous system, it was necessary to evaluate the responsiveness of peripheral resistance vessels and the contributions of vascular geometry and intrinsic vascular smooth muscle myogenic tone to the maintenance of blood pressure.

Blood pressure data collected over the period of 0–4 dietary weeks revealed some dramatic changes among and within the various dietary groups. Animals fed a high sodium diet responded with a rapid increase in blood pressure that was not moderated by a potassium supplement at the end of dietary week 1. At this time, urinary NE excretion was suppressed in the sodium fed group suggesting diminished sympathetic nervous system tone. Neurogenic tone, assessed by the perfused hindlimb procedure, showed no evidence of enhancement at this time and the response to sympathetic nerve stimulation was indistinguishable from that of the Control Diet Group. Exogenous NE dose–response curves were comparable to that of controls, suggesting there was no change in reactivity or geometry of resistance vessels. Nitroprusside vasodilated pressure–flow data substantiated that there were no changes in geometry. The intrinsic myogenic tone of resistance vessels was similarly unaffected at this time. Thus, it appears that acute dietary sodium loading resulted in decreased sympathetic nervous system activity that was appropriate under the conditions of elevated blood pressure but insufficient to reduce the pressure to a level comparable to that of the Control Diet Group. It is unknown what was responsible for the maintenance of this elevated pressure at the end of dietary week 1, but the suppressed rate of urinary NE excretion and otherwise normal peripheral vasculature suggest that some other factors were important.

The inclusion of a potassium supplement in the high sodium diet resulted in data similar to that of the nonsupplemented diet group at the end of dietary week 1. There was one notable exception. The supplemented animals were hyporesponsive to sympathetic nerve stimulation. It must be noted, however, that data relating to intrinsic myogenic tone are scanty and do not allow a firm opinion to be formed about this variable. Available data suggest it is not different from that of the Control Diet Group. Blood pressure and urinary NE excretion data from this group indicate that those animals that subsequently develop severe hypertension do not suppress their urinary NE excretion rate sufficiently to be considered different from that of·the Control Diet Group. These animals also had a tendency toward higher blood pressures than similarly treated animals that did not develop subsequent severe hypertension and did have a significant depression of their urinary NE excretion rate. Thus, the data from the potassium supplemented groups at the end of dietary week 1 suggest decreased sympathetic nervous system activity similar to that of the sodium-loaded nonsupplemented group. The inclusion of potassium in the diet appears to have added a dimension of reduced responsiveness to sympathetic nerve traffic but did not prevent or ameliorate the development of hypertension.

Blood pressure and urinary NE data for dietary weeks 2 and 3 revealed that the high sodium diet group and high sodium, potassium-supplemented groups were each composed of two subgroups: one that developed moderate hypertension and one that developed severe hypertension. Although the pressures developed in the two severely hypertensive subgroups were similar, the inclusion of the potassium supplement in the diet appears to have the effect of displacing the time course of the pressure changes such that they occurred more rapidly. Thus, the highest pressures in the potassium-supplemented animals occurred a full week before that of the high sodium group and had already begun to fall by the time the high sodium group's pressures had reached their maximum. Urinary NE values during this period were very suggestive. By dietary week 2, both the moderately hypertensive subgroups' rates of urinary NE excretion had returned to levels indistinguishable from that of controls, where they remained for the duration of the study. The severely hypertensive subgroups' urinary NE values, however, reflected a tendency not to suppress but to increase that became statistically significant by the end of dietary week 3. It was during this time frame that these two subgroups developed their most severe hypertension. Perhaps the differences in blood pressures between the moderate and severely hypertensive subgroups were due to differences in sympathetic vasomotor tone during this period. By the end of week 4, blood pressures of both severely hypertensive subgroups had fallen to levels slightly greater than that of the moderately hypertensive subgroup and urinary NE excretion rates had returned to levels indistinguishable from that of the Control Diet Group. Thus, it appears that the development of severe hypertension among sodium-loaded animals is accompanied by greater sympathetic nervous system activity, and that as pressures fall in these subgroups, sympathetic tone also falls until both blood pressures and urinary NE excretion are comparable to that of moderately hypertensive subgroups at dietary week 4. Potassium supplements in the severely hypertensive group had the effect of accelerating the time course of the changes in pressure but did not ameliorate or prevent its occurrence.

Perfused hindlimb data obtained at the end of dietary week 4 indicate that the response to sympathetic nerve stimulation in the severely hypertensive, high sodium group was enhanced. Neurogenic tone, however, showed no evidence of enhancement. Intrinsic myogenic tone may have been suppressed at this time, but more data are needed to evaluate this variable. The response to exogenous NE was similar to that of the Control group and vascular geometry did not appear to be affected. These data, along with that of urinary NE excretion, suggest that there was a level of effective neurogenic tone that was lower than at dietary weeks 2 and 3 but still inappropriately high for the elevated blood pressure observed and that intrinsic myogenic tone may have been reduced in this group as in the moderately hypertensive group. These differences could be responsible for the lower level of blood pressure observed at dietary week 4 when compared to the previous week. The pressure at week 4 was still, however, higher than that of the moderately hypertensive sodium-loaded group. The inclusion of potassium in the high sodium diet resulted in a "normalization" of the stimulus–response curve and intrinsic myogenic tone, the net result being a blood pressure that was lower than that of the nonsupplemented, high sodium diet group, and very similar to that of the moderately hypertensive groups.

Perfused hindlimb data from moderately hypertensive animals at the end of dietary week 4 revealed that sodium-loaded animals had hyporesponsive stimulus–response curves and NE dose–response curves indistinguishable from the Control Diet Group. Vascular geometry was not affected, but intrinsic myogenic tone was significantly depressed. Neurogenic tone was likewise significantly depressed when compared to the severely hypertensive sodium-loaded group. These data suggest that the principle differences between the severely hypertensive group and the moderately hypertensive group at dietary week 4 were the attenuated response to sympathetic nerve traffic, diminished effective neurogenic tone, and decreased intrinsic vascular smooth muscle myogenic tone.

V. SUMMARY

During the course of development of sodium-induced hypertension, there are several transients in the determinants of blood pressure, many of which are short-lived. Compensatory decreases in indices of sympathetic nervous system tone such as the urinary excretion of NE appear very quickly but are soon incorporated into other compensatory changes involving response to sympathetic nerve traffic, response to pressor agonists, intrinsic myogenic tone of peripheral resistance vessels, and vascular geometry. Superimposed on these effects of dietary sodium are the effects of dietary potassium, which have been shown to have significant modulating effects on the response of resistance vessels to sympathetic nervous system traffic, perhaps sympathetic nerve traffic itself, and resistance vessel intrinsic myogenic tone. This "plasticity" of the determinants of blood pressure under conditions of dietary sodium loading and the modulating influences of potassium are no doubt responsible for a portion of the confusion that has surrounded studies of sodium-induced hypertension.

ACKNOWLEDGMENTS

The authors wish to express thanks for the expert technical assistance of Mrs. Bobbie Gibson, Mrs. Laurel McNatt, and Mr. Glenn Farrar, and to thank Mrs. Vicki Rambin for her assistance in the preparation of this manuscript. This work was supported in part by a grant from the American Heart Association, Louisiana, Inc.

REFERENCES

Addison, W. (1928). The uses of sodium chloride, potassium chloride, sodium bromide and potassium bromide in cases of arterial hypertension which are amenable to potassium chloride. *Can. Med. Assoc. J.* **18**, 281–285.

Battarbee, H. D., and Meneely, G. R. (1978). The toxicity of common table salt (sodium chloride). *CRC Crit. Rev. Toxicol.* **5**, 355–378.

Battarbee, H. D., Funch, D. P., and Dailey, J. W. (1979). The effect of dietary sodium and potassium upon blood pressure and catecholamine excretion in the rat. *Proc. Soc. Exp. Biol. Med.* **161**, 32–37.

Battarbee, H. D., Dailey, J. W., McNatt, L., and Farrar, G. E. (1980). Dietary sodium induced hypertension and catecholamine excretion in tbe Sprague–Dawley rat. *Physiologist* **23**, 127.

Brody, M. J., Shaffer, R. A., and Dixon, R. L. (1963). A method for the study of peripheral vascular responses in the rat. *J. Appl. Physiol.* **18**, 645–647.

Dahl, L. K., Leitl, G., and Heine, M. (1972). Influence of dietary potassium and sodium/potassium molar ratios on the development of salt hypertension. *J. Exp. Med.* **136**, 318–330.

DeChamplain, J., Farley, L., Cousineau, D., and vanAmeringen, M. R. (1976). Circulating catecholamine levels in human and experimental hypertension. *Circ. Res.* **38**, 109–114.

DeQuattro, V. (1971). Evaluation of increased norepinephrine excretion in hypertension using L-DOPA-^{3}H. *Circ. Res.* **28**, 84–97.

DeQuattro, V., and Chan, S. (1972). Raised plasma catecholamines in some patients with primary hypertension. *Lancet* **1**, 806–809.

Doyle, A. E., and Black, H. (1955). Reactivity to pressor agonists in hypertension. *Circulation* **12**, 974–980.

Doyle, A. E., and Fraser, J. R. E. (1961a). Vascular reactivity in hypertension. *Circ. Res.* **9**, 755–758.

Doyle, A. E., and Fraser, J. R. E. (1961b). Essential hypertension and inheritance of vascular reactivity. *Lancet* **2**, 509–511.

Engleman, K., Portnoy, B., and Sjoerdsma, A. (1970). Plasma catecholamine concentrations in patients with hypertension. *Circ. Res.* **26, 27**, Suppl. 1, 141–146.

Folkow, B. (1971). The haemodynamic consequences of adaptive structure changes of the resistance vessels in hypertension. *Clin. Sci.* **41**, 1–12.

Folkow, B., Grimby, G., and Thulesius, O. (1958). Adaptive structural changes in the vascular walls in hypertension and then relation to the control of peripheral resistance. *Acta Physiol. Scand.* **44**, 255–272.

Folkow, B., Hallback, M., Lundgren, Y., and Weiss, L. (1970). Background of increased flow resistance and vascular reactivity in spontaneously hypertensive rats. *Acta Physiol. Scand.* **80,** 93–106.

Folkow, B., Gurevich, M., Hallback, M., Lundgren, Y., and Weiss, L. (1971). Hemodynamic consequences of regional hypertension in spontaneously hypertensive and normotensive rats. *Acta Physiol. Scand.* **83,** 532–541.

Freis, E. D. (1976). Salt, volume and the prevention of hypertension. *Circulation* **53,** 589–595.

Grollman, A., and Grollman, E. F. (1962). The teratogenic induction of hypertension. *J. Clin. Invest.* **41,** 710–714.

Hoeldtke, R. (1974). Catecholamine metabolism in health and disease. *Metab., Clin. Exp.* **23,** 663–686.

Januszewicz, W., and Wocial, B. (1975). Dopa, catecholamines and their metabolites in essential hypertension. *Clin. Sci. Mol. Med.* **48,** 295s–298s.

Lais, L. T., and Brody, M. J. (1975). Mechanism of vascular hyperresponsiveness in the spontaneously hypertensive rat. *Circ. Res.* **36, 37,** Suppl. 1, 1216–1222.

Lais, L. T., and Brody, M. J. (1978). Vasoconstrictor hyperresponsiveness: An early pathogenic mechanism in the spontaneously hypertensive rat. *Eur. J. Pharmacol.* **47,** 177–189.

Lais, L. T., Shaffer, R. A., and Brody, M. J. (1974). Neurogenic and humoral factors controlling vascular resistance in the spontaneously hypertensive rat. *Circ. Res.* **35,** 764–774.

Langford, H., and Watson, R. L. (1975). *In* "The Epidemiology and Control of Hypertension" (O. Paul, ed.), p. 119. Chapt. II. Dietary and Chemical Factors: Electrolytes and Hypertension. Intercontinental Medical Book Corp. New York.

Louis, W. J., Tabei, R., and Spector, S. (1971). Effects of sodium intake on inherited hypertension in the rat. *Lancet* **2,** 1283–1286.

Louis, W. J., Doyle, A. E., Anavekar, S. N., and Chua, K. G. (1973). Sympathetic activity and essential hypertension. *Clin. Sci. Mol. Med.* **45,** 119s–121s.

Louis, W. J., Anavekar, S., Doyle, A. E., Johnson, C. I., and Geffen, L. B. (1975). The autonomic nervous system and blood pressure regulation in man. *In* "Central Action of Drugs in the Blood Pressure Regulation" (D. S. Davis and J. R. Reed, eds.), pp. 241–250. Pitman, London.

Luft, F. C., Rankin, L. I., Henry, D. P., Bloch, R., Grim, C. E., Wegman, A. E., Murray, R. H., and Weinberger, M. H. (1979). Plasma and urinary norepinephrine values at extremes of sodium intake in normal man. *Hypertension* **1,** 261–266.

McQuarrie, I., Thompson, W. H., and Anderson, J. A. (1936). Effects of excessive ingestion of sodium and potassium salts on carbohydrate metabolism and blood pressure in diabetic children. *J. Nutr.* **11,** 77.

Mendlowitz, M. (1973). Vascular reactivity in systemic arterial hypertension. *Am. Heart J.* **85,** 252–259.

Mendlowitz, M., and Naftchi, N. E. (1958). Work of digital vasoconstriction produced by infused norepinephrine in primary hypertension. *J. Appl. Physiol.* **13,** 247–251.

Mendlowitz, M., Naftchi, N., Gitlow, S. E., Weinreb, H. L., and Wolf, R. L. (1960). The effect of chlorothiazide and its congeners on the digital circulation in normotensive subjects and in patients with essential hypertension. *Ann. N.Y. Acad. Sci.* **88,** 964–974.

Mendlowitz, M., Naftchi, N. E., Bobrow, E. B., Wolf, R. L., and Gitlow, S. E. (1963). The effect of aldosterone on electrolytes and on digital vascular reactivity to 1-norepinephrine in normotensive, hypertensive and hypotensive subjects. *Am. Heart J.* **65,** 93–101.

Meneely, G. R., and Battarbee, H. D. (1976). The high sodium low potassium environment and hypertension. *Am. J. Cardiol.* **38,** 768–786.

Meneely, G. R., Ball, C. O. T., and Youmans, A. (1957). Chronic sodium toxicity: Protective effect of potassium chloride. *Ann. Intern. Med.* **47,** 263.

Miura, Y., Kobayashi, K., Sakuma, H., Tomioka, H., Adachi, M., and Yoshinaga, Y. (1978).

Plasma noradrenaline concentrations and hemodynamics in the early stages of essential hypertension. *Clin. Sci. Mol. Med.* **55**, 645–715.

Mulvaney, M. J., Hansen, P. K., and Aalkjaer, E. (1978). Direct evidence that the greater contractility of resistance vessels in spontaneously hypertensive rats is associated with a narrowed lumen, a thickened media, and an increased number of smooth muscle cell layers. *Circ. Res.* **43**, 854–864.

Murray, R. H., Luft, F. C., Block, R., and Wegman, A. E. (1978). Blood pressure responses to extremes of sodium intake in normal man. *Proc. Soc. Exp. Biol. Med.* **159**, 432–436.

Nichols, M. G., Kiowski, W., Zweifer, A. J., Julius, S., Schork, M. A., and Greenhouse, J. (1980). *Hypertension* **2**, 29–32.

Parfrey, P. S., Wright, P., Goodwin, F. J., Vanderberg, M. J., Holly, J. M., and Evans, S. J. W. (1981a). Blood pressure and hormonal changes following alteration in dietary sodium and potassium in mild essential hypertension. *Lancet* **1**, 59–63.

Parfrey, P. S., Condon, K., Wright, P., Vandenburg, M. J., Holly, J. M. P., Goodwin, F. J., Evans, S. J. W., and Ledingham, J. W. (1981b). Blood pressure and hormonal changes following alteration in dietary sodium and potassium in young men with and without a familial predisposition to hypertension. *Lancet* **1**, 113–117.

Pietinen, P. I., Wong, O., and Altschul, A. M. (1979). Electrolyte output blood pressure, and family history of hypertension. *Am. J. Clin. Nutr.* **32**, 997–1005.

Priddle, W. W. (1931). Observations on the management of hypertension. *Can. Med. Assoc. J.* **25**, 5.

Romoff, M. S., Klusch, G., Campere, V. M., Wang, M., Friedler, R. M., Weidman, P., and Massry, S. G. (1978). Effect of sodium intake on plasma catecholamines in normal subjects. *J. Clin. Endocrinol. Metab.* **48**, 26–31.

Sasaki, N., Mitsubashi, T., and Fakushi, S. (1959). The effects of the ingestion of large amounts of apples on blood pressure in farmers in Akita Prefecture. *Igaku to Seibutsugaku* **51**, 103.

Sivertsson, R. (1970). Hemodynamic importance of structural vascular changes in essential hypertension. *Acta Physiol. Scand., Suppl.* **343**, 6–56.

Sivertsson, R., and Olander, R. (1968). Aspects of the nature of increased vascular resistance and increased "reactivity" to noradrenaline in hypertensive subjects. *Life Sci.* **7**, Part 1, 1291.

Touw, K. B., Haywood, J. R., Shaffer, R. A., and Brody, M. J. (1980). Contribution of the sympathetic nervous system to vascular resistance in conscious young and adult spontaneously hypertensive rats. *Hypertension* **2**, 408–418.

Viktora, J. K., Baukal, A., and Wolff, F. W. (1968). New automated fluorometric methods for estimation of small amounts of adrenaline and noradrenaline. *Anal. Biochem.* **23**, 513–528.

Walker, W. G., Whelton, P. K., Saito, H., Russell, R. P., and Herman, J. (1979). Relationship between blood pressure and renin, renin substrate, angiotensin II, aldosterone and urinary sodium and potassium in 574 ambulatory subjects. *Hypertension* **1**, 287–291.

Watson, R. L., Langford, H. G., Abernathy, J. Barnes, T. Y., and Watson, M. J. (1980). Urinary electrolytes, body weight, and blood pressure. *Hypertension* **2**, Suppl. 1, 193–198.

Weidmann, P., Keusch, G., Flammer, J., Ziegler, W. H., and Reubi, F. C. (1979). Increased ratio between changes in blood pressure and plasma norepinephrine in essential hypertension. *J. Clin. Endocrinol. Metab.* **48**, 727–731.

12

To Salt or Not to Salt, That Is the Question: A Discussion with Digressions

GEORGE R. MENEELY

Some years ago I undertook the formation of a new medical school in the far northwestern part of Louisiana with Dr. Edgar Hull as the founding Dean, and my scientific pursuits perforce began to atrophy. I now find myself somewhat in the position of that unfortunate Englishman who addressed a major conference. Later, one of his listeners remarked, ''Not only had he left the field ten years before, but he hadn't *been* missed!''

An after dinner speaker at a serious scientific meeting confronts a dilemma. He would like to be witty and entertaining, and, at the same time, he would wish to transmit a message of great and memorable moment. It is probably impossible to do both. Not a few such speakers do neither!

I shall pass between the horns of this dilemma by avoiding any attempt to be witty, and, instead of a memorable message, I shall ramble in a diffuse and aimless way through odds and ends of thoughts about salt, which have interested me over the years.

To document this intent, I must tell you an anecdote concerning Alexander Gutman, whom most of us know best as the long-time editor of the *American Journal of Medicine*. He is equally well known for his sharpness of mind and his sharpness of tongue. The occasion was a meeting of the Harvey Society in New

175

THE ROLE OF SALT IN
CARDIOVASCULAR HYPERTENSION

York. As it happened, the occasion was an important anniversary of William Harvey's birth, and the Harveian Society had sent a deputation from England to bring greetings and a gift to the New York Society. It was, thus, an auspicious occasion, and the turnout for it was accordingly large.

Before the formal dinner, cocktails were served, martinis and manhattans, and nothing else. I had given up the consumption of alcohol some time before, having by measure consumed my fair share, and, after a suitable negotiation with the bartender, obtained a tall glass of a more temperate beverage. With this in hand, I encountered Gutman in the crowd. "Meneely, where did you get that marvelous highball?" he enquired. Upon my explanation that it was, in fact, plain ginger ale, his face fell and he moved away, in evident fear of contagion.

Nothing further of note transpired until we were midway through dinner. Gutman was seated, not next to me, but next to me but one. He suddenly leaned forward, and called to me, in the tones for which he was well known, "Meneely, your conversation used to be more interesting when you drank!" Since I still do not drink, and since I have you as a semicaptive audience, you will have the opportunity to see whether Gutman was right.

It is appropriate to look back to the origins of the human use of added salt and reappraise our taste for this material which Hakluyt reported the Icelanders of the sixteenth century called, "the provocation of gluttony. . . ."

No one knows when or how salt came into human use. It will probably never be possible to find out with certainty, but it is certainly a legitimate target for guided guessing. Since salt, sodium chloride, that is, occurs in nature in a fairly pure form especially near the sea, and in efflorescences elsewhere, one may intuit chance lead to experimentation, and the agreeable flavor of added salt soon confirmed its use. It cannot have been long thereafter before the preservative properties of brine became evident.

There is evidence, as we shall see later, that primitive man developed his taste for salt concurrently with his progress from a nomadic to a more settled agricultural existence, that soon thereafter, the preservative properties of salt were observed and exploited. In the tropical and subtropical climates where all this went on, prevention of the decay of foodstuffs must have had important survival value for the tribes that learned this secret.

Widespread use of salted foods may well have played an important role in dissociating the human taste for salt from the need for it. Life expectancy was short in those days, and man was grateful to survive from season to season. The fact that the preservative value of salt depends on its relatively higher toxicity for lower forms of life troubled him little, and he was more concerned with keeping his blood inside him than with the pressure it might attain in his middle age. Over the millennia that have since elapsed, the taste for salt and the need for it underwent a progressive dissociation to the present time, when every cafeteria table supports what once was a prince's ransom of snowy white salt.

Later we will look at the evidence there is more to a taste for salt than the flavorsomeness of it. What is beyond debate is the fact that salt came into human use before, indeed, long before recorded history, but not, perhaps, before a major division in language had occurred.

There have been efforts to adduce, through the evidence from linguistics, that salt came into human use concurrently with the changeover from the hunter–gatherer way of life to the more settled agricultural mode, with heavy dependence on various grains, a herbivorous diet if you will, instead of the earlier meat and animal products diet of feral man, a "carnivorous" diet.

In the Indo-European language family, it is not possible to trace a common word for salt farther back than primitive Greek, and there is no word for salt in the ancient Sanskrit. The same is true of terms for farming. While common roots from nomadic life for the herd, the cattlefold, the herdsman, and the milking time occur in rich profusion, terms such as for the plow, tilling, and other more advanced agricultural activities do not share common roots, suggesting strongly that these, too, were of much later introduction.

The stem seems to be *hal-s* or *sal-s*. It would, thus, appear the word came into language some time after the split of the parent speech, the "Indo-European" or the "stem language" into Asiatic and European divisions.

Of the south European languages, the hal-s = sal-s spreads over to the Italo-Celtic. In the Celtic limb, it is *halen* in Welsh, *salann* in old Irish and similar in Gaelic, Armoric, and Breton. In the Italian limb, it is *sal* in Latin, Spanish, Portugese and Provencal, *sale* in Italian and *sel* in the French. In the north European branch, it is virtually the same from original Teutonic onward, with vagaries in spelling: *solt, salt, salts, salz, sault,* etc. In old Saxon, Anglo-Saxon = old English, old and modern Frisian, middle low German, middle and modern Dutch, old and middle high German and modern German, old Norse, old Icelandic, Swedish, Danish, Moeso-Gothic and Gothic, etc. In the Lituslavonic limb, we have *sali* in old Slavonic.

All of this is small wonder. The Amber Route, for example, ran down from Jutland along the Weser, the Saale, or the Elbe, to and through the Brenner Pass to the head of the Adriatic, and thence by sea to Mycenae. And the Danube was a notable trade route. But these were only Bronze Age routes for traffic in amber, salt, and other valuables, established later, but over the same routes as the migrations that had taken the Indo-European languages from the origin somewhere between the Carpathians and the Caucasus through Eurasia sometime before 2000 B.C. The main language group in the ancient Near East, in, say 2500 B.C., was that of Semitic variants, but beyond, and to the north, were the related dialects or languages of quite different types which were to have a remarkably wide and effective dispersal, for, "by 1000 B.C., to take a convenient round date, they must have been spoken from India in the East to central and western Europe." Hittite drifted to Anatolia, Celtic to central Europe, and the Italic language behind Latin to Italy, and, in later movements, Sanskrit to India, and Greek to the Aegean. Still later, the Germanic languages developed in central Europe in close contact with Celtic and the Slavic tongues.

One of the most fascinating fields of current archeological research is tracking the "tribal migrations" and ancient routes of trade by the techniques of linguistics. Words and pieces of words seem more ephemeral than pieces of pottery or designs on shards, but syllables have a curious and vital tenacity, almost like that of self-replicating deoxynucleic acid. Most of us carry live viruses, for example, herpes simplex, which are incredibly ancient, passed on to us by our forebears, and, daily, we use stem words which may be thousands of years old. All of these languages had their salt, for it was everywhere in Europe by then, valuable, highly prized because it was seldom in sufficient supply to satisfy man's appetite for it.

From first recorded history, indeed from the very first time of writing, salt has been with us, not only as the name of sodium chloride itself, but also in euphemism and as a symbol. The latter usually relates to the flavor of salt, but its preservative properties confer significance on its use as a covenant, an enduring compact.

Aside from the prime meaning of the word, for the substance itself, that is, there are at least 31 different meanings which could be identified with sufficient clarity to impress the lexicographic scholars who assembled the ten volume "New Dictionary on Historical Principles" from which the twelve volume Oxford English Dictionary derives. We know and use many of these meanings, some are unfamiliar, and some seem strange until a different etymology explains an apparently irrational meaning. For example, the word salt can also mean sexual desire or excitement, usually of a bitch in heat. The etymology clarifies: it is from the French, *saute* = leap, assault, etc.

There are, then, the uses of salt with qualifying words, white-salt, great-salt, small-salt, but most of us would not know salt upon salt which means salt made by purifying a poorer grade of foreign imported salt, and, hence, a literary work which really is a plagiarism, "improved" from the writings of another author. One can be in salt, both literally, as a pickle, and figuratively likewise. There are innumerable proverbial and allusive uses, such as "some account the falling of salt upon the table ominous" (Flavel, 1681), and, "if the salt thou chance to spill, token sure of coming ill," which is an old English proverb. How many have noticed the overturned saltcellar in the Last Supper of Leonardo da Vinci?

If we "eat his salt" we have enjoyed his hospitality, or, have we become dependent on him? If we want him for a friend, we must "eat a bushel of salt with him." Quotes George Herbert in Jacula Prudentum, 1640, but Taverner in Erasm, Prov. 30, (1539) quotes "trust no man unless thou has first eaten a bushel of salt with him." Cervantes, in Don Quixote (Book III, Chap. 1) reduces it to a peck, but having eaten only this much, feels only that he "knows him." The idea isn't new, and it wasn't then. It is an ancient Greek proverb.

You may allude to salt on a bird's tail, take things with a grain of salt, or your poetry or prose can reference the bitter saline taste of tears. You can be worth your salt, although this expression is usually used in the negative. The Roman legionaires received an allowance of salt, and, later, instead, they received a sum of money for salt, salarium, hence the word for salary.

You can be salt all through, so long have you been a sailor, or you can be an old salt if you are sufficiently experienced. Figurative uses reference the piquancy of it, "salt of youth," or its pungency, "with salt and sharpness upbraid."

The word salt can stand for a saltcellar, thus, "Limoges enameled salts," and it is used to mark a station at table, thus, "Hee humbly sate below the salt and munch'd his sprat." Ten acres of salts would be a marsh (or perhaps some south Louisiana real estate?). Or it could be seawater entering a fresh river, "the last incursion of the salts was seven years ago." It can be a tip or gratuity, "stop the carriage to ask for salt."

There seems, at this time, no way to trace the earliest human use of salt, and much less so, why it came to be used at all. There are, however, data that bear on this latter point. Since time immemorial, it has been noted that there were populations that did not use salt. The Odyssey, for example, tells of the inlanders of Epirus who did not know the sea and used no salt. In relatively recent times, numerous populations have been found who were unaccustomed to salt. It has, however, been observed repeatedly that such populations, upon introduction to salt, tended to become dedicated users of it.

There is an abundance of evidence that, once it is established, the taste for salt is strong. In an historical note (Meneely, 1954) 30 years ago I wrote,

> . . . once accustomed to its use, the human craving for it is intense and we do not lack for evidence that men took strong views about it. The Teutons waged wars for saline streams. Wives and children were sold into slavery to obtain it. Decapitation or dismemberment was sometimes the penalty for carrying salt out of ancient cities. Governors early employed taxation of salt to raise money and some of the bitterest passages of English history from the sixteenth to the nineteenth century trace the taxation of salt and the misery and misgovernment attending it. In 1758 the Earl of Dundonald wrote, "Every year in England, ten thousand people are seized for salt smuggling and three hundred men are sent to the gallows for contraband trade in salt and tobacco" . . .

I am sorry to report that, after writing this passage of ringing prose, I dove headlong into a trap which had been laid almost a century before. That happens to be a pretty well-populated trap. For example, I have before me at this writing the article on potassium and sodium in biological systems in the current edition of Van Nostrand's Scientific Encyclopedia. It reiterates the error into which I, with many others, had fallen. It has been quoted so often, it is taken to be holy writ. The error is epitomized in one sentence of mine: ''A nomadic diet of flesh and milk did not require any additional salt but as cereal grains and vegetables took their place in the diet, added salt became a necessity.'' That is just plain wrong. It was shown to be wrong in 1853, about 130 years ago.

How this fallacy came to pass is an interesting story. While the earliest of ancient literature and written history records the use of salt, meaning sodium chloride, true scientific knowledge about it was not possible before 1807 when Humphrey Davy isolated it by electrolysis. It is interesting that potassium, not sodium, was the first element to be isolated by electrolysis, in that same year.

Now it had been known for long that herbivorous animals were prone to make long treks to salt licks. Carnivorous animals did not. Among those human populations that did use salt, and that means just about all the civilized peoples of those times, salt was considered to be an essential dietary constituent. It was reasonable to suppose that the herbivores got their salt from the salt licks, and the carnivores got theirs from the herbivores. However, as early as the 1840s, it was shown by direct chemical analysis that the sodium in the herbivorous diet without benefit of salt licks is just about the same as the sodium in the diet of the carnivores. There was, however, a notable difference in the potassium content. An herbivorous diet is a high potassium diet, there is perhaps 12 to 20 times as much potassium in the herbivorous diet as there is of sodium. In contrast, the carnivorous diet has only 4 or 5 times as much potassium as sodium. This correct observation set the stage for the next step in the generation of the fallacy.

First, however, we must digress to note when sodium was first related to human disease. Credit usually goes to Redtenbacher (1850) and Carl Schmidt (1850), and deservedly so, for the full work they did. As so often happens, though, they were not the first. Gamble unearthed a short note in the English literature on the deficit of sodium in the blood in cholera by O'Shaughnessy (1831–1832) published in *Lancet*. If there is an earlier work on sodium in human disease, I do not know of it.

Von Bunge (1874, 1894) the great German biochemist, became fascinated with the herbivore/carnivore story and searched out instances of human populations that were vegetarian and that used salt, and populations of meat and animal product eaters that did not. This convinced him that the high potassium content of the ''agricultural'' or vegetarian diet required the consumption of extra sodium to offset the high potassium content of such a diet, and he published so extensively on the subject that he is quoted and requoted today, as earlier I noted. And he was wrong!

Despite the charm of the herbivores/carnivores concept of how man came to use salt, there really is nothing to support it and a wealth of evidence to negate it. Kaunitz (1956) summarizes the case against von Bunge, its main advocate, thus:

In a book which reveals a remarkably modern outlook, Lehman, in 1853, came to the conclusion that the adding of salt to natural foodstuffs is unnecessary for man. This view seemed to be supported by the fact that most animals, in freedom and in captivity, do well on natural foodstuffs without addition of salt. Although some species (for example, cattle, deer, etc.) consume salt eagerly when they are offered the substance or when they encounter it in salt licks, there is no proof they need it for a healthy life.

Later, however, von Bunge formulated his famous hypothesis that extra dietary salt is needed by populations consuming predominantly vegetable products. The excess salt was presumed to be necessary for the more effective excretion of potassium. Von Bunge arrived at this conclusion on the basis of anthropological studies which he thought indicated that nomadic societies mainly subsisting on meats do not add salt to their food, whereas, once agriculture is developed, salting becomes necessary. He linked this with his observation that the intake of salt is accompanied by the rapid onset of potassium excretion. However, he emphasized that the large amounts of salt usually consumed are out of proportion to what he thought are biological needs. Osborne and Mendel later showed that salt requirements for growth of experimental animals are indeed low; their animals were able to live on traces of salt. Thus, one might have expected that this theory could never have achieved major importance; but, curiously enough, this has not been the case, and it is still cited without further discussion by current textbooks of nutrition and anthropology.

Objections to the theory should by now be all too obvious. So far as the increased potassium excretion after salt intake is concerned, such a reaction occurs unspecifically with many injuries and diseases. Von Bunge himself never offered any proof that the increases potassium excretion is biologically of advantage, although he implied so. Now we might be inclined to the opinion that these potassium losses are disadvantageous.

As for Bunge's anthropological data, he brushed away the objection that some African tribes mainly subsisting on a vegetarian diet use potassium-rich plant ashes rather than salt as a condiment.

The ashes of burned plant material are indeed high in potassium, most usually in the form of potash, which is potassium carbonate. It tastes very bad! In fact, it was called salt of wormwood in the jargon of the alchemists, and the name persists to recent times. As most of you know, ashes of plant origin can be used to make soap by cooking with fats. Since this is a potassium soap, it is a soft soap, well known in days gone bye to our American colonist forebearers.

There are, however, certain plants, especially some growing along the ocean littoral, that yield ashes high enough in sodium chloride to provide a starting material for a sort of do-it-yourself low grade Lite Salt (Ball and Meneely, 1957; Frank and Mickelsen, 1969).

The great Louis Lapicque (1896), French physiologist/physician, he of the chronaxie beloved of medical students, had something important to offer. Lapicque found a large tribe in Africa which made its own salt by lixiviation of the ashes of a particular plant. Lix is the Latin word for ashes, and lixiviation is the slow percolation of water through ashes to dissolve out the soluble material. This tribe performed this function by use of bark filter funnels, and subsequently boiled down the effluent to produce the crystalline material. The particular plant they used was a species of water lily which grew abundantly in certain streams.

They dragged great quantities of these plants up on the bank and allowed them to dry. Then they burned them and lixiviated the ashes in the manner I have described above.

Lo and behold! Upon chemical analysis this "salt" of theirs turned out to be an almost perfectly pure potassium chloride! Lapicque reported it was so pure of potassium, and so low in sodium, that the color in the Bunsen burner flame was a bright purple, with none of the yellow sodium color at all.

Now this was an agricultural tribe. They had no intake of meat or other animal products in the diet of any significance. As Lapicque succinctly summarized, this blew Von Bunge's thesis clear out of the water. Not only did they eat the vegetarian diet high in potassium, but they chose to flavor it with yet more potassium, and flourished on this diet.

Sodium chloride, trader's salt, was freely available to these people, but they preferred their own potassium chloride. They averred that the ordinary trader's salt lacked the zippy flavor to which they were accustomed, and wanted no part of it. In times when their own became scarce, they always saved a little of it to admix with the trader's salt to beef up the flavor of the latter. In this they somewhat antedated the innovation of Lite Salt!

Lapicque concluded that the whole thing was a matter of taste, "salt" was a condiment, not an aliment. He went on to say that this tribe probably discovered the flavorful nature of this plant ash product "by the unconscious experimentation of successive generations" in much the same manner as others had discovered the gustatory enhancement of which pepper, curry, paprika (capsicum), pimento, and other flavorings are capable. He noted that the stimulant effect of caffeine was discovered in a similar way by widely different people in widely different places and among plants not closely related, tea in China, coffee in Abyssinia and Arabia, guarana in the Amazon, and mate by the Paraguayans.

I have not said much about potassium in this presentation. Most of you know we have views on the subject. These we have expressed fully elsewhere (Meneely and Batterbee, 1976). To say it all in a few words, we think we are all living in a high sodium–low potassium environment and we think this is bad for those many people who have an hereditary propensity to develop hypertension whey they eat an excess of salt. We suspect, but have not proved, that the high sodium–low potassium environment may be bad in other ways, because it loads the diet of man with sodium chloride in excess of any intake he or his remote forebearers ever had before, while, at the same time, diminishing his potassium intake below that of any diet that can be projected as possible for feral man. An exception might be the north European littoral oyster eaters, but who knows whether they ate their oysters raw, or in the form of oysters Rockefeller? Their kitchen middens do not tell!

Lapicque was surely correct as far as he went, but he may not have gone far enough. Perhaps the thought was in the back of his head when he drew the parallel to the discovery of so many different sources of the stimulant, caffeine. In any event, he did not voice the idea, but others more recently have.

I believe it was Kaunitz (1956) who first speculated that sodium chloride might have a sort of stimulant effect. There is a gathering body of evidence that sodium chloride may indeed goad the sympathetic nervous system to higher endeavors. Kaunitz has this to say:

> Carefully weighing the available evidence, one cannot escape the conclusion that normal metabolic processes are possible without the adding of salt to natural foodstuffs. Why then do we eat salt? Merely to answer that certain societies like its taste whereas others do not would be trite and superficial. It seems to me that salt intake is probably correlated with emotional stimulation, a fact perhaps more keenly appreciated in the superstitions of the ancients than our own rational approach. In view of the fact that this stimulation may be consciously or unconsciously pleasurable, it may be a causal factor in the craving for salt.

We hope to learn more apropos this subject at this conference. However, I cannot refrain from emphasizing Kaunitz' point with a quotation from Pliny (ca. 65–75).

> We may conclude then, by Hercules! That the higher enjoyments of life could not exist without the use of salt: indeed, so highly necessary is this substance to mankind, that the pleasures of the mind, even, can be expressed by no better term than the word 'salt', such being the name given to all effusions of wit. All the amenities, in fact, of life, supreme hilarity, and relaxation from toil, can find no word in our language to characterize them better than this.

One might try that paragraph over again with the word alcohol, or tobacco, or, for the matter of that, tea or coffee! Pliny makes a ration of salt sound like a fix!

It was learned long ago, first, I think, by repeated injections of what used to be called "adrenalin," that, if the blood pressure were constantly elevated for a few weeks, thereafter it would stay elevated "of its own accord." That is to say, the barostatic pressure control mechanism had been perverted, and was now reset at a new and higher level. Resetting of the barostat by excess salt eating is an insidious process. Suppose one's blood pressure at age 20 is to rise by age 40 from a diastolic of 80 to a diastolic of 100, this is a rate of rise of 1 mm per year. Following such a rise is like watching moss grow. If the mechanism were set in train in youth, it may not be necessary to continue the salt beyond the point where the control mechanism is permanently perverted. We have stopped the excess salt in our rats and found hypertension to persist. Tobian and Dahl have reported similar observations. Somehow, we have spiked the wheels of the autoregulatory mechanism.

The relevance of autoregulation to our theme tonight is that one current theory of the mechanism whereby salt does its harm in the susceptible individual is that an excess intake of it perturbs the autoregulation of the cardiovascular system in a subtle way such that it results in a serial resetting of the barostatic control system at ever higher and higher settings in the manner described by Guyton and his co-workers (1972a,b, 1974; Coleman *et al.*, 1974).

Autoregulation is by no means confined to living systems, nor to the invention of man. Let us digress to note that the Salt Sea, the more ancient name for the lake now generally known in the western world as the Dead Sea, the final receptacle of the River Jordan, manifests autoregulation. In winter, a large quantity of water is poured into it through the beds of the torrents which lead through the mountains to the east and to the west, as well as from the north and the south (Smith, 1911).

> Since it has no outlet, its level is a balance stuck between the amount of water poured into it and the amount given off by evaporation. If more water is supplied than the evaporation can carry off, the lake will rise until the evaporating surface is so much increased as to restore the balance. On the other hand, should the evaporation drive off a larger quantity than the supply, the lake will descend until the surface becomes so small as again to restore the balance.

Autoregulation is government of the body, for the body, by the body, and if we did not autoregulate ourselves, we would instantly die. The behavior of people or a nation can be considered in much the same manner as one views a biological organism, as Berrian and Indik (1962) have shown in their "Theory of Groups" (groups of people, that is). A group must have a boundary, there must be some way to define who is in and who is not, and a group must autoregulate or, as we in biology would say, it must exhibit homeostasis. In the individual human organism, the boundary is provided by the skin. As the late Charles Stockard was wont to remark to his freshman anatomy class, "The purpose of the skin is to keep the outside out and the inside in."

We have paid amazingly little attention to dietary salt in the apparently normal, and especially in the young, for the evidence indicates a greater sensitivity to sodium in youth. The human appetite for salt has become disengaged from the need for it, and the amount employed by a given individual is almost wholly governed by culture, custom, and the food habits ingrained through early life. Recently, in the airport restaurant at Beaumont, I watched with morbid fascination while a father doused his food with an amazing amount of salt, and then, leaned across the table, shaker in hand, and doused his child's dinner with a like amount, enough to show white on the food from where I was sitting, fully 10 feet away.

If Shakespeare had had a working familiarity with positive and negative feedback as the essential elements in servoloop control mechanisms, he might not have written, "and damned be him that first cries, 'Hold, enough'." The late Sir George Pickering was wont to give this cry, with saltcellar held high in hand, especially if he saw that I was watching! But, perhaps I do Shakespeare an injustice. He may have had something more in mind that iambic pentameter broken by a spondee which would rhyme with Macduff. He may indeed have intuited that any system that does not autoregulate will self-destruct, and this is just about what he had in mind for Macbeth.

Stefansson (1946) has this to say on salt and youth in his book "Not By Bread Alone":

> The MacKenzie Eskimos, Roxy told me, believe that what is good for grown people is good for children and enjoyed by them as soon as they get used to it. Accordingly, they teach the use of tobacco when a child is very young. It then grows up to maturity with the idea that it cannot get along without tobacco. But, said Roxy, the whalers have told that many whites get along without tobacco, and he had himself seen white men who never used it, while of the few white women who had been in this part of the Arctic, wives of captains, none used tobacco. [This, remember, was in 1906.]
>
> Now Roxy had heard that white people believe salt is good, and even necessary for children: so they begin early to add salt to the baby's food. The white child then would grow up with the same attitude toward salt that an Eskimo child has toward tobacco. However, said Roxy, since the Eskimos were mistaken in thinking tobacco so necessary, may it not be that the white men are equally mistaken about salt? Pursuing the argument, he concluded that the reason why all Eskimos disliked salted food, though white men like it, is not racial, but due to custom. You could then, break the salt habit with about the same difficulty as the tobacco habit, and you would suffer no ill result beyond the mental discomfort of the first few days or weeks.

Despite the widespread use of salt, there have been a number who doubted the need for it in the quantities that custom dictated. Swift wrote, "I am confident that the frequent use of salt among us is an effect of luxury" and, at one point, he made his imaginary traveler, Gulliver, a convert to doing without it. Stefansson, in another book, "Life among the Eskimos," reported, "It was here that I learned from experience what I already know theoretically, that (added) salt is not necessary for health, and that the desire for it disappears in about three months when one is without it." Thoreau, in "Walden," called it "that grossest of groceries" and thought that if he did without it, he would drink less water. He was right. This fact was first recorded by Pliny. Lord Somerville (1817) recognized that increased dietary salt requires increased water intake.

In our rats, eating various levels of excess sodium chloride, this effect was striking (Meneely et al., 1952). There was an almost perfectly linear correlation between the amount of salt in the diet and the amount of water consumed. The original data from that study are scattered to the four winds, by reason of migrations or the demise of co-workers, and we did not, at the time we had it, think to examine this correlation more deeply, that is to say, on a rat by rat basis, in relation to the rise in blood pressure.

Obviously, the level of water consumption is coupled to the salt intake in the diet, presumably through the mechanism of thirst. Suppose the hereditary propensity to develop salt hypertension were no more complicated than an inefficient coupling of thirst to salt intake. Wouldn't that be a surprise! Here is a free Nobel Prize for one of you, who has a good rat colony and knows how to use it! Water is one of the best diuretics, and certainly the cheapest. Has anyone treated hypertension with increased water intake? It was shown, long ago, that the dropsical state of cardiac patients can be successfully treated with forced fluids, provided, that is, you do not drown the patient in his own pulmonary edema!

There is an entertaining passage in Robinson Crusoe where Daniel Defoe describes the stranded man's efforts to induce Friday to eat salt. This stalwart, "Spat and sputtered at it, washing his mouth with fresh water after it." Had Friday had access to the current medical literature, he would perhaps even more steadfastly have withstood Crusoe's blandishments, grimaces, and sign language.

ACKNOWLEDGMENTS

The author has drawn freely for quotations and early references on an editorial he published in the *American Journal of Medicine* (Meneely *et al.*, 1952). Other quotations are referenced in the text.

REFERENCES

Ambard, L., and Beaujard, E. (1904). Causes de l'hypertension artérielle. *Arch. Gen. Med.* **1**, 520.

Ball, C. O. T., and Meneely, G. R. (1957). Observations on dietary sodium chloride. *J. Am. Diet. Assoc.* **33**, 366.

Berrien, F. K., and Indik, B. P. (1962). *Trans. N.Y. Acad. Sci.* [2] **24**, 528.

Coleman, T. G., Cowley, A. W., Jr., and Guyton, A. C. (1974). Experimental hypertension and the long-term control of arterial pressure. *MTP Int. Rev. Sci., Physiol. Ser. One* **1**, 259-297.

Frank, R. L., and Mickelsen, O. (1969). Sodium potassium chloride mixture as table salt. *Am. J. Clin. Nutr.* **22**, 464-479.

Guyton, A. C., Coleman, T. G., Cowley, A. W., Jr., *et al.* (1972a). Arterial pressure regulation: Overriding dominance of the kidneys in long-term regulation and in hypertension. *Am. J. Med.* **52**, 584-594.

Guyton, A. C., Colemen, T. G., Granger, H. J. (1972b). Circulation: Overall regulation. *Annu. Rev. Physiol.* **34**, 13.

Guyton, A. C., Coleman, T. G., Cowley, A. W., Jr., *et al.* (1974). A systems analysis approach to understanding long-range arterial blood pressure control and hypertension. *Circ. Res.* **35**, 159-176.

Hubbell, R. B., Mendel, L. B., and Wakeman, A. J. (1937). A new salt mixture for use in experimental diets. *J. Nutr.* **14**, 273.

Kaunitz, H. (1956). Causes and consequences of salt consumption. *Nature (London)* **178**, 1141.

Lapicque, L. (1896). Documents enthnographiques sur l'alimentation minérale. *Antrhopologie* **7**, 35.

Lord Somerville (1817). Ref. cit., E. Hughes, "Studies in Administration and Finance." Univ. of Manchester Press, Manchester.

Meneely, G. R., and Batterbee, H. D. (1976). The high sodium-low potassium environment and hypertension. *Am. J. Cardiol.* **38**, 768.

Meneely, G. R. (1954). Salt. *Am. J. Med.* **16**, 1.

Meneely, G. R., Tucker, R. G., and Darby, W. J. (1952). Chronic sodium chloride toxicity in the albino rat. 1. Growth on a purified diet containing various levels of sodium chloride. *J. Nutr.* **48**, 489.

O'Shaughnessy, W. B. (1831–1832). Experiments on the blood in cholera. *Lancet* **1**, 490.

Plinius (ca. 65–75). "Gaius Secundus: Naturalis Historia."

Redtenbacher, W. (1850). Beobachtungen am Harne bei Lungenentzundungen. *Z. Ges. Arzte Wien* **1**, 373.

Schmidt, C. (1850). "Charakteristik der epidemischen Cholera gegenuber werwandten Transudationsanomalieer, Eine physiologisch-Chemische Untersuchung." Leipzig and Mitau.

Smith, W. R. (1911). "Salt: Ancient History and Religious Symbolism," Encyclopedia Britannica, 11th ed., Vol. 24, p. 87. Cambridge Univ. Press, London and New York.

Smith, W., ed. (1865). The salt sea. *In* "A Concise Dictionary of the Bible," p. 834. Little, Brown, Boston, Massachusetts.

Stefansson, V. (1946). "Not By Bread Alone." Macmillan, New York.

von Bunge, G. (1874). *Z. Biol.* **10**, 295.

von Bunge, G. (1894). "Physiologische Chemie," 3rd ed. Vogel, Leipzig.

General Sources

Braidwood, R. J. (1952). From cave to village. *Sci. Am.* **187**, 62.

Buck, C. D. (1949). "A Dictionary of Selected Synonyms in the Principal Indo-European Languages." Univ. of Chicago Press, Chicago, Illinois.

Eskew, G. L. (1948). "Salt, the Fifth Element." J. G. Ferguson and Associates, Chicago, Illinois.

Holmberg, A. R. (1950). "Nomads of the Long Bow: The Sirinono of Eastern Boliva," Inst. Soc. Anthropol., Publ. No. 10, p. 35. Smithsonian Institution, Washington, D.C.

Kaufman, D. W. (1960). "Sodium Chloride." Van Nostrand-Reinhold, Princeton, New Jersey.

Keary, C. F. (1921). "The Dawn of History." Scribner's, New York.

Kroeber, A. L. (1941–1942). Culture element distributions. XV. Salt, dogs, tobacco. *Anthropol. Rec.* **6**, 1.

"Oxford English Dictionary, The" (1933). Twelve volume reissue of A New English Dictionary on Historical Principles. Oxford Univ. Press, London and New York.

Pigott, S. (1961). "The Dawn of Civilization." McGraw-Hill, New York.

II

Sodium Excretion and the Factors Affecting It

13

Regulation of Sodium Excretion, Renal Function, and Arterial Pressure: Role of the Renin–Angiotensin–Aldosterone and Kallikrein–Kinin Systems

ROBERT E. McCAA

THE ROLE OF SALT IN
CARDIOVASCULAR HYPERTENSION

Copyright © 1982 by Academic Press, Inc.
All rights of reproduction in any form reserved.
ISBN 0-12-267280-1

I. INTRODUCTION

The importance of the adrenal glands in the regulation of sodium and potassium metabolism was firmly established in 1926 when Banting and Gairns demonstrated that bilateral adrenalectomy resulted in a decrease in serum sodium concentration and an increase in serum potassium concentration in experimental animals. Marine and Baumann in 1927 demonstrated that the symptoms of bilateral adrenalectomy could be delayed by the administration of sodium or accelerated by the administration of potassium. In 1927, Hartman *et al.* demonstrated that an extract from the adrenal cortex contained a factor with high sodium-retaining activity that prolonged the life of adrenalectomized animals. Luetscher and Deming (1950) found a high concentration of a "sodium-retaining factor" in urine from patients with edema. In subsequent studies, Luetscher and associates demonstrated that the urinary "sodium-retaining factor" was high when sodium intake was restricted, normal in patients with hypopituitarism, and undetectable in patients with Addison's disease.

In 1953, Simpson and Tait, using paper chromatographic techniques, reported the successful separation of the "sodium-retaining factor" from cortisone. Since this steroid possessed a much greater effect on the renal handling of sodium and potassium than any other known substance, it was called "electrocortin." The isolation and purification of electrocortin from beef adrenal glands led to the characterization of its structure. It was a naturally occurring biologically active steroid with an aldehyde group and accordingly given the definitive name "aldosterone."

Since the identification of the major sodium-retaining steroid hormone, aldosterone, 28 years ago, numerous investigative studies have demonstrated that aldosterone plays a primary role in maintaining the overall adequacy of the circulatory system. A hypodynamic state of the circulation is usually followed within minutes by increased aldosterone secretion, and a hyperdynamic state of the circulation results in decreased aldosterone secretion. Despite the vast importance of aldosterone in overall circulatory control, the regulation of aldosterone biosynthesis and the role of aldosterone in the development and maintenance of hypertension still remain the subject of intense debate.

Although the importance of aldosterone in the regulation of fluid and electrolyte metabolism is well recognized, it is essential to remember that experimental animals and man escape from the sodium-retaining effects of aldosterone within hours after continuous administration of the steroid hormone. During the past decade, several investigative studies have indicated that the renin–angiotensin and kallikrein–kinin systems may also play important roles in regulating sodium excretion, renal function, and arterial blood pressure. This chapter presents a review of recent experimental studies from our laboratory with special emphasis on the roles of aldosterone, angiotensin II, and kinins on the long-term regulation of urinary sodium excretion, renal function, and arterial blood pressure in sodium-deficient animals.

II. METHODS

The studies in this review were designed to evaluate the role of the renin–angiotensin–aldosterone and kallikrein–kinin systems in the long-term regulation of urinary sodium excretion, renal function, and arterial blood pressure in sodium-deficient dogs. Our studies were designed to suppress renin release with the β-adrenergic blocking agent, propranolol, to block the action of angiotensin II at the receptor sites with angiotensin II inhibitory analogs, and to inhibit the conversion of angiotensin I to angiotensin II with the angiotensin I converting enzyme inhibitor, captopril.

Our studies differ from those of other investigators in that they are long-term in nature, often lasting for several days or weeks. The animal experiments presented in this review were performed in intact unanesthetized mongrel dogs with chronic indwelling catheters in the femoral artery and vein. The venous catheter was used to maintain continuous infusion of various pharmacologic agents at a constant rate from a syringe infusion pump. Continuous 24-hr arterial blood pressure measurements were obtained from the arterial catheter by a pressure transducer and a recorder. The animals were housed in separate metabolic cages during the control, experimental, and recovery stages of the study. The experimental animal preparation used in these studies and the procedure for collection and analysis of the blood samples for steroids and peptides by radioimmunoassay have been described in complete detail in previous publications (McCaa *et al.*, 1972, 1973, 1974, 1978).

III. RESULTS

A summary of the responses of urinary sodium excretion, plasma aldosterone concentration, and arterial blood pressure after 10 days of continuous administration of propranolol, angiotensin II inhibitory analogs, and captopril in sodium-deficient animals is illustrated in Fig. 1.

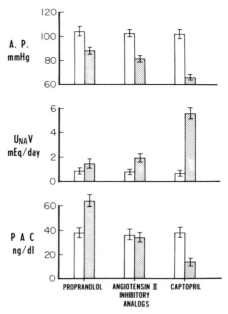

Fig. 1. Response of arterial blood pressure (AP), urinary sodium excretion ($U_{Na}V$) and plasma aldosterone concentration (PAC) in sodium-deficient dogs after continuous infusion of propranolol, angiotensin II inhibitory analogs, or captopril for 10 days. Vertical lines indicate ± SE.

A. Effects of Propranolol on Urinary Sodium Excretion, Plasma Aldosterone Concentration, and Arterial Blood Pressure

Conscious sodium-deficient dogs were maintained on continuous propranolol infusion (200 mg/day) for 21 days to determine the response of arterial blood pressure, plasma aldosterone concentration, and urinary sodium excretion during suppression of renin secretion by β-adrenergic blockade. In response to β-adrenergic blockade in sodium-deficient dogs, plasma renin activity decreased from 3.63 ± 0.42 to 1.12 ± 0.26 ng/ml per hour ($p < 0.001$), arterial blood pressure decreased from 100 ± 3 to 84 ± 2 mm Hg ($p < 0.001$), plasma aldosterone concentration increased from 36.8 ± 6.9 to 73.6 ± 8.7 ng/dl ($p < 0.001$) and urinary kallikrein activity increased from 19.7 ± 3.9 to 41.3 ± 4.8 EU/day ($p < 0.001$). Also, during β-adrenergic blockade with propranolol, serum sodium and potassium concentration increased from 143 ± 0.5 to 145 ± 0.5 (NS, $p > 0.01$) and 4.3 ± 0.5 to 5.6 ± 0.5 ($p < 0.001$) mEq/liter, respectively, while urinary sodium and potassium excretion increased from 0.59 ± 0.25 to 1.12 ± 0.32 ($p < 0.01$) and 34.7 ± 4.8 to 39.7 ± 5.1 ($p < 0.01$) mEq/day, respectively.

In sodium-deficient dogs, β-adrenergic blockade with propranolol produced parallel decreases in plasma renin activity and arterial blood pressure. Also, there was a slight increase in urinary sodium excretion during propranolol administration (Fig. 1). The increase in plasma aldosterone concentration during β-adrenergic blockade was associated with a highly significant sustained increase in serum potassium concentration induced by propranolol administration. It is well established that propranolol and other β-adrenergic blocking agents induce a massive efflux of intracellular potassium ions from red blood cells (Ekman et al., 1969) and from muscle cells in man (Manninen, 1970). The increase in urinary kallikrein activity observed during propranolol administration is probably due to the marked increase in aldosterone secretion since considerable experimental evidence indicates a high positive correlation between kallikrein activity and changes in activity of sodium retaining steroids (Geller et al., 1972; Margolius et al., 1974, 1976; McCaa et al., 1978).

B. Effects of Angiotensin II Inhibitory Analogs on Urinary Sodium Excretion, Plasma Aldosterone Concentration, and Arterial Blood Pressure

Long-term infusion of two potent angiotensin II inhibitory analogs [Sar^1, Ala^8]angiotensin II and [Sar^1,Ile^8]angiotensin II, effectively lowered arterial blood pressure and increased urinary sodium excretion in sodium-deficient dogs (Fig. 1). In response to continuous infusion of angiotensin II inhibitory analogs in sodium-deficient dogs, arterial blood pressure decreased from 103 $\pm$ 4 to 78 $\pm$ 2 mm Hg ($p < 0.001$) while urinary sodium excretion increased from 0.61 $\pm$ 0.23 to 1.8 $\pm$ 0.31 mEq/day ($p < 0.001$). During long-term continuous infusion of [Sar^1,Ala^8]angiotensin II in sodium-deficient dogs, plasma aldosterone concentration failed to change significantly from control levels. Indeed, chronic continuous infusion of [Sar^1,Ile^8]angiotensin II resulted in a significant increase in plasma aldosterone concentration in sodium-deficient dogs (McCaa, 1977). The agonistic properties of the angiotensin II inhibitory analogs on the adrenal glomerulosa cells have been observed by several other investigators in experimental animals (Steele and Lowenstein, 1974; Williams et al., 1974; Beckerhoff et al., 1975; Bravo et al., 1975, 1976; McCaa, 1977) and in man (Hollenberg et al., 1976; Sealey et al., 1976) and have led some investigators (Steele and Lowenstein, 1974; Williams et al., 1974; Bravo et al., 1975) to postulate that significant functional differences exist between the receptors in the vascular smooth muscle and the adrenal glomerulosa cells.

C. Effects of Captopril on Urinary Sodium Excretion, Plasma Aldosterone Concentration, and Arterial Blood Pressure

Although propranolol and the angiotensin II inhibitory analogs significantly decreased arterial blood pressure and increased urinary sodium excretion in sodium-deficient dogs, the hypotensive and natriuretic response to inhibition of angiotensin I converting enzyme with captopril was considerably greater (Fig. 1). The response of arterial blood pressure, urinary sodium excretion, and plasma aldosterone concentration to continuous captopril administration in sodium-deficient dogs is illustrated in Fig. 2. In response to long-term captopril administration in sodium-deficient dogs, arterial blood pressure decreased from 103 ± 5 to 67 ± 2 mm Hg ($p < 0.001$), urinary sodium excretion increased from 0.65 ± 0.26 to 4.8 ± 1.2 mEq/day ($p < 0.001$) and plasma aldosterone concentration decreased from 36.4 ± 6.8 to 14.2 ± 3.4 ng/dl ($p < 0.001$). When captopril administration was discontinued, arterial blood pressure, urinary sodium excretion, and aldosterone secretion returned to levels that existed before treatment.

D. Effects of Captopril on Renal Blood Flow and Glomerular Filtration Rate

To evaluate changes in renal hemodynamics during captopril administration, we determined effective renal plasma flow and glomerular filtration rate in sodium-deficient animals during inhibition of angiotensin I converting enzyme (kininase II) with captopril. The response of arterial blood pressure, effective renal plasma flow, and glomerular filtration rate to long-term administration of captopril in conscious sodium-deficient dogs is illustrated in Fig. 3. In response

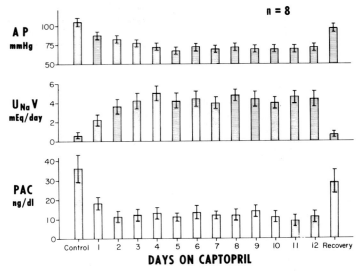

Fig. 2. Response of arterial blood pressure (AP), urinary sodium excretion ($U_{Na}V$), and plasma aldosterone concentration (PAC) to long-term administration of captopril (400 mg/day) in conscious dogs maintained on dietary sodium restriction (5 mEq Na^+/day). Vertical lines indicate $\pm SE$.

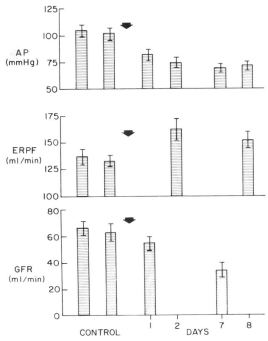

Fig. 3. Response of arterial blood pressure (AP), effective renal plasma flow (ERPF), and glomerular filtration rate (GFR) to long-term administration of captopril (400 mg/day) in conscious dogs maintained on dietary sodium restriction (5 mEq Na$^+$/day). Vertical lines indicate ±SE.

to long-term administration of captopril in sodium-deficient dogs, arterial blood pressure decreased from 103 ± 5 to 70 ± 3 mm Hg ($p < 0.001$), effective renal plasma flow increased from 136 ± 6 to 154 ± 8 ml/min ($p < 0.01$), and glomerular filtration rate decreased from 65 ± 9 to 36 ± 7 ml/min ($p < 0.001$). Also, during captopril administration, afferent and efferent arteriolar resistances decreased markedly. When captopril administration was discontinued, arterial blood pressure, effective renal plasma flow and glomerular filtration rate returned to levels that existed before treatment (McCaa *et al.*, 1978).

E. Effects of Captopril on the Kallikrein–Kinin System

In recent years, evidence has accumulated to indicate that the kallikrein-kinin–prostaglandin system may be involved in the regulation of arterial blood pressure. Since captopril inhibits the formation of the potent vasopressor octapeptide, angiotensin II, and prevents the degradation of the potent vasodepressor nonapeptide, bradykinin, we evaluated the response of blood kinins, urinary kinin excretion, and urinary kallikrein activity in sodium-deficient dogs during long-term captopril administration (McCaa *et al.*, 1978). The response of blood kinin concentration, urinary kinin excretion, and urinary kallikrein activity to long-term captopril administration in sodium-deficient dogs is illustrated in Fig. 4. During long-term captopril administration, the concentration of kinins in the blood increased from 0.17 ± 0.02 to 0.41 ± 0.04 ng/ml ($p < 0.001$), urinary kinin excretion increased from 7.2 ± 1.5 to 31.4 ± 3.2 μg/day ($p < 0.001$), and urinary kallikrein activity decreased from 23.6 ± 3.1 to 5.3 ± 1.2 EU/day ($p < 0.001$). Since urinary kallikrein activity decreased markedly during long-term continuous captopril administration, the increase in circulating and renal concentration of kinins must result from a decrease in the rate of degradation of the kinins. This significant increase in circulating and renal concentration of kinins during long-term administration of captopril suggests that the hypotensive and natriuretic actions of the inhibitors of angiotensin I converting enzyme (kininase II) could be due in part to inhibition of angiotensin II formation and in part to the accumulation of kinins.

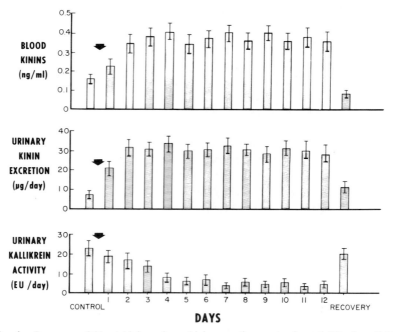

Fig. 4. Response of blood kinin, urinary kinin excretion, and urinary kallikrein activity to long-term administration of captopril (400 mg/day) in conscious dogs maintained on dietary sodium restriction (5 mEq Na+/day). Vertical lines indicate ±SE.

F. Long-Term Effects of Aldosterone and Angiotensin II on Urinary Sodium Excretion during Captopril Administration

While our studies demonstrate that inhibition of angiotensin I converting enzyme (kininase II) with captopril in sodium-deficient dogs results in decreased circulating and renal concentrations of angiotensin II and increased circulating and renal concentrations of kinins, the precise role of the renin–angiotensin and kallikrein–kinin systems in mediating the decrease in arterial blood pressure and increase in urinary sodium excretion remains to be elucidated. To evaluate the roles of aldosterone and angiotensin II in mediating the changes in arterial blood pressure and urinary sodium excretion in sodium-deficient dogs during captopril administration, sodium-deficient dogs were maintained on aldosterone infusion at the rate of 10 μg/kg/day. After 2 weeks of continuous aldosterone infusion, the animals were administered captopril in addition to the continuous aldosterone infusion. The response of arterial blood pressure, urinary sodium excretion, and plasma aldosterone concentration to continuous aldosterone and captopril administration in sodium-deficient dogs is illustrated in Fig. 5. In sodium-deficient

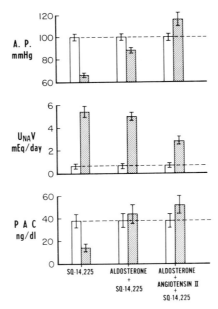

Fig. 5. Response of arterial blood pressure (AP), urinary sodium excretion ($U_{Na}V$), and plasma aldosterone concentration (PAC) after 7 days of captopril administration (400 mg/day), aldosterone (10 μg/kg/day) plus captopril (400 mg/day), and aldosterone (10 μg/kg/day), angiotensin II (25 ng/kg/min), and captopril (400 mg/day) in conscious dogs maintained on dietary sodium restriction (5 mEq Na$^+$/day). Vertical lines indicate $\pm$SE.

animals maintained on continuous aldosterone infusion to prevent plasma aldosterone concentration from decreasing during inhibition of angiotensin I converting enzyme (kininase II), urinary sodium excretion increased to levels that were not significantly different from levels observed in sodium-deficient animals in which plasma aldosterone concentration decreased to near sodium-replete levels after captopril administration. Thus, these data indicate that the increase in urinary sodium excretion in response to inhibition of angiotensin I converting enzyme (kininase II) with captopril in sodium-deficient dogs is independent of changes in plasma aldosterone concentration.

In additional experiments, sodium-deficient dogs were maintained on continuous aldosterone infusion at the rate of 10 μg/kg/day and continuous angiotensin II infusion at the rate of 25 ng/kg/min to prevent plasma concentrations of aldosterone and angiotensin II from decreasing during inhibition of angiotensin I converting enzyme (kininase II). The response of urinary sodium excretion during captopril administration in sodium-deficient animals maintained on continuous aldosterone and angiotensin II infusion is illustrated in Fig. 5. In sodium-deficient animals maintained on fixed plasma concentrations of aldosterone and angiotensin II, captopril administration caused an increase in urinary sodium excretion but to less than 50% of the levels observed in untreated sodium-deficient animals administered captopril. These data support the concept for an important intrarenal role of the renin–angiotensin system to conserve sodium and fluid during sodium deficiency.

G. Effects of Angiotensin II on Urinary Sodium Excretion during Captopril Administration

The marked responses of arterial blood pressure, urinary sodium excretion, plasma aldosterone concentration, and renal hemodynamics to angiotensin II in sodium-deficient dogs during inhibition of angiotensin I converting enzyme (kininase II)(McCaa, 1979) led us to investigate the importance of the renin-angiotensin system in the conservation of sodium during sodium deficiency.

To evaluate quantitatively the role of angiotensin II in mediating the hypotensive and natriuretic actions of captopril, the response of arterial blood pressure, urinary sodium excretion, and plasma aldosterone concentration to angiotensin II infusion was determined in sodium-deficient dogs maintained on captopril (McCaa, 1980). The results are illustrated in Fig. 6. Sodium-deficient dogs were maintained on continuous captopril infusion (400 mg/day) for 7 days. After 7 days of captopril infusion, arterial blood pressure decreased from 102 ± 3 to 68 ± 4 mm Hg ($p < 0.001$), urinary sodium excretion increased from 0.69 ± 0.24 to 7.8 ± 1.6 mEq/day ($p < 0.001$), and plasma aldosterone concentration decreased from 37.8 ± 6.5 to 16.3 ± 3.6 ng/dl ($p < 0.001$). During the next 7 days, the animals were maintained on captopril infusion at the rate of 400 mg/day

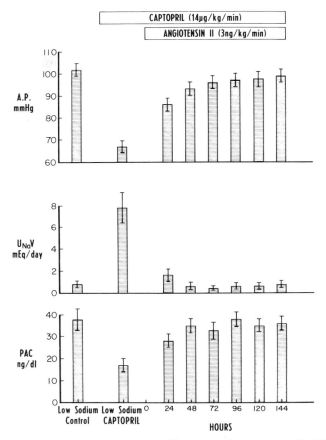

Fig. 6. Response of arterial blood pressure (AP), urinary sodium excretion ($U_{Na}V$), and plasma aldosterone concentration (PAC) to continuous angiotensin II infusion (3 ng/kg/min) for 6 days in sodium-deficient dogs maintained on captopril (400 mg/day). Vertical lines indicate ±SE.

and angiotensin II infusion (3 ng/kg/min). In response to angiotensin II infusion (3 ng/kg/min), arterial blood pressure increased from 68 ± 4 to 86 ± 3 mm Hg ($p < 0.001$), urinary sodium excretion decreased from 7.8 ± 1.6 to 1.7 ± 0.9 mEq/day ($p < 0.001$), and plasma aldosterone concentration increased from 16.3 ± 3.6 to 27.5 ± 5.2 ng/dl ($p < 0.001$) within 24 hr after beginning angiotensin II infusion. During the next 48 hr of continuous angiotensin II infusion, arterial blood pressure increased to 96 ± 3 mm Hg, urinary sodium excretion decreased to 0.53 ± 0.21 mEq/day, and plasma aldosterone concentration increased to 34.3 ± 6.4 ng/dl. Continuous infusion of angiotensin II at the rate of 3 ng/kg/min restored arterial blood pressure, urinary sodium excretion, and plasma aldosterone concentration to levels that were not significantly different from those observed in untreated sodium-deficient dogs, indicating that the hypotensive and natriuretic actions of inhibitors of angiotensin I converting enzyme (kininase II) are due to the inhibition of angiotensin II formation and not to increased circulating and renal concentration of kinins. When angiotensin II infusion was increased to higher rates in sodium-deficient dogs maintained on captopril, arterial blood pressure, urinary sodium excretion, and plasma aldosterone concentration increased markedly. However, at the higher rates of angiotensin II infusion the increase in urinary sodium excretion was due to pressure-induced diuresis and natriuresis.

IV. DISCUSSION

Sodium deficiency induced by dietary sodium restriction or removal of sodium from the body by any of several means is associated with parallel increases in activity of the renin–angiotensin system and aldosterone biosynthesis. During sodium deficiency, urinary sodium excretion decreases markedly. The studies presented in this chapter will demonstrate that changes in urinary sodium excretion during dietary sodium restriction are independent of changes in the steroid hormone, aldosterone, but highly dependent on the activity of the renin–angiotensin system.

We have used three pharmacologic agents to evaluate the role of the renin–angiotensin system in the regulation of aldosterone biosynthesis and the control of renal function and arterial blood pressure during sodium deficiency in experimental animals: the β-adrenergic blocking agent, propranolol, to suppress renin release, the angiotensin II inhibitory analog, [Sar^1,Ala^8]angiotensin II, to block the action of angiotensin II at the receptor sites, and the angiotensin I converting enzyme inhibitor, captopril, to inhibit the formation of angiotensin II. Although all three pharmacologic probes induced hypotensive and natriuretic actions in sodium-deficient animals, inhibition of angiotensin I converting enzyme (kininase II) with captopril produced a greater effect on arterial blood pressure, urinary sodium excretion, and aldosterone secretion. Indeed, during inhibition of angiotensin I converting enzyme (kininase II) with captopril, plasma angiotensin II concentration, plasma aldosterone concentration, and arterial blood pressure decreased markedly while urinary sodium excretion increased tenfold and remained elevated during continuous captopril treatment. It is of interest to note that urinary sodium excretion increased to similar levels during inhibition of angiotensin II formation with captopril in sodium-deficient animals pretreated with aldosterone and maintained on continuous aldosterone infusion to prevent a fall in plasma aldosterone concentration. These experiments demonstrate that the changes in urinary sodium excretion in sodium-deficient animals during inhibition of angiotensin II formation with captopril are totally independent of changes in the steroid hormone, aldosterone.

It is well established that angiotensin II, the most potent vasopressor octapeptide, is produced by the enzymatic removal of a dipeptide from the biologically inactive decapeptide, angiotensin I, by angiotensin I converting enzyme, while the vasodepressor peptides, bradykinin and kallidin, are inactivated by the enzymatic removal of a dipeptide by kininase II. Angiotensin I converting enzyme and kininase II are the same protein, peptidyldipeptide hydrolase (dipeptidyl carboxypeptidase)(Erdos and Yang, 1970). In experimental animals, angiotensin I converting enzyme inhibitors inhibit the biological action of angiotensin I and potentiate the biological action of bradykinin. Since inhibition of angiotensin II formation and increased circulating and renal concentration of kinins both produce hypotensive and natriuretic actions in experimental animals, some investigators believe that the increase in urinary sodium excretion during captopril could be due, at least in part, to the accumulation of kinins. Indeed, in our studies, circulating and renal kinin concentrations increased during long-term captopril administration in sodium-deficient animals while urinary kallikrein activity decreased markedly, indicating that the increase in circulating and renal kinin concentration was due to a decrease in the rate of degradation of the kinins and not to increased kallikrein activity. Yet, the effects of increased circulating and renal concentrations of kinins on arterial blood pressure and urinary sodium excretion remain to be determined.

Since the hypotensive and natriuretic actions of angiotensin I converting enzyme inhibition (kininase II) occurred independently of changes in aldosterone secretion, we evaluated the role of the renin–angiotensin and kallikrein–kinin systems on the control of renal function, sodium excretion, and arterial blood pressure in experimental animals. Sodium-deficient animals were maintained on continuous captopril infusion for 10 days. During this time, arterial blood pressure and plasma aldosterone concentration decreased and urinary sodium excretion increased to steady-state levels. Also, during continuous captopril infusion, circulating and renal angiotensin II concentrations decreased to near undetectable levels while circulating and renal kinin concentrations increased to new steady-state levels. Angiotensin II was added to the infusate so that the animals were receiving captopril at the rate of 14 μg/kg/min and angiotensin II at the rate of 3 ng/kg/min. Despite the sustained increase in circulating and renal concentration of kinins in sodium-deficient dogs maintained on captopril infusion, angiotensin II at the low rate of 3 ng/kg/min restored arterial blood pressure, urinary sodium excretion, and plasma aldosterone concentration to the level that existed in untreated sodium-deficient dogs. In addition, angiotensin II infusion restored renal blood flow and glomerular filtration rate to levels observed in untreated sodium-deficient dogs. These studies indicate that the hypotensive and natriuretic actions of inhibitors of angiotensin I converting enzyme (kininase II) are due to inhibition of angiotensin II formation and not to increased circulating and renal concentrations of kinins.

Thus, our studies indicate that changes in urinary sodium excretion during sodium deficiency are highly dependent on the activity of the renin–angiotensin system. Although the action of angiotensin II on the adrenal glomerulosa cells to stimulate aldosterone biosynthesis is well established, the sodium-retaining effect of angiotensin II results from a direct intrarenal action of angiotensin II. Since there is little evidence that angiotensin II has a direct effect on the tubules to promote active sodium reabsorption, it appears that the mechanism by which angiotensin II acts to control sodium excretion during sodium deficiency is by increasing both efferent and afferent arteriolar resistance (Guyton, 1980; Navar *et al.*, 1981).

ACKNOWLEDGMENT

These studies were supported by USPHS Grant HL 09921 from the National Institutes of Health.

REFERENCES

Banting, F. G., and Gairns, S. (1926). Suprarenal insufficiency. *Am. J. Physiol.* **44,** 100–113.

Beckerhoff, R., Uhlschmid, G., Furer, J., Nussberger, J., Schmied, U., Vetter, W. J., and Siegenthaler, W. (1975). In vivo effects of angiotensin antagonists on plasma aldosterone in the dog. *Eur. J. Pharmacol.* **34,** 363–367.

Bravo, E. L., Khosla, M. C., and Bumpus, F. M. (1975). Vascular and adrenocortical responses to a specific antagonist of angiotensin II. *Am. J. Physiol.* **228,** 110–114.

Bravo, E. L., Khosla, M. C., and Bumpus, F. M. (1976). Comparative studies of the humoral and arterial pressure responses to Sar^{1}Ala^8, Sar^{1}Ile^8 and Sar^{1}Thr^{8}angiotensin II in the trained unanesthetized dog. *Prog. Biochem. Pharmacol.* **12,** 33–40.

Ekman, A., Manninen, V., and Salminin, S. (1969). Ion movements in red cells treated with propranolol. *Acta Physiol. Scand.* **74,** 333–334.

Erdos, E. G., and Yang, H. Y. T. (1970). "Handbook of Experimental Pharmacology," pp. 298–323. Springer-Verlag, Berlin and New York.

Geller, R. G., Margolius, H. S., Pisano, J. J., and Keiser, H. R. (1972). Effects of mineralocorticoids, altered sodium intake and adrenalectomy on urinary kallikrein in rats. *Circ. Res.* **31,** 857–861.

Guyton, A. C. (1980). "Arterial Pressure and Hypertension." Saunders, Philadelphia, Pennsylvania.

Hartman, F. A., MacArthur, C. G., and Hartman, W. E. (1927). A substance which prolongs the life of adrenalectomized cats. *Proc. Soc. Exp. Biol. Med.* **25,** 69–70.

Hollenberg, N. K., Williams, G. H., Burger, B., Ishikawa, I., and Adams, D. F. (1976). Blockade and stimulation of renal, adrenal and vascular angiotensin II receptors with 1-Sar, 8-Ala angiotensin II in normal man. *J. Clin. Invest.* **57,** 39–46.

Luetscher, J. A., Jr., and Deming, Q. B. (1950). Treatment of nephrosis with cortisone. *J. Clin. Invest.* **29,** 1576–1587.

McCaa, R. E. (1977). Role of the renin-angiotensin system in the regulation of aldosterone biosynthesis and arterial pressure during sodium deficiency. *Circ. Res.* **40**, I-157–I-162.

McCaa, R. E. (1979). Studies in vivo with angiotensin I converting enzyme (kininase II) inhibitors. *Fed. Proc., Fed. Am. Soc. Exp. Biol.* **38**, 2783–2787.

McCaa, R. E. (1980). Specificity of converting enzyme inhibition. *In* "Enzymatic Release of Vasoactive Peptides" (F. Gross and G. Vogel, eds.), pp. 383–399. Raven Press, New York.

McCaa, R. E., McCaa, C. S., Read, D. G., Bower, J. D., and Guyton, A. C. (1972). Increased plasma aldosterone concentration in response to hemodialysis in nephrectomized man. *Circ. Res.* **31**, 473–480.

McCaa, R. E., McCaa, C. S., Cowley, A. W., Jr., Ott, C. E., and Guyton, A. C. (1973). Stimulation of aldosterone secretion by hemorrhage in dogs after nephrectomy and decapitation. *Circ. Res.* **22**, 356–362.

McCaa, R. E., McCaa, C. S., and Guyton, A. C. (1974). Role of angiotensin II and potassium in the long-term regulation of aldosterone secretion in intact conscious dogs. *Circ. Res.* **36/37**, Suppl. 1, 57–67.

McCaa, R. E., Hall, J. E., and McCaa, C. S. (1978). The effects of angiotensin I-converting enzyme inhibitors on arterial blood pressure and urinary sodium excretion—Role of the renal renin-angiotensin and kallikrein-kinin systems. *Circ. Res.* **43**, Suppl. 1, 32–39.

Manninen, V. (1970). Movements of sodium and potassium ions and their tracers in propranolol-treated red cells and diaphragm muscle. *Acta Physiol. Scand.* **355**, Suppl. I, 1–76.

Margolius, H. S., Horwitz, D., Geller, R. G., Alexander, R. W., Gill, J. R., Jr., Pisano, J. J., and Keiser, H. R. (1974). Urinary kallikrein in normal subjects: Relationships to sodium intake and to sodium retaining steroids. *Circ. Res.* **35**, 812–819.

Margolius, H. S., Horwitz, D., Pisano, J. J., and Keiser, H. R. (1976). Relationships among urinary kallikrein, mineralocorticoids, and human hypertensive disease. *Fed. Proc., Fed. Am. Soc. Exp. Biol.* **35**, 203–206.

Marine, D., and Baumann, E. J. (1927). Duration of life after suprarenalectomy in cats and attempts to prolong it by injections of solutions containing sodium salts, glucose and glycerol. *Am. J. Physiol.* **81**, 86–100.

Navar, L. G., Jirakulsomchok, D., Bell, P. D., and Huang, W. C. (1981). Converting enzyme inhibition results in equivalent reductions in afferent and efferent arteriolar resistances in sodium restricted dogs. *Fed. Proc., Fed. Am. Soc. Exp. Biol.* **40**, No. 3, 516.

Sealey, J. E., Wallace, J. M., Case, D. B., and Laragh, J. H. (1976). Inhibition of aldosterone secretion by converting enzyme blockade contrasted with the agonist/antagonist effect of an angiotensin II analogue. *Endocrinology* **98**, 160 (abstr.).

Simpson, S. A., and Tait, J. F. (1953). Physico-chemical methods of detection of a previously unidentified adrenal hormone. *Mem. Soc. Endocrinol.* **2**, 9–24.

Steele, J. M., Jr., and Lowenstein, J. (1974). Differential effects of angiotensin II analogue on pressor and adrenal receptors in the rabbit. *Circ. Res.* **35**, 592–600.

Williams, G. H., McConnell, L. M., Raux, M. C., and Hollenberg, N. K. (1974). Evidence for different angiotensin II receptors in the rat adrenal glomerulosa and rabbit vascular smooth muscle cells. *Circ. Res.* **34**, 384–390.

14

The Role of the Renin–Angiotensin and Prostaglandin Systems in Salt-Sensitive and Non-Salt-Sensitive Hypertension in Man

TOSHIRO FUJITA, CATHERINE S. DELEA, AND
FREDERIC C. BARTTER

THE ROLE OF SALT IN
CARDIOVASCULAR HYPERTENSION

I. INTRODUCTION

It is widely believed that excessive sodium intake plays a role in the development of hypertension in man (Dahl and Love, 1954; Meneely and Dahl, 1961). Conversely, it has been clearly demonstrated that loss of salt produced by diuretics is associated with a decrease of blood pressure in hypertensive patients (Dustan *et al.*, 1959; Wilson and Freis, 1959).

In previous studies (Fujita *et al.*, 1980; Kawasaki *et al.*, 1978), patients with idiopathic hypertension were classified as "salt-sensitive" (SS) or "non-salt-sensitive" (NSS) as estimated from the rise in blood pressure with increases in sodium intake (Fig. 1). On a high-salt diet, the SS hypertensive patients retained more sodium and gained more weight, with greater increases in blood pressure, than did the NSS patients. There were no statistically significant differences between the two groups in plasma electrolyte concentrations or glomerular filtration rate. We have presented evidence (Fujita *et al.*, 1980) that pressor and depressor substances may be involved in the impaired sodium excretion and the resultant higher blood pressure with sodium loads in the salt-sensitive patients. However, the role of dietary salt in the pathophysiology of hypertension has not been explained.

Knowledge of the role of prostaglandins in the control of renal function and blood pressure has advanced rapidly since their presence in the kidney was first

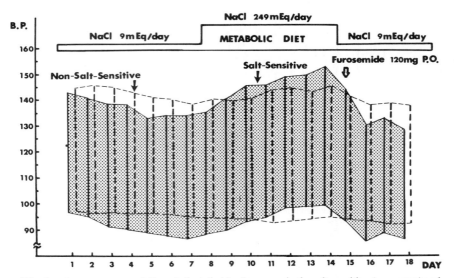

Fig. 1. Average mean systolic and diastolic blood pressure in the salt-sensitive (gray areas) and the non-salt-sensitive (clear areas) patients during changes of sodium intake and after furosemide. (Reproduced by permission from the *American Journal of Medicine*, Fujita *et al.*, 1980.)

demonstrated. Renal prostaglandins have been thought to increase renal sodium loss. PGE_2 causes sodium loss and renin secretion when injected into the renal artery (Tannenbaum *et al.*, 1975; Yun *et al.*, 1977). Given intravenously to dogs and rabbits, it lowers blood pressure. In contrast, $PGF_{2\alpha}$ has no effect on either urinary sodium excretion or on renin secretion, and raises blood pressure (Yun *et al.*, 1977; Yun, 1979).

II. METHODS

Twelve patients with idiopathic hypertension (8 men, 4 women) were studied in the metabolic ward of the Clinical Center, National Institutes of Health. Outpatient blood pressures ranged from 150 to 180 mm Hg systolic and from 90 to 115 mm Hg diastolic. Patients with primary aldosteronism, pheochromocytoma, renal vascular disease, diabetes mellitus, or Cushing's syndrome were excluded by urinalysis, rapid-sequence intravenous pyelograms, measurements of plasma potassium and creatinine concentrations, plasma renin activity, and plasma aldosterone and norepinephrine concentrations. None of them had "malignant" hypertension. All of the patients in this study had "normal-renin" hypertension as defined in this clinic (Mitchell *et al.*, 1977).

All antihypertensive medications had been discontinued at least 2 weeks prior to admission. The subjects took a constant "metabolic" diet containing each day 9 mEq of sodium and 70 mEq of potassium. Patients were studied for 7 days on this diet, then for 7 days with 240 mEq of sodium chloride added daily ("high-sodium"), and finally for 4 days again on the low-sodium diet (Fig. 2). On the

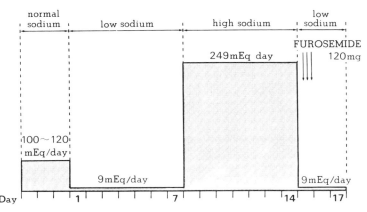

Fig. 2. Protocol of study of hypertensive patients. A constant metabolic diet was used with addition of sodium chloride at the specified dosages.

first day of the second period on the low-sodium diet, furosemide, 40 mg three times a day, was given orally.

Body weight was measured each morning after the patient had voided at 0700. Blood pressure was measured by sphygmomanometer every 4 hr. Mean blood pressure, calculated for every 4-hr reading (day and night) as diastolic pressure plus one-third of pulse pressure, for the seventh day of the low-sodium and the high-sodium regimens and the third day after furosemide, was used for statistical comparison of the effects of dietary sodium and furosemide on blood pressure. A simple average of the 4 hourly mean blood pressures was used to estimate the mesor for each 24-hr period (Bartter *et al.*, 1976a). As in the previous study (Fujita *et al.*, 1980), patients whose average mean blood pressure value on day 7 of the high-sodium regimen exceeded by 10% or more that on day 7 of the low-sodium regimen were classified as "salt-sensitive," those whose average mean blood pressure fell, did not change, or increased by less than 10%, as "non-salt-sensitive."

A. Plasma Renin Activity and Plasma Aldosterone Concentration

Plasma renin activity and aldosterone concentration were measured at 0700 with the patient supine on the last day of the low-sodium period, the high-sodium period, and the furosemide-plus-low-sodium period. Plasma renin activity was measured by radioimmunoassay of the angiotensin I generated at pH 6.0, by a modification of the method of Katz and Smith (1972). Plasma aldosterone concentration was measured by radioimmunoassay (Kurtz and Bartter, 1976).

B. Urinary Prostaglandins

Urine samples were collected in 24-hr lots, kept cold in a refrigerator throughout the collection period, and measured for volume; two samples were frozen for analysis. Samples on days 6 and 7 of each period and on the day furosemide was administered were analyzed for prostaglandins.

A 2.0-ml aliquot of urine to which 1500 cpm of $[^3H]PGE_2$ and 1200 cpm of $[^3H]PGF_{2\alpha}$ (New England Nuclear) had been added (to monitor recoveries) was adjusted to pH 3.0–3.5 with 1.0 N HCl and extracted twice with 4.0 ml of redistilled ethyl acetate (Baker Analyzed Reagent). Extracts were evaporated to dryness under air in a water bath at 25°C, and then reconstituted in 0.2 ml of benzene:ethyl acetate:methanol (60:40:10) to which, after vortex mixing, 0.6 ml of benzene:ethyl acetate (60:40) were added. Each sample was added to a column (Kontes Chromaflex Column) packed with a 2.0 ml slurry of 0.5 g silicic acid in benzene:ethyl acetate (60:40), and thus separated into eluates containing PGA, PGB, neutral lipids, and fatty acids, which were discarded, and the PGEs, which were eluted with 12 ml of benzene:ethyl acetate:methanol (60:40:2). The final fraction, containing the PGFs, was eluted with 5.0 ml benzene:ethyl acetate:methanol (60:40:30). Both fractions were dried under air, and then dissolved in 1.0 ml Tris buffer. An aliquot of 0.3 ml from each was removed for determination of the recovery of PGE_2 and $PGF_{2\alpha}$ during extraction and purification. The recovery of PGE_2 was 48 $\pm$ 4% (mean $\pm$ SEM), that of $PGF_{2\alpha}$, 76 $\pm$ 5%. The remaining sample was divided into two, 0.3-ml aliquots for analysis in duplicate for PGE_2 and $PGF_{2\alpha}$.

The aliquots in duplicate and unlabeled PGE_2 or PGF_2 standards were incubated in 0.5 ml of 0.01 M Tris buffer (pH 7.4) containing antibodies (Steranti Research Limited, England) plus 15,000 cpm [^{3}H]PGE_2 or 12,000 cpm [^{3}H]-$PGF_{2\alpha}$ for 22 hr at 4°C. Separation of antibody bound to free antigen was achieved by shaking with cold solution of 0.9 ml of a charcoal–dextran mixture. The samples were counted with addition of a liquid scintillator in a Packard Liquid Scintillation Counter. All samples were calculated by means of the Rodbard Computer Program for Radioimmunoassays. At a 1 : 500 dilution of PGE_2 antiserum, 0.1 ml binds 40% of 15,000 cpm [^{3}H]PGE_2. Cross-reactivity with PGE_1 is 41%. At a 1 : 1200 dilution of $PGF_{2\alpha}$ antiserum, 0.1 ml binds 50% of 12,000 cpm [^{3}H]$PGF_{2\alpha}$. Cross-reactivity with $PGF_{1\alpha}$ is 30%. Although the antibody does not distinguish between PGE_1 and PGE_2, it has been demonstrated previously that PGE_2 and not PGE_1 is produced by the kidney. Therefore, it was assumed that under the conditions of these experiments, the PGE_2 antiserum was measuring PGE_2. Logit transformation of the standard curves resulted in linear functions between 0.1 and 10 ng PGE_2/ml or $PGF_{2\alpha}$/ml incubation medium.

C. Plasma Norepinephrine

Plasma norepinephrine concentration was measured on day 7 of the low-sodium diet and on days 3 and 4 of the high-sodium diet, by a method previously described (Fujita *et al.*, 1980).

D. Data Handling

All data are expressed as mean $\pm$ standard error of the mean (SEM), and differences were evaluated by Student's paired t or unpaired t as appropriate. Differences were considered significant when the p value was less than 0.05.

III. RESULTS

Six patients were categorized as SS, and 6 as NSS by our criteria (Fujita *et al.*, 1980) (Fig. 3). There was no significant difference in either age or sex distribution (both, 4 males and 2 females). Also, there were no significant differences in either systolic or diastolic blood pressures, or in secondary effects of the hyper-

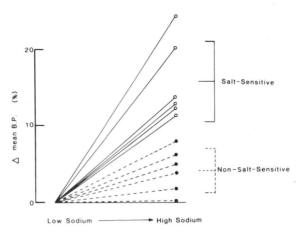

Fig. 3.   The response of mean average blood pressure to the high-sodium regimen for the 6 SS and 6 NSS patients chosen for urinary prostaglandin measurements.

tension, as revealed by the concentrations of either electrolytes or creatinine in serum, or in the incidence of left ventricular hypertrophy or retinopathy.

The average mean blood pressures for the SS patients ingesting the low-sodium diet, the high-sodium diet, or the furosemide-plus-low-sodium diet were 102.3 ± 3.9 (SE), 116.2 ± 4.1, and 99.2 ± 3.8 mm Hg, respectively (Table I). Corresponding averages of mean blood pressure for the NSS patients were 111.5 ± 2.2, 115.3 ± 2.0, and 108.7 ± 1.6 mm Hg, respectively. The mean blood pressure of SS patients ingesting the low-sodium diet and that of the same patients after administration of furosemide differed significantly (both $p < 0.05$) from the corresponding means for the NSS patients (Table I) although the average values for the mean blood pressures on the high-sodium diet did not differ significantly between the groups. The mean percentage increment of mean blood pressure between the low-sodium and high-sodium values, as analyzed by paired t test, differed significantly ($p < 0.01$) between the groups [15.6 ± 2.1, (SS) versus 4.1 ± 1.2, (NSS), $p < 0.05$](Fig. 2). The mean percentage decrement of average blood pressure between the high-sodium and the furosemide values, analyzed by paired t test, differed significantly ($p < 0.01$) between the groups [(15.4 ± 1.1 (SS) versus 6.5 ± 1.6, (NSS)].

The urinary sodium on the seventh day of the low-sodium diet was significantly greater in the NSS than in the SS patients [10.2 ± 1.6 (NSS) versus 4.5 ± 2.7 mEq/day (SS), $p < 0.01$], although the changes in body weight were not significantly different between the two groups [-1.62 ± 0.32 (NSS) versus -1.58 ± 0.20 kg (SS), N.S.]. The SS patients retained significantly ($p < 0.02$) more sodium during the 7 days of high-sodium diet than did the NSS patients,

TABLE I

Mean Blood Pressure (mm Hg) during Three Experimental Periods

	Low sodium	High sodium	Furosemide
Non-salt-sensitive (6)	111.5 ± 2.2 ⟷ $p < 0.05$	115.3 ± 2.0 ⟷ $p < 0.01$	108.7 ± 1.6
	↑ $p < 0.05$ ↓ $p < 0.01$	↑ N.S. ↓ $p < 0.01$	↑ $p < 0.05$ ↓
Salt-sensitive (6)	102.3 ± 3.0 ⟷ $p < 0.01$	116.2 ± 4.1 ⟷	99.2 ± 3.8

and gained significantly ($p < 0.01$) more weight than the NSS patients [1.29 ± 0.28 (SS) versus 0.49 ± 0.16 kg (NSS)]. An estimate of the mean cumulative sodium retention (Na intake minus urinary Na) over the 7 days of the high-sodium diet was 431 ± 76 mEq for the SS and 166 ± 42 mEq for the NSS patients ($p < 0.02$). Furthermore, "escape" from sodium retention occurred on day 3 in the NSS patients (Fig. 4) as opposed to day 5 in the SS patients.

A. Plasma Renin Activity and Plasma Aldosterone Concentration

With the low-sodium diet, plasma renin activity (PRA) was higher in the NSS than in the SS patients [5.5 ± 1.1, ng/ml per hour (NSS) versus 2.8 ± 0.5 (SS), $p < 0.05$], as was plasma aldosterone concentration (PAC)[39.4 ± 9.1 (NSS)

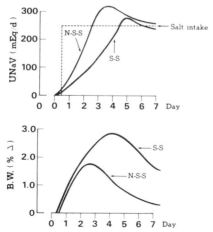

Fig. 4. Curves for average of urinary sodium excretion by NSS and SS patients (upper) and corresponding curves for mean body weight of the same patients (lower curve).

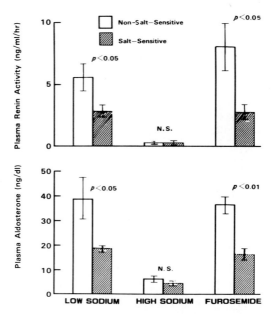

Fig. 5. Plasma renin activity and plasma aldosterone concentration on day 7 of the low-sodium and high-sodium regimens, and on day 3 of the furosemide regimen.

versus 18.0 ± 1.4 ng/dl (SS), $p < 0.05$, (Fig. 5)]. On the seventh day of the high-sodium diet, all these values had been suppressed to the same low values [PRA 0.2 ± 0.1 (NSS) versus 0.2 ± 0.1 (SS), and PAC 7.2 ± 1.7 (NSS) versus 4.8 ± 0.9 (SS)]. Thus, the decrement in PRA and PAC with salt loading was greater in the NSS patients than in the SS ones ($p < 0.01$). With furosemide, PRA reached significantly ($p < 0.05$) higher values (mean, 8.0 ± 1.9 ng/ml/hr) in the NSS patients than in the SS patients (mean, 2.7 ± 0.6 ng/ml/hr), as did PAC (mean, 36.8 ± 3.6 ng/dl (NSS) versus 16.8 ± 2.2 (SS), $p < 0.01$). Thus the increment in PRA and PAC with furosemide was greater in the NSS patients ($p < 0.01$). The response of PRA and PAC to the low-sodium diet and furosemide in NSS patients was similar to that of normal subjects, and the response in the SS patients was below normal (Mitchell *et al.*, 1977).

B. Urinary Prostaglandins

Because of the known relationship of prostaglandins to the renal handling of sodium and to the renin–angiotensin-aldosterone system, we measured urinary $PGF_{2\alpha}$ in 12 patients (6 SS and 6 NSS) (1) at the end of the low-sodium period, (2) at the end of the high-sodium period, and (3) on the day of treatment with furosemide.

There was no significant difference between groups as regards urinary $PGF_{2\alpha}$ (Fig. 6). At the end of the low-salt period, mean urinary $PGF_{2\alpha}$ was 1.22 ± 0.18 (SS) versus 1.47 ± 0.11 $\mu g/day$ (NSS). It was not changed with the high-sodium regimen, but rose after furosemide to 1.84 ± 0.18 (SS) versus 2.09 ± 0.22 $\mu g/day$ (NSS). It is thus unlikely that changes in renal $PGF_{2\alpha}$ are related to the difference between SS and NSS patients.

With the low-sodium diet, urinary PGE_2 was significantly ($p < 0.01$) higher in the NSS than in the SS patients [1.04 ± 0.07 (NSS) versus 0.66 ± 0.04 $\mu g/day$ (SS) (Fig. 6)]. In the NSS patients, urinary PGE_2 decreased significantly from day 7 of the low-sodium diet to day 7 of the high-sodium diet (1.04 ± 0.07 $\mu g/day$ low-Na to 0.62 ± 0.05 high-Na, $p < 0.01$ by paired t), but urinary PGE_2 did not change with the high-sodium regimen in the SS patients. With furosemide, urinary PGE_2 increased significantly in the NSS patients (0.62 ± 0.05, high-Na, to 1.55 ± 0.25 $\mu g/day$, furosemide, $p < 0.01$, by paired t) but did not change in the SS patients. When all patients were considered as one

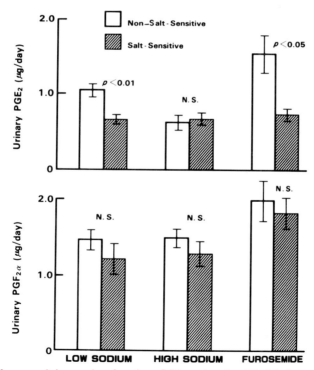

Fig. 6. Upper panel shows values for urinary PGE_2 on days 6 and 7 of the low-sodium and the high-sodium regimens, and on day 1 of the furosemide regimen. Lower panel shows values for urinary $PGF_{2\alpha}$.

group, urinary PGE$_2$ was positively correlated with PRA ($r = 0.34$, $p < 0.05$) and PAC ($r = 0.51$, $p < 0.01$).

C. Plasma Norepinephrine

Plasma norepinephrine increased on day 3 in the SS patients ($p < 0.01$), whereas it did not change in the NSS patients (Fujita *et al.*, 1980) (Fig. 7).

IV. DISCUSSION

A ranking of hypertensive subjects according to the response of the 24 hr averages of mean blood pressure to salt loading after limitation of sodium intake for 7 days suggests a continuum of such responses, ranging from 0 to 23 mm Hg (0 to +24%) above the values for the low-sodium diet (Fig. 3). For a study of related variables, we have divided these patients into two groups, according to the blood-pressure response to the salt load: those with a response of 10% or more are termed "salt-sensitive" (SS) and those with one of less than 10% are termed "non-salt-sensitive" (NSS) (Fig. 3). Although it has been suggested that subjects with so-called "normal-renin, essential" hypertension are homogeneous in their hormonal patterns (Laragh, 1973), the present study indicates that they

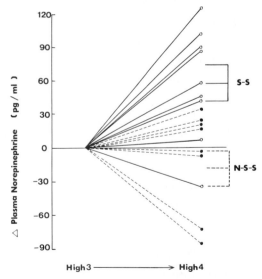

Fig. 7. Increment in plasma norepinephrine between day 3 (taken as 0) and day 4 for all patients on the high-sodium regimen.

can be divided readily into two groups by differences in their salt-sensitivities. The NSS patients, who showed a smaller decrement in blood pressure than the SS patients with the low-sodium diet, had higher PRA and PAC values than did the SS patients. With a high-sodium diet, the NSS patients (renin suppressing normally) gained less weight and excreted more sodium than the SS patients (renin showing delayed suppression), whose blood pressure was higher after salt loading. Similar findings were reported by Tuck and associates (1976), suggesting a division of patients with "normal-renin, essential" hypertension according to the decline of plasma renin activity during the first 2 hr of saline infusion (2 liters). Some of them showed a delayed decrease of plasma renin activity and a further rise of blood pressure, and the others showed a normal decrease of PRA without a further rise of blood pressure.

The finding of the higher values of PRA and PAC in NSS than in SS patients after sodium deprivation might suggest that the higher activity of the renin–angiotensin system in NSS hypertension contributes to the maintenance of the relatively higher blood pressure on a low-sodium diet and with furosemide (Laragh, 1978). It is supported by the finding that captopril-induced fall in blood pressure was significantly greater in NSS than in SS patients on a 30 mEq salt intake (Fujita *et al.*, 1981).

The greater decrement in PRA and PAC in the NSS patients might be invoked to explain their greater sodium loss during the period of high-sodium intake. It may be, however, that differences in renal function not related to the renin–angiotensin–aldosterone system are responsible for the differences of sodium excretion between the two groups. As noted, the NSS patients lost more sodium in the urine on the seventh day of the low-sodium diet than did the SS patients, despite their higher plasma aldosterone concentration. After the low-sodium diet, urinary PGE_2 was significantly higher in the NSS than in the SS patients. If renal PGE does indeed promote sodium excretion, as has been suggested (Tannenbaum *et al.*, 1975; Yun *et al.*, 1977; Gross and Bartter, 1973), the increased renal PGE production in the NSS patients on the low-sodium diet may have operated to facilitate sodium loss, despite their higher PAC. Alternatively, the lower plasma norepinephrine in the NSS patients on day 3 of the high-sodium diet may have facilitated "escape" in these patients (Gill and Bartter, 1966).

There was a positive correlation of urinary PGE_2 with PRA and with PAC. Since PGE_2, infused into the renal arteries (Yun *et al.*, 1977) or incubated with renal slices (Whorton *et al.*, 1980), stimulates renin release, and since urinary PGE is an index of renal (and not plasma) prostaglandins, the higher renal PGE_2 may have served as a stimulus to renin release in these patients. Therefore, the higher values for urinary PGE_2 in the NSS patients after the low-sodium period and with furosemide may explain in part the higher values for PRA and PAC in these NSS patients (Frölich *et al.*, 1976; Bartter *et al.*, 1976b).

V. SUMMARY

Twelve patients with idiopathic hypertension were studied while ingesting a low-sodium diet for 7 days, then a high-sodium diet for 7 days, and finally after the oral administration of furosemide. They were classified as "salt-sensitive" (SS) or "non-salt-sensitive" (NSS) according to the responses of their blood pressure to the sodium load. The percentage increments of mean blood pressure in NSS patients with salt loading were significantly ($p < 0.01$) less than in SS patients ($6.5 \pm 1.6\%$ versus $15.4 \pm 1.1\%$). With the low-sodium diet, NSS patients had less decrease in blood pressure, and showed significantly higher plasma renin activity (PRA) and plasma aldosterone concentration (PAC) than the SS patients. With furosemide, NSS patients showed significantly higher PRA and PAC. Results suggest that the higher activity of the renin–angiotensin system observed in NSS patients either on a low-sodium diet or with furosemide may contribute to the maintenance of the higher blood pressure during sodium deprivation.

There was no significant difference between groups as regards urinary $PGF_{2\alpha}$. After the low-sodium diet, urinary PGE_2 was significantly higher in NSS than in SS patients. With furosemide, urinary PGE_2 increased significantly in the NSS patients but did not change in SS patients. For all patients, considered together, urinary PGE_2 was positively correlated with PRA and PAC. The evidence suggests that the higher values of urinary PGE_2 in NSS patients following administration of either a low-sodium diet or furosemide may contribute to the greater sodium loss, and the higher PRA and PAC also seen in these patients.

REFERENCES

Bartter, F. C., Delea, C. S., Baker, W., Halberg, F., and Lee, J. K. (1976a). Chronobiology in the diagnosis and treatment of mesor-hypertension. *Chronobiologia* **3**, 199–213.

Bartter, F. C., Gill, J. R., Frölich, J. C., Bowden, R. E., Hollifield, J. E., Radfar, N., Keiser, H. R., Oates, J. A., and Taylor, A. A. (1976b). Prostaglandins are overproduced by the kidneys and mediate hyperreninemia in Bartter's syndrome. *Trans. Assoc. Am. Physicians* **89**, 77–91.

Dahl, L. K., and Love, R. A. (1954). Evidence for relationship between Na (chloride) intake and human essential hypertension. *Arch. Intern. Med.* **94**, 525–531.

Dustan, H. P., Cumming, G. R., Corcoran, A. C., and Page, I. H. (1959). A mechanism of chlorothiazide enhanced effectiveness of antihypertensive ganlioplegic drugs. *Circulation* **19**, 360–365.

Frölich, J. C., Hollifield, J. W., Dormois, J. C., Seyberth, H. J., Michelakis, A. M., and Oates, J. A. (1976). Suppression of plasma renin activity by indomethacin in man. *Circ. Res.* **39**, 447–452.

Fujita, T., Henry, W. L., Bartter, F. C., Lake, C. R., and Delea, C. S. (1980). Factors influencing blood pressure in salt-sensitive patients with hypertension. *Am. J. Med.* **69**, 334–344.

Fujita, T., Yamashita, N., and Yamashita, K. (1981). Effects of angiotensin converting enzyme inhibition on blood pressure and plasma renin activity in essential hypertension. *Am. Heart J.* **101,** 259-263.

Gill, J. R., and Bartter, F. C. (1966). Adrenergic nervous system in sodium metabolism. II. Effects of guanethidine on the renal response to sodium deprivation in normal man. *N. Engl. J. Med.* **275,** 1466-1470.

Gross, J. B., and Bartter, F. C. (1973). Effects of prostaglandins E_1, A_1 and F_2 on renal handling of salt and water excretion. *Am. J. Physiol.* **225,** 218-224.

Katz, F. H., and Smith, J. A. (1972). Radioimmunoassay of angiotensin I. Comparison of two renin activity methods and use for other measurements of the renin system. *Clin. Chem. (Winston-Salem, N.C.)* **18,** 528-533.

Kawasaki, T., Delea, C. S., and Bartter, F. C. (1978). The effect of high-sodium and low-sodium intakes on blood pressure and other related variables in human subjects with idiopathic hypertension. *Am. J. Med.* **64,** 193-198.

Kurtz, A. B., and Bartter, F. C. (1976). Radioimmunoassays for aldosterone and deoxycorticosterone. *Steroids* **28,** 133-142.

Laragh, J. H. (1973). Vasoconstriction-volume analysis for understanding and treating hypertension: The role of renin and aldosterone profiles. *Am. J. Med.* **55,** 261-274.

Laragh, J. H. (1978). The renin system in essential, renovascular and adrenocortical hypertension. An overview. *Adv. Nephrol.* **7,** 157-189.

Meneely, G. R., and Dahl, L. K. (1961). Electrolytes in hypertension: The effects of sodium chloride. *Med. Clin. North Am.* **45,** 271-283.

Mitchell, J. R., Taylor, A., Pool, J., Lake, C. R., Rollins, D. E., and Bartter, F. C. (1977). Renin-aldosterone profiling in hypertension. *Ann. Intern. Med.* **87,** 596-612.

Tannenbaum, J., Splawinski, J. A., Oates, J. A., and Nies, A. S. (1975). Enhanced renal prostaglandin production in the dog. I. Effect on renal function. *Circ. Res.* **36,** 197-203.

Tuck, M. L., Williams, G. H., Dluhy, R. G., Greenfield, M., and Moore, T. J. (1976). A delayed suppression of the renin-aldosterone axis following saline infusion in human hypertension. *Circ. Res.* **39,** 711-717.

Whorton, A. R., Lazar, J. D., Smigel, M. D., and Oates, J. A. (1980). Prostaglandin-mediated renin release from renal cortical slices. *Adv. Prostaglandin Thromboxane Res.* **7,** 1123-1129.

Wilson, I. M., and Freis, E. D. (1959). Relationship between plasma and extracellular fluid volume depletion and the antihypertensive effect of chlorothiazide. *Circulation* **20,** 1028-1036.

Yun, J. C. H., Kelly, G., Bartter, F. C., and Smith, H., Jr. (1977). Role of prostaglandins in the control of renin secretion in the dog. *Circ. Res.* **40,** 459-464.

Yun, J. C. H. (1979). On the control of renin release. *Nephron* **23,** 72-78.

15

The Role of Sodium in DOCA-Induced Hypertension in Pigs

ROGER J. GREKIN, DAVID M. COHEN,
STEPHEN P. DYBUS, JOHN MITCHELL,
MARY D. GRIGORIAN, AND DAVID F. BOHR

I. INTRODUCTION

Concurrent administration of salt and mineralocorticoids causes hypertension in a wide variety of experimental and clinical conditions. Renal sodium retention appears to play an important role in the genesis of the hypertension and salt restricted animals are resistant to the hypertensive effects of mineralocorticoids (Hall and Hall, 1969; Tobian, 1960; Dahl *et al.,* 1963; Kassirer *et al.,* 1970).

We have characterized the hemodynamic, electrolyte, and endocrine changes that result from the administration of deoxycorticosterone acetate (DOCA) in pigs in an attempt to establish the pathogenesis of the hypertension. We have also

221

measured these same variables during sodium restriction in animals with established DOCA hypertension to determine the role of salt in the maintenance of the hemodynamic and electrolyte changes.

II. METHODS

Male feeder pigs weighing 18–20 kg were obtained from a local farm and housed in 4 × 4 ft metabolic cages throughout the studies. Animals grew approximately 0.5 kg per day. Standard diet consisted of Purina Pig Growena (112 mEq Na and 191 mEq K/kg) *ad libitum* and tap water. Operative preparation consisted of thoracic placement of an electromagnetic flowprobe (Zepeda Instruments, Seattle, Washington) around the ascending aorta and insertion of two Herd–Barger tygon catheters, one in the aortic arch and one in the central venous pool through the azygous vein (Miller *et al.*, 1979).

Aortic and venous pressures and cardiac output were measured daily. Total peripheral resistance was calculated by dividing mean arterial pressure by cardiac output. Water and food intake were measured, and urine and fecal output were collected daily. Fecal samples were homogenized, and 1-g aliquots were ashed and then digested in 1 N nitric acid for measurement of sodium and potassium. Plasma samples were obtained daily from 5 days prior to implantation until 5 days after implantation, and every fifth day thereafter. Arterial blood samples were collected in 5-ml plastic tubes containing 50 μl lithium heparin and centrifuged at room temperature. Sodium and potassium concentrations were measured in food, urine, feces, and plasma using a National Instrument Laboratories flame photometer (IL 443) with an automatic constant ratio (1:200) diluter (Turner). Plasma concentrations of aldosterone, DOC, and renin activity were measured using radioimmunoassays as previously described (Cohen *et al.*, 1971; Mayes *et al.*, 1970; Grekin *et al.*, 1980).

DOCA was administered by subcutaneous implantation of DOCA-impregnated silastic (100 mg/kg body wt) (Miller *et al.*, 1979). Control animals received similar implantations of silastic without DOCA. Implantations were made in the left flank under light thiamylal sodium (Surital, Parke-Davis) anesthesia.

Animals with established DOCA hypertension of 4 to 6 weeks duration were placed on a powdered "normal sodium" diet for 4–12 days (112 mEq Na, 253 mEq K/kg) in preparation for a switch to powdered low sodium diet (10.1 mEq Na/kg)(Cohen *et al.*, 1980). All measurements were continued during the 3-week period on the low sodium diet.

Comparison of variables between groups was made using Student's t test. Comparisons within groups utilized the paired-t test.

III. RESULTS

Mean arterial pressure was approximately 100 mm Hg before implantation in all pigs. All animals receiving DOCA had an increase in mean arterial pressure within 3 days of implantation. The rise in pressure was significant compared to control animals 48 hr after implantation ($p < 0.005$). Pressure continued to rise steadily during the first 10 days following implantation. Thereafter, pressure stabilized at approximately 130 mm Hg. Control animals had no change in arterial pressure throughout the course of study (Fig. 1).

Previous studies have shown that the hemodynamic changes associated with the rise in pressure are heterogeneous (Miller *et al.*, 1979). Some animals have increases in total peripheral resistance without a change in cardiac output. Other animals have a rise in cardiac output while peripheral resistance is unchanged. Most commonly there is a rise in both cardiac output and peripheral resistance. Examples of these patterns are graphically represented in Fig. 2.

Plasma DOC levels rose from a mean of 112 ± 37 ng/dl prior to implantation to a mean of 1677 ± 172 ng/dl 24 hr later. DOC levels fell gradually thereafter, but remained elevated for as long as 3 months. Plasma renin activity was suppressed following administration of DOCA, falling to levels significantly below control by the third day after implantation, and becoming unmeasurable by day 20. Serum concentration of aldosterone in DOCA-treated pigs was approximately 50% of control after day 6 postimplantation.

Sodium intake and urinary output were stable in control pigs throughout the

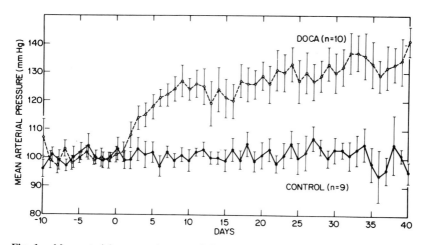

Fig. 1. Mean arterial pressure (mean $\pm$ SEM) in DOCA-treated and control pigs. (Reprinted from Grekin *et al.*, 1980, by permission of the American Heart Association.)

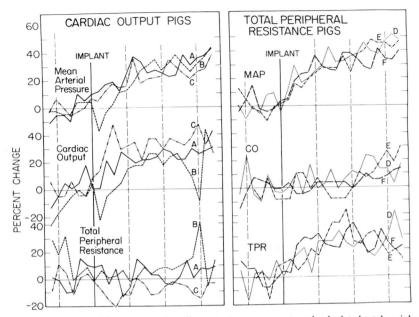

Fig. 2.   Mean arterial pressure and cardiac output measurements and calculated total peripheral resistance in six selected DOCA-treated pigs. Pigs in the left panel had a rise in arterial pressure associated solely with increased cardiac output. Pigs in the right panel had pressure rises associated exclusively with increased peripheral resistance. (Reprinted from Miller *et al.*, 1979, by permission of the American Heart Association.)

study. DOCA-treated animals had a transient decrease in urinary sodium concentration lasting 3 days. During the first 2 days following implantation, the decrease in urine sodium was significant ($p < 0.002$) when compared to control animals. Thereafter urinary sodium excretion returned to the levels of control animals. The mean sodium retention was 114 mEq per animal during the first 2 days following implantation.

Recent studies have demonstrated a decrease in fecal sodium excretion following DOCA implantation (Grigorian *et al.*, 1980). Mean fecal sodium excretion fell from 0.71 ± 0.11 mEq/kg body wt before implantation to 0.24 ± 0.04 mEq/kg body wt 24 hr after the procedure. This decrease was sustained throughout the course of study. Control animals had no change in fecal sodium excretion.

Serum sodium concentration was measured in six control pigs and seven DOCA-treated animals throughout the course of study. As shown in Fig. 3, serum sodium concentration in DOCA-treated pigs was not different from controls before and for 5 days following implantation. By day 10, sodium concentration rose significantly ($p < 0.05$, paired-t), and thereafter was higher in the

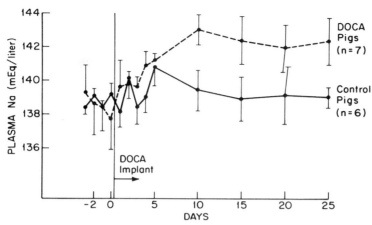

Fig. 3. Plasma sodium concentration in DOCA-treated and control pigs. The increase in plasma sodium concentration in DOCA-treated pigs between day 5 and day 10 is significant ($p < 0.05$).

experimental animals than in controls ($p < 0.05$). This difference remained constant at 3 mEq/liter.

All DOCA-treated pigs became hypokalemic; mean plasma K concentration fell from 4.11 ± 0.07 before implant to 3.44 ± 0.07 on the first day postimplant ($p < 0.001$). Thereafter plasma potassium concentration steadily decreased to 2.81 ± 0.11 by day 15. No changes were seen in potassium intake or urinary potassium excretion to account for the hypokalemia. Although fecal potassium measurements in DOCA-treated pigs demonstrated a mild increase in fecal potassium, formal potassium balance calculations (dietary intake − urinary + fecal output) revealed a slightly more positive potassium balance in DOCA-treated pigs than in controls. This difference was not statistically significant.

As demonstrated in Fig. 4, DOCA-treated animals had a marked increase in water intake, beginning on the fourth day after implant and increasing steadily until the fifteenth day. The rise in water intake from day 3 to day 10 closely paralleled the rise in plasma Na concentration. Urine volume rose along with water intake. The increase in water intake in DOCA-treated animals was significant compared to controls after day 8 ($p < 0.001$).

When placed on a sodium-restricted diet, pigs showed two distinctly different blood pressure responses. Blood pressure fell to nearly normal levels in five DOCA-treated pigs. In four other animals with more severe hypertension ($p < 0.01$), only a small fall in pressure was seen (Fig. 5).

For those animals with a fall in blood pressure, concomitant falls in total peripheral resistance were seen; mean resistance was $77 \pm 3\%$ of the pre-low sodium value. No change in cardiac output was seen. Animals with no fall in

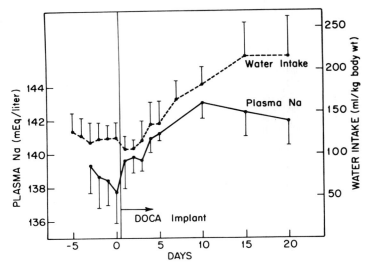

Fig. 4. Plasma sodium concentration and daily water intake in 7 DOCA-treated pigs. Increases in plasma sodium concentration and water intake are parallel during the first 10 days following implantation.

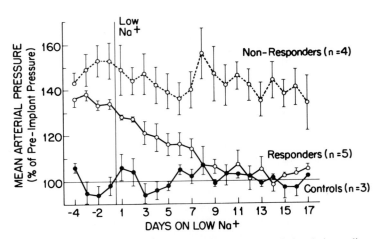

Fig. 5. Mean arterial pressure in DOCA-hypertensive and control pigs during sodium restriction. Pressure returned to control levels in five DOCA-hypertensive animals (responders). Four other animals had no significant change in arterial pressure during sodium restriction (nonresponders). (Reprinted from Cohen *et al.*, 1980, by permission of the American Heart Association.)

pressure on low sodium diet had no change in either cardiac output or peripheral resistance.

Urine sodium excretion fell to 15.3 ± 6.1 mEq/day by the fifth day following the start of the low sodium diet. Mean positive sodium balance fell from 75.8 ± 26.6 mEq/day on standard diet to 10.4 ± 2.7 mEq/day during the low sodium diet. There were no differences in U_{Na} and Na balance between animals that remained hypertensive and those that became normotensive.

Serum sodium concentration fell in DOCA-treated animals during administration of a low sodium diet (Fig. 6). Serum potassium concentration also returned to normal in DOCA-treated animals during the low sodium diet. Mean serum potassium concentration increased from 2.9 ± 0.1 mEq/liter on the standard diet to 4.2 ± 0.1 mEq/liter after 3 days of sodium restriction ($p < 0.001$).

The marked increase in water intake was reversed during the low sodium diet. Mean water intake was 308 ± 23 ml/kg/day on the standard diet, and fell steadily to 60 ± 9 ml/kg/day by day 14 of sodium restriction ($p < 0.001$) (Fig. 6). Urine volume decreased in parallel with water intake, and no change in water balance was observed.

IV. DISCUSSION

The mechanism whereby mineralocorticoid excess causes sustained hypertension has not been established. Sodium appears to play an essential role, and

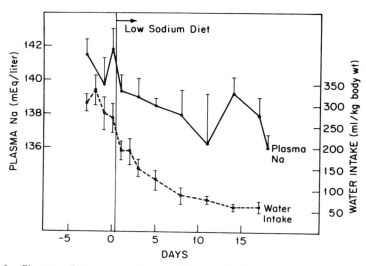

Fig. 6. Plasma sodium concentration and daily water intake in 4 DOCA-treated pigs during sodium restriction. Both plasma sodium concentration and water intake decreased to control levels during sodium restriction.

increased salt intake is frequently required for the development of hypertension (Hall and Hall, 1969; Ledingham, 1954; Dahl *et al.*, 1963). Several experiments have also demonstrated reversal of the hypertension with salt restriction (Musilova *et al.*, 1966; deChamplain *et al.*, 1968). A major effect of DOCA is to promote renal sodium retention, and this effect has been observed in every species that has been studied (Tobian, 1960; Kassirer *et al.*, 1970; Wenting *et al.*, 1977). Whether or not this sodium retention is the proximate cause of the hypertension, however, still remains to be established. Norman *et al.* (1975) have demonstrated that dialysis induced sodium retention leads to elevated arterial pressure in the absence of mineralocorticoids. Other studies, however, suggest that DOCA may cause hypertension in nephrectomized animals, supporting an extrarenal mechanism as being responsible for the hypertension (Langford and Snavely, 1959).

Our hemodynamic studies suggest that simple volume expansion followed by autoregulation cannot explain the hypertension in all animals. Animals with initial rises in blood pressure accompanied by increased peripheral resistance and no change in cardiac output must have some other sequence which causes hypertension. The heterogeneity of the hemodynamic response argues that the primary response to DOCA induced changes is one of increased arterial pressure rather than a specific change in cardiac output or peripheral resistance. This concept is supported by the observation that β-blockade in mineralocorticoid hypertensive dogs blocks the rise in cardiac output but does not alter the rise in blood pressure (Bravo *et al.*, 1977; Conway and Hatton, 1978).

The return of arterial pressure to normal in five DOCA-treated pigs following salt restriction indicates a major role of sodium retention in the maintenance of hypertension. It does not, however, exclude the possibility that extrarenal effects of DOCA also play an important role in increasing the blood pressure. By restricting salt severely in growing pigs, we have, in effect, produced relative salt depletion. This is because the control pigs require a positive sodium balance of 75 mEq of sodium per day to support their growth. Salt restricted pigs can only retain 10 mEq/day, resulting in effective sodium depletion. Important hypertensive effects of DOCA may well be masked during sodium depletion, even if these effects are mediated through mechanisms unrelated to salt retention.

The persistence of hypertension in four animals despite sodium restriction may be secondary to irreversible changes induced by the elevated pressure. Such changes have been observed in other studies, in which mineralocorticoid levels are returned to normal, and the term metacorticoid hypertension has been used to describe it (Sturtevant, 1958). We have speculated that those animals that remain hypertensive on sodium restriction have sustained structural vascular changes (Cohen *et al.*, 1980). The higher blood pressures seen in these animals support that speculation, as does the observation that each of these animals had its initial rise in blood pressure associated with primary rises in total peripheral resistance.

In contrast, three of four animals whose blood pressure returned to normal had primary rises in blood pressure associated with an increase in cardiac output (Cohen *et al.*, 1980).

The late rise in plasma sodium concentration in DOCA-treated animals is different from our previous observations (Grekin *et al.*, 1980). We ascribe this difference to the improved accuracy of plasma sodium determinations in the present study. We are not certain of the mechanism whereby plasma sodium concentration begins to rise after urinary sodium retention has been completed. The initial sodium retention is accompanied by isotonic amounts of water retention maintaining plasma sodium concentration constant (Grekin *et al.*, 1980). The subsequent rise in sodium concentration corresponds with "escape," when urine sodium excretion returns to basal levels. Perhaps the natriuretic mechanisms leading to escape promote a small increase in free water loss as well, resulting in mild hypernatremia.

The polydipsia associated with DOCA-induced hypertension is not a result of primary renal water loss. Preliminary experiments in which DOCA-hypertensive pigs have been subjected to water restriction have shown that they are capable of producing a concentrated urine and retaining water. Under these circumstances, however, they demonstrate marked increases in plasma sodium concentration (J. Mitchell *et al.*, unpublished observations). We believe that the hypernatremia may be stimulating the thirst center directly, causing the profound polydipsia seen in these animals. As can be seen in Fig. 4, the time course of the onset of polydipsia parallels the rise in serum sodium concentration. The time course of the decrease in water intake following salt restriction also parallels the return of serum sodium concentration to normal, although not as closely as during the onset of polydipsia.

Potassium balance studies, including careful fecal and urinary measurements, clearly demonstrate that DOCA-treated pigs do not have a loss of potassium. The hypokalemia in pigs is, therefore, secondary to a DOCA-induced shift of potassium into the intracellular compartment. A similar shift also takes place in mineralocorticoid treated rabbits (Dawborn and Ross, 1967). It is of interest to speculate that intracellular shifts of potassium may be a major cause of hypokalemia in other species, even though kaliuresis is also observed.

The rapid reversal of hypokalemia with sodium restriction strongly argues against a direct effect of DOCA in causing the intracellular shift of potassium. A more likely explanation might be the effect of alkalosis on intracellular potassium distribution. Alkalosis is a consistent feature of mineralocorticoid excess, and results from increased renal hydrogen ion excretion (Kassirer *et al.*, 1970). Preliminary results in our laboratory confirm the development of alkalosis in DOCA-treated pigs (J. Mitchell *et al.*, unpublished observations). Systemic alkalosis promotes an exchange of intracellular hydrogen for extracellular potassium (Burnell *et al.*, 1956) possibly causing hypokalemia. During sodium restriction, when only small amounts of sodium are being delivered to the distal exchange sites of renal tubules, hydrogen ion excretion would be expected to decrease, and systemic pH and potassium would both then return to normal.

There was complete reversal of both hypokalemia and polydipsia in all animals regardless of blood pressure response. These abnormalities, therefore, appear to result directly from DOCA-induced sodium retention.

V. SUMMARY

Sodium, potassium, and water balances were measured in growing male pigs during the development of DOCA-induced hypertension. Elevated blood pressure was seen in all pigs within 3 days of implantation of DOCA impregnated silastic strips. Transient sodium retention occurred during the first 48 hr following implantation, characterized by a decrease in urine and fecal sodium output. Urinary sodium output increased to preimplant levels by the third day after implantation, but fecal sodium content was decreased throughout the experimental period. Plasma sodium rose gradually in the experimental group, reaching levels significantly higher than control animals by day 10. Hypokalemia occurred during the first week following implantation. No significant change in potassium balance was observed during the interval, and no kaliuresis occurred. Hypokalemia appears to be caused by an intracellular shift of potassium. Experimental animals also developed marked polydipsia and polyuria and the onset of polydipsia closely followed the rise in serum sodium concentration.

Nine DOCA-treated hypertensive animals were studied during administration of a diet containing 20 mEq sodium per day. Blood pressure fell to normal in five animals and remained elevated in four. Fall in blood pressure, when it occurred, was associated with a fall in total peripheral resistance whereas cardiac output remained constant. Serum potassium concentration returned to normal in all animals during sodium restriction. Water intake fell dramatically during low sodium intake, again paralleling the change in plasma sodium concentration.

Hypokalemia and increased water turnover appear to result from DOCA-induced sodium retention, rather than from direct effects of DOCA. The failure of low sodium diet to produce a fall in arterial pressure in some animals is not explained by the present studies.

REFERENCES

Bravo, E., Tarazi, R., and Dustan, H. (1977). Multifactorial analysis of chronic hypertension induced by electrolyte-active steroids in trained, unanesthetized dogs. *Circ. Res.* **40,** Suppl I, I140–I145.
Burnell, J. M., Villamil, M. F., Uyeno, B. F., and Scribner, B. H. (1956). The effect in humans of

extracellular pH change on the relationship between serum potassium concentration and in-tracellular potassium. *J. Clin. Invest.* **35**, 935–939.

Cohen, D. M., Grekin, R. J., Mitchell, J., Rice, W. H., and Bohr, D. F. (1980). Hemodynamic, endocrine, and electrolyte changes during sodium restriction in DOCA hypertensive pigs. *Hypertension* **2**, 490–496.

Cohen, E. D., Grim, C. E., Conn, J. W., Blough, W. M., Guyer, R. B., Kem, D. C., and Lucas, C. P. (1971). Accurate and rapid measurement of plasma renin activity by radioimmunoassay. *J. Lab. Clin. Med.* **77**, 1025–1038.

Conway, J., and Hatton, J. (1978) Development of deoxycorticosterone acetate hypertension in the dog. *Circ. Res.* **43** Suppl. I, I82–I86.

Dahl, L. K., Heine, M., and Tassinari, L. (1963). Effects of chronic salt ingestion. Role of genetic factors in both DOCA-salt and renal hypertension. *J. Exp. Med.* **118**, 605–617.

Dawborn, J. K., and Ross, E. J. (1967). The effect of prolonged administration of aldosterone on sodium and potassium turnover in the rabbit. *Clin. Sci.* **32**, 559–570.

deChamplain, J., Krakoff, L. R., and Axelrod, J. (1968). Relationships between sodium intake and norepinephrine storage during the development of experimental hypertension. *Circ. Res.* **23**, 479–491.

Grekin, R. J., Terris, J. M., and Bohr, D. F. (1980). Electrolyte and hormonal effects of deoxycorticosterone acetate in young pigs. *Hypertension* **2**, 326–332.

Grigorian, M. E., Grekin, R. J., Mitchell, J., Buiteweg, J., Cohen, D. M., and Bohr, D. F. (1980). Differential effects of deoxycorticosterone acetate (DOCA) on renal and gastrointestinal handling of electrolytes in pigs. *Physiologist* **23**, 65, Abstr. No. 338.

Hall, C. E., and Hall, O. (1969). Interaction between desoxycorticosterone treatment, fluid intake, sodium consumption, blood pressure, and organ changes in rats drinking water, saline, or sucrose solution. *Can. J. Physiol. Pharmacol.* **47**, 81–86.

Kassirer, J. P., London, A. M., Goldman, D. M., and Schwartz, W. B. (1970). On the pathogenesis of metabolic alkalosis in hyperaldosteronism. *Am. J. Med.* **49**, 306–315.

Langford, H. G., and Snavely, J. R. (1959). Effect of DCA on development of renoprival hypertension. *Am. J. Physiol.* **196**, 449–450.

Ledingham, J. M. (1954). Hypertension and disturbances of tissue water, sodium and potassium distribution associated with steroid administration in adrenalectomized rats. *Clin. Sci.* **13**, 543–553.

Mayes, D., Furayama, S., Kem, D. C., and Nugent, C. A. (1970). A radioimmunoassay for plasma aldosterone. *J. Clin. Endocrinol. Metab.* **30**, 681–685.

Miller, A. W., Bohr, D. F., Schork, A. M., and Terris, J. M. (1979). Hemodynamic responses to DOCA in young pigs. *Hypertension* **1**, 591–597.

Musilova, H., Jelinek, J., and Albrecht, I. (1966). The age factor in experimental hypertension of the DCA type in rats. *Physiol. Bohemoslov.* **15**, 525–531.

Norman, R. A., Coleman, T. G., Wiley, T. L., Jr., Manning, R. D., Jr., and Guyton, A. C. (1975). Separate roles of sodium ion concentration and fluid volumes in salt-loading hypertension in sheep. *Am. J. Physiol.* **229**, 1068–1072.

Sturtevant, F. M. (1958). The biology of metacorticoid hypertension. *Ann. Intern. Med.* **49**, 1281–1293.

Tobian, L. (1960). Interrelationships of electrolytes, juxtaglomerular cells and hypertension. *Physiol. Rev.* **40**, 280–312.

Wenting, G. J., Man in't Veld, A. J., Verhoeven, R. P., Derkx, F. H. M., and Schalekamp, M. A. D. H. (1977). Volume pressure relationships during development of mineralocorticoid hypertension in man. *Circ. Res.* **40**, Suppl. I, I163–I170.

16

Some Characteristics of Hormonal and Salt Hypertension

CHARLES E. HALL AND SHIRLEY HUNGERFORD

I. INTRODUCTION

Adrenal regeneration hypertension (ARH) is an experimental disorder induced in rats by (1) enucleation of the adrenal glands, (2) mononephrectomy, and (3) the imposition of a high salt intake. All three were originally believed to be essential components (Skelton, 1959), but the latter is now known to be dispensable (Hall *et al.*, 1967). There is no doubt, however, that a high salt intake

233

greatly enhances development and exacerbates the condition. The optimal conditions for development of the syndrome are thus precisely those under which the mineralocorticoid adrenocortical hormone deoxycorticosterone (DOC) most effectively elicits very similar phenomena. Hence, it is not surprising that the regenerating adrenal glands should be suspected of hypersecreting deoxycorticosterone, a prime suspect in the etiology of ARH. Although evidence has been presented in support of that view (Brownie and Skelton, 1965; Brown et al., 1972), contrary opinions have also appeared (Grekin et al., 1972; Hauger-Klevene and Vecsei, 1976). There are also several respects in which the two disorders differ. Among these are (1) deoxycorticosterone-treated rats invariably develop saline polydipsia, whereas rats with regenerating adrenals do not always do so; (2) deoxycorticosterone hypertension is enhanced by, but is not dependent on mononephrectomy, which is essential to the development of ARH in rats drinking 1% NaCl solution; and (3) hypokalemia develops in DOCA-treated rats, but not in those with ARH. Recently, it has been shown that captopril, which effectively prevents or reverses a variety of experimental forms of hypertension, neither prevents the development of DOC hypertension in rats nor reverses the established condition (Douglas et al., 1979). Therefore, it seemed worthwhile to explore the effect of the drug on the course of ARH.

Deoxycorticosterone and salt-induced hypertension is often regarded as an accelerated form of salt hypertension, since the steroid enhances Na consumption and reduces its excretion. Another way of accelerating the development of salt hypertension is to increase the quantity of salt consumed, which can be done by adding sugar to saline solutions given rats to drink (Hall and Hall, 1964). The effect of captopril on this form of accelerated salt hypertension (ASH) was also explored.

The naturally occurring adrenal corticoids share a C-21 hydroxyl grouping, which is generally believed to be a requisite for mineralocorticoid activity. It was therefore surprising to learn that 19-norprogesterone was a potent hypertensogen (Komanicky and Melby, 1979), since the parent steroid, progesterone, is antimineralocorticoid (Landau et al., 1958; Sharp and Leaf, 1966) and antihypertensogenic (Armstrong, 1959; Laidlaw et al., 1964). Particularly baffling was the report that it caused adrenal enlargement, but failed to cause cardionephromegaly. A study was undertaken to examine the properties of this unusual steroid.

The fact that the 19-nor configuration could convert an antimineralocorticoid, natriuretic steroid, progesterone, into one having hypertensive activity comparable to that exhibited by the most potent mineralocorticoids raised a number of questions. Several androgens such as methylandrostenediol, methyltestosterone (Brownie et al., 1970), and testosterone (Colby et al., 1970) have been shown to cause hypertension in mononephrectomized, salt-loaded rats, accompanied by extreme atrophy of the adrenal glands. The latter display impaired 11-β-hydroxylation, leading to accumulation of 11-deoxycorticosterone, to which the hypertensive effect has been attributed. The last experiment compared the hypertensogenic properties of testosterone and 19-nortestosterone.

II. MATERIALS AND METHODS

Sprague–Dawley female rats were used in all of the studies. They were maintained individually caged in an environmentally controlled room, lighted 8 A.M.–8 P.M. Purina Laboratory Chow was fed *ad libitum*.

Conscious systolic blood pressures were obtained each week using the tail-cuff method. Successive pressures were taken until three consecutive values agreeing to within 15 mm Hg were obtained. These were averaged to obtain the value recorded, all other measurements being disregarded. Values above 150 mm Hg were regarded as hypertensive. Heart rates were taken through needle electrodes placed bilaterally through thoracic skin. The equipment consisted of a Mark IV Physiograph interfaced with a PE 300 Programmed Electrosphygmomanometer and a DD 350 Digital Display Unit (Narco Biosystems, Houston, Texas). Blood electrolytes were measured on a flame photometer (Model 343, Instrumentation Laboratories, Lexington, Mass.), and blood proteins with a protein meter (American Optical Co., Buffalo, N.Y.).

When fluid measurements were made, they were taken on three consecutive days weekly, and the average considered to be representative for the week.

Organs taken for weight and histology were removed at autopsy and placed in neutral 10% formalin. When fixed, they were removed, trimmed, blotted, and weighed on an analytical balance. Statistical comparisons utilized Student's double-tailed, unpaired t test.

A. Experiment 1

Thirty female Sprague–Dawley rats, 80–95 g, were divided into three equal groups. All animals were right mononephrectomized under ether anesthesia. Groups 1 and 2 were given a 5% sucrose 1% NaCl solution to drink, whereas group 3 received 5% sucrose solution. Fluid consumption was measured each week. The animals of group 1 received 100 mg/kg/day of captopril in physiological saline intraperitoneally in a single injection. Those of group 2 received only vehicle, and those of group 3 were not injected. The animals were killed with ether on the thirty-third day and various organs taken for weight and histology.

B. Experiment 2

Eighteen rats 80–95 g were divided into three equal groups. All animals were right nephroadrenalectomized and given 1% NaCl solution to drink. Those of groups 1 and 2 were left adrenal enucleated; those of group 3 sham operated. Beginning on the third postoperative day and daily thereafter, animals of group 1 each received 100 mg/kg/day of captopril in a single intraperitoneal injection. Animals of groups 2 and 3 each received only vehicle. Fluid consumption was measured. The animals were killed with ether on the thirty-third day.

C. Experiment 3

Twenty-six rats 80–100 g were divided into two groups of 14 and 12, respectively. All animals were right mononephrectomized and given 1% NaCl solution to drink. Animals of group 1 each received 1 mg/day of 19-norprogesterone in 0.1 ml sesame oil subcutaneously: those of group 2 received only the oil. Fluid intake was measured each week. A blood sample was taken on the twenty-eighth day by cardiac punture for plasma protein and serum Na^+ and K^+ measurement. The animals were then killed with ether and organs taken for study.

D. Experiment 4

Twenty-four rats weighing 80–100 g were divided into three equal groups. They were right mononephrectomized and given 1% NaCl solution to drink. Animals of groups 1 and 2 each received, respectively, 10 mg/day, in 0.2 ml of sesame oil subcutaneously, of testosterone, or 19-nortestosterone (Sigma Chemical Co.). Fluid consumption was measured only in the final week. On the thirty-sixth day a blood sample was taken by cardiac puncture for analysis. The animals were then killed with ether and autopsied.

III. RESULTS

A. Experiment 1

In general, captopril-treated rats drank less sucrose–saline solution than untreated animals (Fig. 1). The greatest volume consumption was exhibited by controls, drinking only sucrose solution (Fig. 2). In both groups drinking sucrose–saline, blood pressure rose at comparable rates during the first 2 weeks, but untreated rats continued to develop higher pressures during the following 2 weeks, by which time 70% were hypertensive (Table I). In eight rats, captopril reduced saline intake and all of these remained normotensive, seven having lower blood pressures terminally than they had initially. Two rats, however, displayed extreme saline polydipsia, and these ultimately became hypertensive despite drug treatment (Fig. 2); one of these was hypertensive from the second week onward, reaching the highest pressure of any rat in the experiment, 222 mm

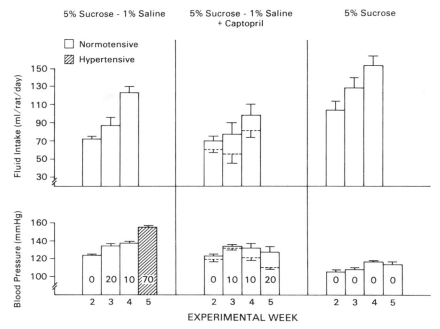

Fig. 1. Effect of captopril on sucrose–saline consumption and salt hypertension. The bars represent an average of the weekly values over the entire period. In controls drinking sucrose, fluid intake and blood pressure were not correlated. The three saline consuming rats remaining normotensive drank more than four of those that became hypertensive. Only when captopril reduced saline intake did it prevent hypertension.

TABLE I

Cardiovascular–Respiratory Findings in Rats Drinking Sucrose–Saline or Sucrose Solution: Effect of Captopril on the Former

Treatment	Week	No. rats[b]		Arterial pressure (mm Hg)	Heart rate (beats/min)	Respiration rate (breaths/min)
Sucrose–saline	1	10	(0)[a]	$124 \pm 1^{b,c}$	460 ± 6	98 ± 4
	2	10	(2)	135 ± 2^{b}	414 ± 8	98 ± 3
	3	10	(4)	138 ± 2^{b}	398 ± 8	98 ± 3
	4	10	(7)	155 ± 2^{b}	401 ± 10^{b}	88 ± 4
Sucrose–saline	1	10	(0)	123 ± 2^{b}	451 ± 7	102 ± 5
+ captopril	2	10	(0)	134 ± 2^{b}	419 ± 8	99 ± 4
	3	10	(1)	134 ± 2^{b}	416 ± 11	88 ± 3^{b}
	4	10	(2)	127 ± 7	429 ± 10	88 ± 3
Sucrose	1	10	(0)	106 ± 2	458 ± 22	103 ± 3
	2	10	(0)	108 ± 2	458 ± 22	104 ± 4
	3	10	(0)	117 ± 1	421 ± 5	100 ± 3
	4	10	(0)	114 ± 2	428 ± 12	88 ± 3

[a] Figures in parentheses indicate no. of hypertensives.
[b] Significantly different from controls ($p < 0.05$ or better).
[c] Mean $\pm$ SEM.

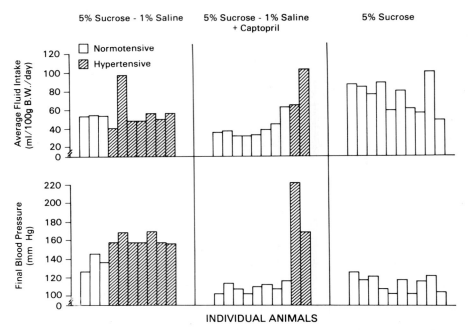

Fig. 2. Fluid consumption of individual rats averaged over the entire experiment and final blood pressures. Note that captopril prevented hypertension only when fluid intake was diminished.

Hg. The other one reached 169 mm Hg. These were the only two in their group having vascular lesions. Control animals remained normotensive.

Organ weights revealed that group 1 animals displayed cardionephromegaly. Captopril prevented cardiac but not kidney enlargement, and caused adrenomegaly (Table II).

B. Experiment 2

Captopril treatment had no discernible effect on either fluid consumption, the development of hypertension (Fig. 3), or the degree of cardionephromegaly (Table III) developed by adrenal-enucleate rats.

C. Experiment 3

Steroid treatment had no effect on growth rate, but caused a marked saline polydipsia (Fig. 4), and a progressive increase in blood pressure to hypertensive levels (Fig. 5).

Blood analysis revealed that rats treated with 19-norprogesterone developed a relative hypoproteinemia, hypernatremia, and hypokalemia (Table IV). They

TABLE II

Effect of Drinking Fluid and Captopril on Body and Organ Weight[a]

Data	Sucrose–saline		Sucrose[b]
	Vehicle[b]	Captopril[b]	
Body wt (g)			
Initial	86 ± 2[c]	89 ± 2	86 ± 2
Final	193 ± 4	189 ± 6	197 ± 4
Organ wt (mg/100 g body wt)			
Adrenals	30.5 ± 1.0	36.4 ± 1.4 (37.0 ± 1.2[d])	33.2 ± 0.9
Thymus	153 ± 6	104 ± 14[c] (108 ± 14[d])	152 ± 7
Heart	374 ± 13[d]	367 ± 34 (324 ± 9)	313 ± 5
Kidney	725 ± 21[d]	788 ± 59[c] (727 ± 14[d])	544 ± 11

[a] Figures in parentheses are averages from normotensives in group.

[b] Number of rats: 10.

[c] Mean ± SEM.

[d] Significantly different from control value ($p < 0.05$).

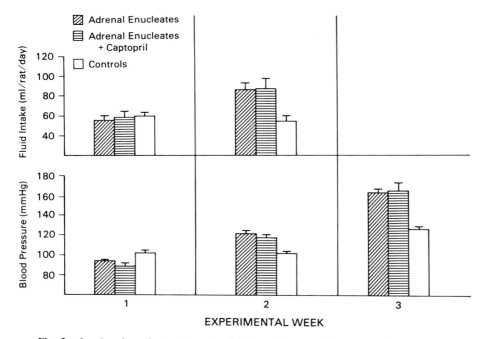

Fig. 3. In adrenal-enucleate rats, captopril had no effect on saline consumption or on blood pressure; ARH developed despite drug treatment.

TABLE III

Body and Organ Weight of Experimental and Control Animals

Weight	Adrenal enucleates		Controls[a]
	No drug[a]	Captopril[a]	
Body wt (g)			
Initial	89 ± 3[b]	90 ± 2	89 ± 3
Final	158 ± 5	158 ± 5	154 ± 5
Organ wt (mg/100 g body wt)			
Adrenals	17.1 ± 1.4[c]	16.3 ± 1.4[c]	23.2 ± 0.6
Heart	441 ± 25[c]	409 ± 8[c]	343 ± 10
Kidney	1114 ± 86[c]	1004 ± 56[c]	792 ± 15

[a] Number of rats: 6.

[b] Mean ± SEM.

[c] Significantly different from controls ($p < 0.01$ or better).

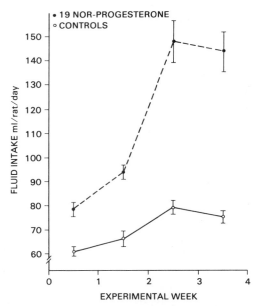

Fig. 4.   Rapid onset of marked saline polydipsia in 19-norprogesterone-treated rats. (From Hall *et al.*, 1981; reprinted by permission.)

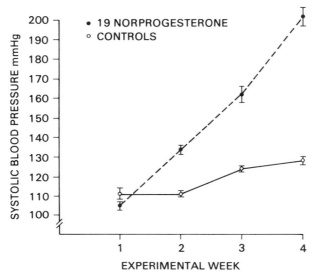

Fig. 5. Induction of arterial hypertension by 19-norprogesterone. (From Hall *et al.*, 1981; reprinted by permission.)

also exhibited cardionephromegaly, but no change in adrenal or thymus weight (Table V). Several of the hypertensives exhibited degenerative vascular lesions in hearts and kidneys (Table VI), like those seen in rats made hypertensive by potent mineralocorticoids.

D. Experiment 4

Testosterone-treated rats developed hypertension, but those given 19-nortestosterone remained entirely normotensive (Fig. 6).

TABLE IV

Effect of 19-Norprogesterone on Blood Protein, Sodium, and Potassium Concentration[a]

Data	19-Norprogesterone[b]	Controls[c]	p
Plasma protein (g/dl)	8.08 ± 0.11[d]	8.40 ± 0.07	0.03
Serum Na$^+$	138.9 ± 0.6	137.3 ± 0.4	0.04
Serum K$^+$	4.11 ± 0.14	4.67 ± 0.10	0.01

[a] From Hall *et al.* (1981); reprinted by permission.

[b] Number of rats: 13.

[c] Number of rats: 12.

[d] Mean $\pm$ SEM.

TABLE V

Body and Organ Weights of 19-Norprogesterone-Treated and Control Rats[a]

Data	19-Norprogesterone[b]	Controls[c]	p
Body wt (g)			
Initial	92 ± 2[d]	92 ± 2	NS
Final	237 ± 6	236 ± 4	NS
Organ weight (mg/100 g body wt)			
Kidney	856 ± 70	616 ± 28	< 0.005
Heart[e]	440 ± 15	311 ± 9	< 0.001
Thymus	149 ± 14	185 ± 12	NS
Adrenals	27.5 ± 1.2	26.7 ± 0.7	NS

[a] From Hall *et al.* (1981); reprinted by permission.
[b] Number of rats: 14.
[c] Number of rats: 12.
[d] Mean ± SEM.
[e] Ventricles only.

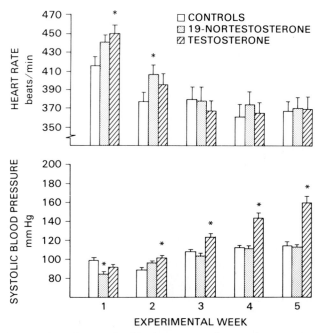

Fig. 6. Comparative changes in blood pressure of control, testosterone-, and 19-nortestosterone-treated rats.

TABLE VI

Observed Incidence of Renal and Cardiac Lesions in Experimental and Control Rats

Lesions		Experimentals[a,e]	Controls[b]
Cardiac lesions	% Incidence	50	0
	Severity[c]	0.79 ± 0.26^d (1.6 ± 0.3)	0
Nephrosclerosis	% Incidence	42.6	0
	Severity	0.86 ± 0.33 (2.4 ± 0.2)	0

[a] Number of rats: 14.

[b] Number of rats: 12.

[c] Arbitrarily graded on a scale of 0 to 3+ severity. From Hall *et al.* (1981); reprinted by permission.

[d] Mean ± SEM.

[e] Figures in parentheses reflect severity of lesions in animals having them: the preceding figure being derived from the entire group.

IV. DISCUSSION

Clearly, captopril in a dosage that reduced saline consumption in 80% of treated rats and prevented the development of salt hypertension in them had neither effect in animals undergoing adrenal regeneration. This indicates that whatever the fundamental mechanisms are in the two experimental conditions, they are qualitatively different, and that ARH is more than merely an accelerated form of salt hypertension. Strikingly, in ASH, 20% of treated rats behaved differently from 80% of them, as they also did in a confirmatory experiment of the disorder (C. E. Hall and S. Hungerford, unpublished observations). In these minority cases, animals developed a particularly high volume consumption of saline despite treatment with captopril, and an early fulminant form of hypertension. This suggests the possibility of more than one mechanism for hypertension in this disorder, one of which depends on the participation of angiotensin II and is therefore blocked by the enzyme inhibitor, the other being independent of such involvement. In the confirmatory experiment previously alluded to, it was found that the unusual minority hypertensive response was associated with a markedly elevated serum renin activity, identifying these as forms of high renin hypertension.

Treatment with 19-norprogesterone resulted in exactly the same responses as treatment with potent mineralocorticoids such as aldosterone, DOC, or 19-nor-DOC: including marked saline polydipsia, hypernatremia, hypokalemia, hypertension, and vascular lesions. Cardionephromegaly was evident, but not adrenomegaly: these changes are exactly opposite to those reported to occur with a lower dosage of the steroid (Komanicky and Melby, 1979).

In studies reported elsewhere (Hall *et al.*, 1981) we have, in fact, found

19-norprogesterone to be a potent mineralocorticoid. The absence of the 21 hydroxyl grouping, considered as requisite for that activity, necessitates a reassessment of structural requirements for a mineralocorticoid, unless it develops that the C-21 methyl group is hydroxylated endogenously to yield 19-nordeoxycorticosterone. In man, endogenous conversion of progesterone to deoxycorticosterone has been reported (Winkel *et al.*, 1980), but whether the rat can convert the 19-nor derivative is uncertain.

The parent steroid, progesterone, has both antimineralocorticoid saluretic (Landau *et al.*, 1955; Sharp and Leaf, 1966) and antihypertensive actions (Armstrong, 1959; Laidlaw *et al.*, 1964). If these actions of progesterone were inherent properties of its primary activity as a gestagen, 19-norprogesterone should be even more effective in both respects, since it has 4–8 times the gestagenic potency of the parent steroid (Djerassi *et al.*, 1953). Since the antimineralocorticoid and antihypertensive actions are reversed rather than enhanced in 19-norprogesterone, it is evident that they are not dependent on luteoid potency.

The same C-10 demethylation that enhances the gestagenic potency of progesterone, simultaneously reversing its antimineralocorticoid and antihypertensive properties, both weakens the androgenic activity of testosterone (Wilds and Nelson, 1953) and abolishes its hypertensive and sodium-retaining effects. In this instance, therefore, the subsidiary sodium-retaining and hypertensive effects may reflect the primary androgenic activity.

V. SUMMARY

The angiotensin converting enzyme inhibitor, captopril, was ineffective in protecting against adrenal regeneration hypertension as well as the saline polydipsia accompanying this condition. In accelerated salt hypertension the response was quite different. In 80% of the rats, both saline polydipisia and hypertension were prevented. Twenty percent of the animals, however, were refractory; in these, saline intake was excessive; fulminant hypertension developed and severe vascular lesions were found.

In a second type of experiment, the hypertensive effect of 19-norprogesterone was explored in mononephrectomized, salt-loaded rats. The occurrence of saline polydipsia and hypertension was confirmed. Adrenomegaly, however, was absent and both cardio- and nephromegaly were present, along with severe vascular lesions, hypokalemia, and hypernatremia.

Progesterone does not have hypertensive effects in mammals, and yet 19-norprogesterone does; 19-nordeoxycorticosterone has about the same hypertensive potency as deoxycorticosterone.

Testosterone has also been shown to cause hypertensive vascular disease in mononephrectomized, salt-loaded rats. A comparison was made between the hypertensive potency of testosterone and 19-nortestosterone in such rats. The former caused hypertension, but the latter was completely inert at comparable dosage (10 mg/rat/day). It is thus apparent that the hypertensive efficacy of the 19-norconfiguration, evident in certain pregnene steroids, does not extend to those in the androstene series.

ACKNOWLEDGMENTS

These studies were carried out under a grant HL 09911 from the National Institutes of Health. These studies are to be published in part in *Endocrinology* and in the *Journal of Steroid Biochemistry*.

Drs. C. E. Gomez-Sanchez and E. P. Gomez-Sanchez were responsible for synthesizing the 19-norprogesterone and suggesting the experiment. They have also established the mineralocorticoid potency of the steroid.

Captopril was generously supplied by Dr. Z. P. Horovitz of the Squibb Institute of Medical Research.

REFERENCES

Armstrong, J. G. (1959). Hypotensive action of progesterone in experimental and human hypertension. *Proc. Soc. Exp. Biol. Med.* **102,** 452–455.

Brown, R. D., Gaunt, R., Gisoldi, E., and Smith, N. (1972). The role of deoxycorticosterone in adrenal-regeneration hypertension. *Endocrinology* **91,** 921–924.

Brownie, A. C., and Skelton, F. R. (1965). The metabolism of progesterone 4-^{14}C by adrenal homogenates from rats with adrenal regeneration hypertension. *Steroids* **6,** 47–68.

Brownie, A. C., Colby, H. D., Gallant, S., and Skelton, F. R. (1970). Some studies on the effect of androgens on adrenal cortical function of rats. *Endocrinology* **86,** 1085–1092.

Colby, H. D., Skelton, F. R., and Brownie, A. C. (1970). Testosterone-induced hypertension in the rat. *Endocrinology* **86,** 1093–1111.

Djerassi, C., Miramontes, L., and Rosencranz, G. (1953). Steroids. XLVIII. 19-Norprogesterone, a potent progestational hormone. *J. Am. Chem. Soc.* **75,** 4440–4442.

Douglas, H., Langford, H. G., and McCaa, R. E. (1979). Response of mineralocorticoid hypertensive animals to an angiotensin 1 converting enzyme inhibitor. *Proc. Soc. Exp. Biol. Med.* **161,** 86–87.

Grekin, R. J., Dale, S. L., Gaunt, R., and Melby, J. C. (1972). Steroid secretion by the enucleated rat adrenal. Measurements during salt retention and development of hypertension. *Endocrinology* **91,** 1166–1171.

Hall, C. E., and Hall, O. (1964). Salt hypertension: Facilitated induction in two rat strains. *Tex. Rep. Biol. Med.* **22,** 529–549.

Hall, C. E., Holland, O. B., and Hall, O. (1967). Benign and malignant hypertension following adrenal enucleation in the rat. Relationship to salt intake, response to hydrochlorothiazide, and similarity to essential hypertension. *J. Exp. Med.* **126,** 168–177.

Hall, C. E., Gomez-Sanchez, C. E., Hungerford, S., and Gomez-Sanchez, E. P. (1981). On the mineralocorticoid and hypertensive effects of 19-nor-progesterone. *Endocrinology* **109,** 1168–1175.

Hauger-Klevene, J., and Vecsei, P. (1976). Deoxycorticosterone measured by a radioimmunoassay *in vivo* in rats undergoing adrenal-regeneration. *Clin. Sci. Mol. Med.* **51,** Suppl. 3, 299–301S.

Komanicky, P., and Melby, J. C. (1979). 19-Nor-progesterone produces hypertension in the rat. *ASCI Hypertension* **27,** 467A.

Laidlaw, J. C., Yendt, E. R., Bird, C. E., and Gornall, A. G. (1964). Hypertension due to renal artery occlusion simulating primary aldosteronism. *Can. Med. Assoc. J.* **90,** 321–325.

Landau, R. L., and Lugibihl, K. (1958). Inhibition of the sodium-retaining influence of aldosterone by progesterone. *J. Clin. Endocrinol. Metab.* **18,** 1237–1245.

Sharp, G. W. G., and Leaf, A. (1966). Mechanisms of action of aldosterone. *Physiol. Rev.* **46,** 593–633.

Skelton, F. R. (1959). Adrenal regeneration and adrenal-regeneration hypertension. *Physiol. Rev.* **39,** 162–182.

Wilds, A. L., and Nelson, N. A. (1953). The facile synthesis of 19-nor-testosterone and 19-nor-androstenedione from estrone. *J. Am. Chem. Soc.* **75,** 5366–5369.

Winkel, C. A., Milewich, L., Parker, C. R., Jr., Grant, N. F., Simpson, E. R., and MacDonald, P. C. (1980). Conversion of plasma progesterone to deoxycorticosterone in men, nonpregnant and pregnant women and adrenalectomized subjects. Evidence for steroid 21-hydroxylase activity in nonadrenal tissues. *J. Clin. Invest.* **66,** 803–812.

17

Importance of the Antinatriuretic Effects of Angiotensin and Aldosterone in Hypertension

DAVID B. YOUNG, YI-JEN PAN, JOHN E. HALL, AND THOMAS E. LOHMEIER

I. INTRODUCTION

Sodium and hypertension. Angiotensin, aldosterone, and sodium. Angiotensin, aldosterone, and hypertension. So provocatively are these elements intertwined that their interrelationships have attracted the devoted interest of many

247

of us for decades. A quantity of data has arisen from our interest but often those data merely demonstrated how complicated is the entanglement of these factors. Is there a thread of logic we can use to explain the relationships, that we can follow through the clinical reports, a thread that also weaves through the experimental studies of angiotensin, aldosterone, sodium, and hypertension? And if there is a consistent logic present, does it reflect on the nature of hypertension in the general case? I wish to pursue these questions by analyzing several of the interrelationships separately and then attempt to integrate the infromation around a consistent theme of arterial pressure regulation. While special emphasis will be placed on the importance of the relationship between angiotensin and aldosterone and their sodium retaining effects in hypertension, I also must consider several associated functions of importance in arterial pressure control.

II. SODIUM EXCRETION

A. Arterial Pressure

In any discussion of sodium and arterial hypertension, an obvious anatomical and functional relationship must be considered: In the general case, the kidney is attached to the arterial system. Just as there is no way to escape the obviousness of the anatomical relationship, the functional significance of the relationship between arterial pressure and renal function cannot be avoided. Arterial pressure does affect directly several aspects of renal function including sodium excretion. Selkurt *et al.* (1949), Shipley and Study (1951), Thompson and Pitts (1952), Baer *et al.* (1970), Thompson and Dickinson (1976), and many others demonstrated over the last 30 years that sodium excretion increases as arterial pressure is increased in anesthetized dogs, rabbits, and rats. This phenomenon is well known; however, I wish to stress the quantitative aspects of the relationship. Shown in Fig. 1 is the relationship between renal perfusion pressure and sodium excretion which has been compiled from the normalized data of the studies mentioned above. Notice that sodium excretion falls to zero at a perfusion pressure of approximately 50 mm Hg and rises to the normal value at the normal level of mean arterial pressure, 100 mm Hg. Raising perfursion pressure by only 10 mm Hg above normal will result in a 60–75% increase in sodium excretion. It is interesting to note that in all the studies cited, the data were highly consistent in this range around the normal arterial pressure level: Baer and Selkurt both reported a 60% increase in sodium excretion from 100 to 110 mm Hg; Thompson and Pitts, 62%; and Thompson and Dickinson, 75%.

The relationship described from these acute studies performed in anesthetized, surgically prepared animals demonstrates that arterial pressure has a powerful effect on sodium excretion. However, work recently completed in our laboratory

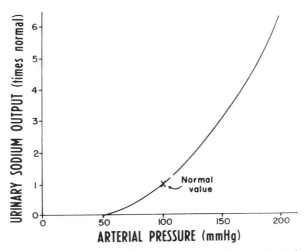

Fig. 1. Presented here is the relationship between renal perfusion pressure in mm Hg versus sodium excretion expressed as per cent of the control value (rate of excretion when perfusion pressure equals 100 mm Hg). Data from Baer *et al.* (1970), Selkurt *et al.* (1949), Shipley and Study (1951), Thompson and Pitts (1952), and Thompson and Dickinson (1976) were normalized and used to construct the relationship.

by Pan *et al.* (1978) demonstrates that these older studies underestimate the actual physiological effect by severalfold. Pan's work differs from the previous experiments in that the data were gathered from conscious animals for several days after the level of perfusion pressure to the kidney was changed. The work was done with dogs whose bladders were split into two hemibladders, each drained by a catheter which was implanted through the bladder wall. The urethra was ligated. Therefore, the urine from each kidney could be collected for extended periods in containers carried by the dogs in a jacket. The animals also had an externally adjustable clamp around the aorta between the renal arteries, and catheters implanted via the femoral artery in the aorta above and below the clamp. Following recovery from the surgery, perfusion pressure to the more caudal kidney could be reduced by tightening the clamp. As a result, the two kidneys would be exposed to identical conditions with respect to circulating hormones, ions, temperature, and neural input; the only difference would be perfusion pressure, which differed by a controlled amount. Using this powerful preparation, Pan was able to analyze the effects of changes in perfusion pressure on renal function in conscious dogs for periods of several days. Three to four days were required for sodium excretion to stabilize at a new level following a change in pressure. Shown in Fig. 2 are data taken on the sixth day following adjustment of the constrictor. The data are expressed as the pressure gradient between the two kidneys versus the ratio of sodium excretion from the two.

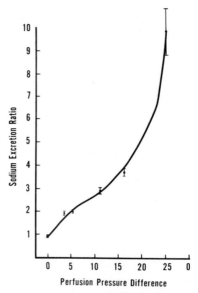

Fig. 2. Presented in this figure is the steady-state relationship between perfusion pressure difference between the two kidneys of dogs and the ratio of sodium excretion from the two kidneys. The perfusion pressure difference was induced by tightening an externally adjustable clamp on the aorta between the two renal arteries.

Notice that at a pressure gradient of about 5 mm Hg, there is a twofold difference in excretion. Whereas the acute effect of a 10 mm Hg change in perfusion pressure was a 60 to 75% change in excretion (Fig. 1), the steady-state effect is a threefold change in excretion.

The renal mechanisms responsible for the dramatic effect of small changes in perfusion pressure on sodium excretion are of interest but lie beyond the goal of this presentation. One point is worth reemphasizing; that is, the two kidneys received identical input from the rest of the body except for perfusion pressure. Therefore, the intrarenal mechanisms responsible for the natriuresis were driven solely by variations in arterial pressure.

B. Angiotensin

Angiotensin II is described frequently as the most potent vasoconstrictor substance known. The peptide's existence was verified by its action on vascular smooth muscle, and for two decades, concentrations of angiotensin in plasma were quantified by determining its pressor effect in bioassay procedures. In view of its history, it is not surprising that its renal effects received little attention until about 10 years ago when William Waugh (1972) demonstrated that small amounts of angiotensin II infused into the renal artery sharply inhibited sodium excretion. Since then, several studies have been conducted in our laboratory in an effort to define angiotensin's direct role in regulation of sodium excretion.

Beginning in 1975, Fagard *et al.* (1978) investigated the effects of slight elevations in renal artery angiotensin II concentration on renal function in anesthetized dogs. Angiotensin was infused directly into the renal artery during 20 min periods in four doses ranging from 125 to 1000 pg/kg/min. These rates gave calculated increases in angiotensin II concentration from two to ten times the normal sodium replete values. Sodium excretion was affected in a very consistent manner, as can be seen in Fig. 3. Even at the lowest rate of infusion, which gave a calculated increase of approximately 100% in arterial angiotensin II levels, sodium excretion fell by $17 \pm 3\%$ ($p < 0.05$), and at higher rates of infusion of angiotensin, sodium excretion was reduced to one-half normal. Fagard's study clearly demonstrated the powerful acute effects of angiotensin in concentrations within the physiological range on sodium excretion and other renal variables important in long-term control of blood pressure.

Fagard's study was a direct approach to the question of the importance of angiotensin II in regulation of sodium excretion and renal function. Their results and conclusions received strong support from two later experiments designed to look at the same subject in a different way. Hall *et al.* (1977) and Lohmeier *et al.* (1977) blocked the renal renin–angiotensin system and measured renal function in dogs that had elevated plasma renin concentrations. In both studies, the competitive angiotensin antagonist [Sar[1], Ile[8]]angiotensin II, was infused into the

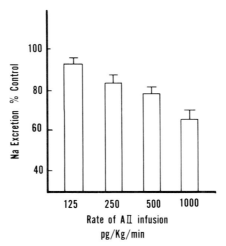

Fig. 3.   The effect of renal arterial infusion of angiotensin II at low rates on sodium excretion in the anesthetized dog. Means and standard errors of the mean are indicated.

renal artery of dogs for up to 90 min. In sodium depleted, anesthetized dogs studied by Hall, renal blood flow, glomerular filtration rate, urine flow, and sodium excretion all increased sharply as a result of blocking the intrarenal effects of angiotensin II. Sodium excretion increased more than fourfold from 0.087 ± 0.002 to 0.380 ± 0.001 μEq/min/g kidney weight, while urine flow increased more than 50%. None of the changes was the result of alterations in plasma aldosterone concentration since its concentration remained unchanged throughout the study.

Lohmeier *et al.* (1977) performed a similar study in which the dogs were conscious and any possible contribution of changes in aldosterone was eliminated by prior adrenalectomy followed by continuous replacement of aldosterone and hydrocortisone at constant levels. Their results, a portion of which are shown in Fig. 4, also indicate the blockade of the renal effects of angiotensin II results in marked increased in excretion of sodium and water, as well as increases in renal blood flow and glomerular filtration rate.

For understanding the contribution of the renal effects of angiotensin in hypertension, the value of the data from the previously mentioned experiments was limited somewhat by the fact that all of the experiments were carried out acutely over a period of only a few minutes, and hypertension is a long-term abnormality. Therefore, we carried out several other experiments to study the renal effects of angiotensin over a longer period of time. Young *et al.* (1980) infused angiotensin II at a rate of 10 ng/kg/min into dogs for 8 days and noted decreased sodium excretion only on the first day of infusion. The decrease in excretion was to 50% of the control level even though arterial pressure *increased* to 135% of normal. At the end of 8 days of infusion, when arterial pressure stabilized at

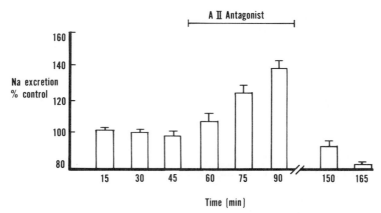

Fig. 4. Presented here are the effects of the competitive angiotensin II antagonist [Sar[1],Ile[8]]angiotensin II on sodium excretion in adrenalectomized conscious dogs. Means and standard errors of the mean are presented.

160% of control, sodium excretion had returned to the normal rate. In Pan's study of the effects of perfusion pressure on sodium excretion, the highest pressure gradient achieved was 25 mm Hg, approximately 25%. At that gradient there was a tenfold difference in sodium excretion between the two kidneys. In this study, the 60% increase in perfusion pressure would have resulted in a massive increase in sodium excretion if renal function had not been altered by the infusion of angiotensin. Therefore, even though sodium retention was evident only on the first day of infusion of angiotensin II, the peptide continued to exert a powerful effect on sodium excretion for the duration of the study. The observed antinatriuretic effect probably was not due to increases in aldosterone concentration since, in several experiments under nearly identical conditions, McCaa (1977) showed that continued angiotensin II infusion in dogs results in large increments in the concentration of aldosterone in plasma only on the first day of infusion.

Hall *et al.* (1978) conducted a study similar to the one by Young *et al.* described previously. In addition to finding a pattern of sodium excretion nearly identical to that described above, they noted that prolonged intravenous angiotensin II caused a sharp fall in renal plasma flow but no change in filtration rate.

DeClue *et al.* (1978) studied the long-term effects of angiotensin on renal function in dogs by manipulating sodium intake while holding angiotensin levels constant by continuous intravenous infusion of 5 ng of angiotensin II/kg/min. They varied sodium intake over approximately a 100-fold range in four steps from less than 5 to more than 500 mEq/day. The animals were permitted several days to come into sodium balance at each step. In the dogs receiving angiotensin, arterial pressures rose 39 mm Hg as the sodium intake was increased, while in the control group that was subjected to the identical sodium load but with no angiotensin infusion, arterial pressure rose only 3 mm Hg. As in previous experiments, aldosterone concentration was not affected significantly by the sustained angiotensin infusion. Once again, this study demonstrates that angiotensin exerts a powerful antinatriuretic effect that must be overcome by increases in renal perfusion pressure in order for the system to return to sodium balance.

Interpretation of the results of experiments employing long-term intravenous infusion of angiotensin to study its renal effects are complicated by the possibility that the angiotensin may indirectly affect renal function. Recently, Lohmeier and Cowley (1979) have completed a study that more clearly identifies the direct intrarenal role of angiotensin in long-term control of sodium excretion. They infused 1 ng of angiotensin II/kg/min into the renal artery of dogs for 10 days. Since 75% of the angiotensin II is cleared by the kidney, this rate of infusion had negligible effects outside the renal circulation. However, the renal effects of this low level of infusion were striking (Fig. 5). Sodium excretion fell to approximately 60% of the control level on the first day of infusion before returning to the

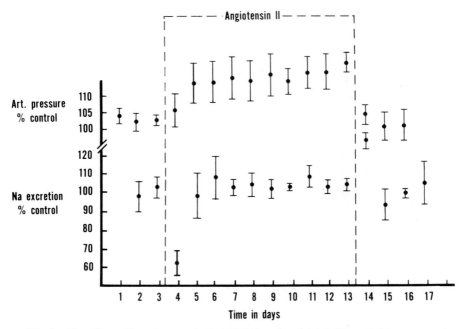

Fig. 5.   The effects of long-term renal-arterial infusion of angiotensin II on arterial pressure and sodium excretion are presented in this figure. Note that the low rate of infusion, 1 ng/kg/min caused no initial increase in arterial pressure. Means and standard errors of the mean are shown.

normal rate by the second day of the study. Glomerular filtration rate fell to less than 90% of control for the first 7 days of the study. Return to sodium balance was associated with a 15 mm Hg increase in arterial pressure, once again demonstrating the interactions between angiotensin, sodium excretion, and arterial pressure.

Data from the experiments reviewed thus far can be used to predict the effects of high levels of angiotensin in hypertensive states. It would be even more helpful, however, to study directly angiotensin's renal effects in established forms of hypertension. Several such investigations are now under way, one of which has been completed by Bengis *et al.* (1978) who inhibited angiotensin formation for several days with an orally administered converting enzyme inhibitor in one-kidney Goldblatt hypertensive rats. Blockade resulted in a 33% increase in sodium excretion and a 15% decrease in arterial pressure. Cessation of converting enzyme inhibition reversed the increase in excretion and fall in arterial pressure.

The results of these studies, carried out in eight different experimental models, all sharply point out the potency of the direct antinatriuretic effect of angiotensin.

Regardless of whether the experiment involved infusion of physiological amounts of the peptide for periods of minutes, hours, days, or weeks, or whether they consisted of blocking the effects of the endogenous renin–angiotensin system, the data led to a common conclusion: The direct action of angiotensin II on renal function is of major importance in controlling the rate of sodium excretion.

Stated another way, these investigations have demonstrated that angiotensin II alters the normal relationship between the level of renal perfusion pressure and the rate of sodium excretion: at a given level of arterial pressure, increasing angiotensin II concentration will decrease sodium excretion. This relationship was demonstrated repeatedly in the experiments described. The initial effect of infusion of angiotensin was a drastic reduction in sodium excretion. In each of the long-term experiments, the effect of changes in angiotensin concentration on the relationship between renal perfusion pressure and sodium excretion was compensated for by an offsetting change in the level of arterial pressure.

C. Aldosterone

Aldosterone's sodium retaining properties are widely appreciated and do not need extensive review here. However, I would like to present some information regarding the apparent mineralocorticoid escape seen in some forms of hypertension. Shown in Fig. 6 are arterial pressures from a group of adrenalectomized dogs (Young and Guyton, 1977) that received aldosterone replacement at four levels, 16, 48, 91, and 216 µg/day, 48 µg/day being the approximate normal value for the 22 kg dogs. Each level was maintained for 10 days, enough time for the animals to come into electrolyte balance on the 30 mEq/day sodium intake. Apparently, the dogs had escaped from the salt-retaining effects of the supranormal levels of aldosterone and had returned to daily sodium balance. However,

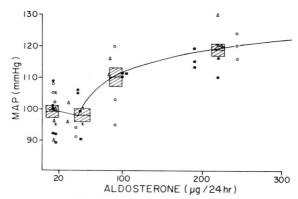

Fig. 6. The steady-state relationship between rate of aldosterone administration and mean arterial pressure in adrenalectomized dogs. (From Young and Guyton, 1977.)

the increase in rate of infusion of aldosterone from the normal level to 91 μg/day was accompanied by a 10 mm Hg rise in mean arterial pressure; further increasing the rate of infusion of aldosterone to 4.5 times normal was attended by an additional increase in pressure to 119 mm Hg. Considering the data presented in Fig. 2 concerning the effect of perfusion pressure on sodium excretion, it is apparent that renal function continued to be strongly affected by the elevated aldosterone levels even though the dogs had returned to sodium balance. If the sodium-retaining effect had, in fact, waned, then sodium excretion from the kidneys perfused at these elevated arterial pressures would be expected to be many times the normal 30 mEq/day.

Recently, Pan and Young (1978) have completed an investigation of the renal effects of chronic high physiological levels of administration of aldosterone in the dog. Infusion of approximately 5 times the normal level of aldosterone resulted in an increase in arterial pressure of approximately 30% from the control level of 87 mm Hg. By the fourth day of infusion, the animals had returned to daily sodium balance. However, glomerular filtration rate and filtered sodium load remained 15–20% above control for the duration of the 16 day infusion period (Fig. 7); the mineralocorticoid continued to exert its sodium-retaining effect on the postglomerular portion of the nephron. Furthermore, this effect must account for the fact that the kidneys perfused at pressures 30% above

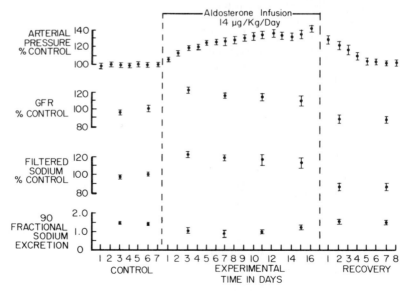

Fig. 7. Effects of continuous infusion of aldosterone at approximately five times the normal rate on arterial pressure, GFR, filtered sodium, and fractional excretion of sodium in dogs. Mean and standard errors of the mean are presented.

normal did not excrete sodium at a rate ten times greater than the control value, as would be predicted from the data presented in Fig. 2.

III. SODIUM AND HYPERTENSION

To this point the presentation has focused on the renal handling of sodium and the effects of arterial pressure, angiotensin, and aldosterone on renal function. For sodium to have a role in hypertension, it must have a cardiovascular effect. A number of studies carried out in Jackson, Mississippi, and elsewhere over the last

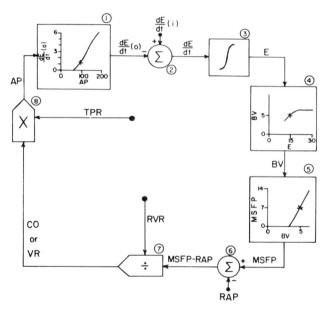

Fig. 8. Basic feedback control loop for regulation of fluid volume and arterial pressure. *Block 1* represents the relationship between arterial pressure and rate of renal excretion of extracellular fluid (E). The relationship is similar to that shown in Figs. 1 and 2. *Block 2* is a summation of the rate of excretion of E and the rate of intake. The result of the summation is the rate of change of E which when integrated over a period of time (*Block 3*) yields the value of extracellular volume, E. *Block 4* represents the relationship between E and blood volume, BV. In *Block 5* the relationship between blood volume and mean systemic filling pressure, MSFP, is determined. *Block 6* represents the subtraction of right atrial pressure from MSFP which yields the driving pressure for movement of blood back to the heart. Division of this driving pressure by the resistance to venous return (RVR) in *Block 7* yields the rate of flow of blood back to the heart, which is also equal to cardiac output, CO. Multiplication of CO by total peripheral resistance, TPR, at *Block 8* yields arterial pressure which is then used in *Block 1* to determine the rate of fluid excretion. See Guyton (1980) for a more complete discussion of the feedback system.

two decades has illustrated the mechanisms of its cardiovascular actions. I would like to review briefly these studies.

A simple, direct experimental model was developed in Jackson to analyze the role of sodium in hypertension. First used by Douglas *et al.* (1964) nearly 20 years ago, the model consists of the dog with 70% of its renal mass surgically removed. On a normal sodium intake the dog is normotensive. However, at increased levels of sodium, arterial pressure increases. Investigation of the events leading to the increase in arterial pressure revealed the following sequence: When sodium intake is increased, the reduced renal mass is incapable of excreting sodium at the rate of intake. A positive sodium balance results, which in turn leads to increased blood volume, increased mean circulatory filling pressure, pressure gradient for venous return, cardiac output, peripheral resistance, and arterial pressure. The positive balance continues to drive the other variables to higher levels until renal perfusion pressure increases to a point such that sodium excretion increases to match the level of intake. When balance is achieved, arterial pressure stabilizes although the other variables mentioned may go through transient changes before they achieve stable values. This series of studies has illustrated two important principles: (1) A positive sodium balance will lead to increased blood volume which will result in an increase in arterial pressure by various combinations of changes in cardiac output and total peripheral resistance. (2) A positive sodium balance will continue until renal perfusion pressure rises to a point that raises sodium excretion to the level of intake. These two principles form the basis of a simple negative feedback control loop for regulation of arterial pressure which has been described extensively by Guyton and co-workers (Guyton, 1980) and is illustrated in Fig. 8. Although this scheme is stripped of all hormonal, neural and local vascular regulatory mechanisms, it does represent the critical loop from renal function to sodium balance to hemodynamics and back to renal function that is of central importance in the control of fluid volume and arterial pressure.

IV. ANGIOTENSIN, ALDOSTERONE, SODIUM, AND HYPERTENSION

To analyze the interrelationship between angiotensin and aldosterone with sodium in hypertension, we prepared experimental models of angiotensin- and aldosterone-induced hypertensions. The emphasis was to study the effects of the hormones on the complete renal and cardiovascular systems so that we could analyze clearly the complex interrelated events that led to the hypertension.

Angiotensin-induced hypertension was achieved in dogs by infusing continuously iv 10 ng angiotensin II/kg/min (Young *et al.*, 1980). Sodium intake was held at 200 mEq/day, approximately 5 times normal. Shown in Fig. 9 are mean

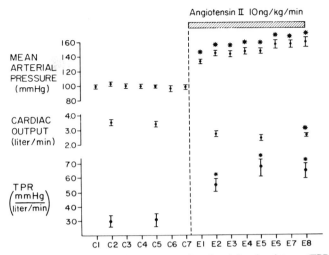

Fig. 9. Mean arterial pressure, cardiac output, and total peripheral resistance (TPR) data during the 7-day control period (labeled C1–C7) and the 8 days of angiotensin II infusion (labeled E1–E8). Means and standard errors of the mean are indicated. Statistically significant changes from control values are denoted by asterisk. (From Young *et al.*, 1980.)

arterial pressure, cardiac output (measured by dye dilution), and total peripheral resistance during the control period (days C1–C7) and during infusion of angiotensin (days E1–E8). Arterial pressure averaged between 96 and 103 mm Hg during the control period. Ten minutes after the beginning of infusion of angiotensin II at a rate of 10 ng/kg/min, the pressure increased to an average of 135 ± 3 mm Hg, and 24 hr later (day E1 in the figure) the arterial pressure remained nearly unchanged at 133 ± 3 mm Hg. By day 8 of infusion of angiotensin, arterial pressure had stabilized at a level of 160 ± 7 mm Hg. Cardiac output averaged 3.5 ± 0.2 liters/min and 3.4 ± 0.2 liters/min during the control period and fell to 2.7 ± 0.2 liters/min by the second day of infusion of angiotensin II, and further to 2.4 ± 0.2 liters/min ($0.05 < p < 0.10$) on day 5 and 2.6 ± 0.1 liters/min ($p < 0.01$) on the final day of the study.

Total peripheral resistance (TPR) was calculated from the mean arterial pressure and cardiac output. The data expressed as mm Hg/liter/min are shown at the bottom of Fig. 9. The two control measurements were 30 ± 2 units and 31 ± 3 units on days 2 and 5. Angiotensin II brought about a large increase in TPR to 55 ± 4 units ($p < 0.001$) on the second day of infusion, and further to 67 ± 6 units ($p < 0.001$) and 65 ± 5 units ($p < 0.001$) on days 5 and 8 of infusion.

Shown in Fig. 10 are the renal function data from the study. Twenty-four hour urine volume did not change from the control range of from approximately 500 to 700 ml/day until the fourth day of angiotensin infusion; however, water excretion

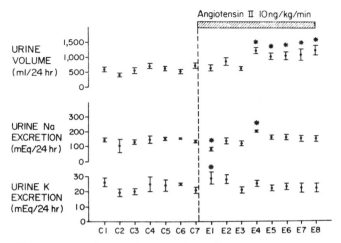

Fig. 10. Urine volume, urinary sodium excretion, and urinary potassium excretion data; abbreviations and symbols as in Fig. 9. (From Young *et al.*, 1980.)

was significantly elevated for the last 5 days of the study, being greater than 1000 ml/day.

The center panel of the figure presents data for sodium excretion during the study. On the first day of infusion, excretion fell to 50% of control even though arterial pressure had increased by 35 mm Hg. Recalling once again the information presented in Fig. 2, the 50% reduction in excretion in the face of such an increase in perfusion pressure demonstrates the powerful antinatriuretic effect of angiotensin. Daily balance was attained by the fifth day of infusion, at perfusion pressures 50–60 mm Hg greater than the control values.

A significant kaliuresis was observed on the initial days of angiotensin II infusion; potassium excretion increased from 21 ± 2 mEq/day on the last control day to 29 ± 4 mEq/day ($p < 0.05$) and 28 ± 3 mEq/liter ($0.10 < p < 0.05$) on the first 2 days of the infusion of angiotensin. For the rest of the study, the dogs were in potassium balance.

Presented in Fig. 11 are data for body weight, ^{22}Na space, and blood volume. Body weight remained nearly constant during the control period, the group average staying between 19.0 and 19.2 kg. Angiotensin infusion resulted in a first day increase of 0.5 kg ($p < 0.01$), an increase that persisted through the fourth day of the hypertension before body weight returned to the control range. Sodium space and blood volume remained nearly constant throughout the experiment.

In summary, angiotensin infusion together with a high sodium intake produced a form of hypertension characterized hemodynamically by intense vascular constriction. The changes in arterial pressure and peripheral resistance were similar

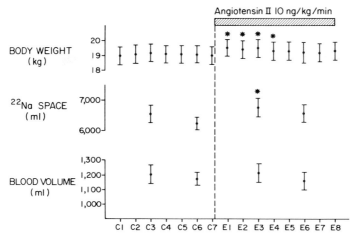

Fig. 11. Body weight, ^{22}Na space, and blood volume data; abbreviations and symbols as in Fig. 9. (From Young *et al.*, 1980.)

to those observed by others studying this model of hypertension. Volume retention was slight and transient while cardiac output decreased significantly. A striking alteration in renal function followed infusion of angiotensin, as demonstrated by the 50% reduction in sodium excretion immediately following adminstration of angiotensin even though arterial pressure increased 35 mm Hg. Balance was achieved when the renal perfusion pressure rose to 50 to 60 mm Hg above the control level.

Aldosterone-induced hypertension was established (Pan and Young, 1978) in a group of dogs by continuous iv infusion of 14 μg/kg/day, approximately five times the normal level. Sodium intake was maintained at a level approximately five times normal also.

Shown in Fig. 12 are arterial pressure and volume measurements made during the course of the 31 day study. During the 16 day infusion of aldosterone, arterial pressure rose from 87 to 117 mm Hg, a 35% increase. Iothalamate space (second panel), which is a measure of extracellular volume, increased by approximately 10%, as did blood volume (third panel).

Cardiac output (not shown) was measured by dye dilution. No consistent change from the control value of 2.9 liters/min could be detected as a result of infusion of aldosterone.

Electrolyte excretion data are presented in Fig. 13. In the upper panel, note that sodium excretion fell drastically on the first day of aldosterone infusion and then gradually rose as arterial pressure and renal perfusion pressure increased. Balance was reached when arterial pressure rose to 130–135% of the control level.

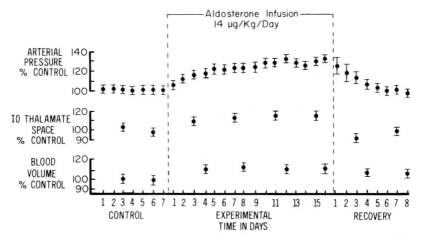

Fig. 12. Effect of infusion of aldosterone at approximately five times the normal rate on arterial pressure, iothalamate space, and blood volume in dogs. Means and standard errors of the means are shown.

In summary, this model of aldosterone hypertension was characterized by sodium and volume retention, increased blood volume, unchanged cardiac output, and increased peripheral resistance. Altered renal function was apparent, particularly regarding the relationship between perfusion pressure and sodium excretion. Sodium balance was not achieved until perfusion pressure reached 135% of the control level.

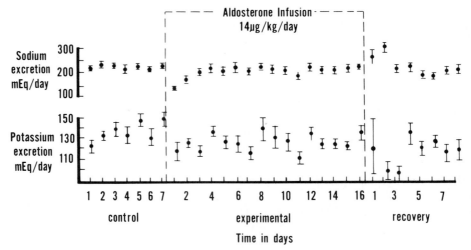

Fig. 13. Effect of aldosterone infusion on sodium and potassium excretion in the same experiment referred to in Fig. 12.

V. SUMMARY

With the information presented here, can we answer the questions posed in the Introduction? Is there a consistent logic that relates sodium, angiotensin, aldosterone, and arterial pressure? From the data contained in the presentation, several statements can be made: First, renal perfusion pressure profoundly affects renal sodium excretion, probably increasing sodium excretion by 300% with a 10 mm Hg rise in steady-state mean arterial pressure. Second, angiotensin II and aldosterone strongly affect sodium excretion. If renal perfusion pressure remains constant, small increments in the levels of these hormones can reduce sodium excretion to a mere fraction of the control value. To overcome the antinatriuretic effects of these agents, renal perfusion pressure must rise above the control level. Stated another way, angiotensin and aldosterone alter the normal relationship between arterial pressure and sodium excretion so that to achieve a given rate of sodium excretion, perfusion pressure must be greater than normal in the presence of elevated concentrations of these hormones. Third, if daily sodium excretion is less than the rate of intake, the positive sodium balance will lead to a variable sequence of events that will bring about an increase in arterial pressure. Arterial pressure will continue to rise until sodium excretion matches sodium intake. The sequence of events may involve an elevated fluid volume and blood volume as is the case in reduced renal mass plus sodium loading hypertension and in aldosterone-induced hypertension, or it may be intense vascular constriction with normal fluid and blood volume as in angiotensin-induced hypertension. The events leading to the elevated pressure are operational details that vary in the different models of hypertension. What is consistent in the various models is that the relationship between arterial pressure and sodium excretion has been altered so that a higher than normal arterial pressure is required to achieve a rate of excretion equal to the rate of intake. In the reduced renal mass model, the alteration in function was achieved surgically; in the angiotensin and aldosterone models, the function was changed by the high levels of the hormones.

The thread that weaves through the information presented is that angiotensin and aldosterone affect the relationship between arterial pressure and sodium excretion. Furthermore, it is this specific renal effect that makes these agents causative factors in hypertension, for their antinatriuretic effects are overcome by sustained increases in arterial pressure.

Does this conclusion reflect on the nature of arterial pressure control and hypertension in general? In Fig. 2, data were presented that makes clear the fact that if renal function is normal, a slight elevation in arterial pressure will lead to massive increases in sodium and water excretion. Clearly, for a state of sustained hypertension to exist, renal function with respect to sodium excretion must be altered, as is the case in aldosterone- and angiotensin-induced hypertensions. Arterial systems in the general case are connected to kidneys; if arterial pressure is above normal for a sustained period, then the normal relationship between arterial pressure and sodium excretion has been altered.

REFERENCES

Baer, P. G., Navar, L. G., and Guyton, A. C. (1970). Renal autoregulation, filtration rate and electrolyte excretion during vasodilation. *Am. J. Physiol.* 219, 619–625.

Bengis, R. G., Coleman, T. G., Young, D. B., and McCaa, R. E. (1978). Long-term blockade of angiotensin formation in various normotensive and hypertensive rat models using converting enzyme inhibitor (SQ 14225). *Circ. Res.* 43, I-45-I-53.

DeClue, J. W., Guyton, A. C., Cowley, A. W., Jr., Coleman, T. G., Norman, R. A., Jr., and McCaa, R. E. (1978). Subpressor angiotensin infusion, renal sodium handling and salt induced hypertension in the dog. *Circ. Res.* 43, 503–512.

Douglas, B. H., Guyton, A. C., Langston, J. B., and Bishop, V. S. (1964). Hypertension caused by salt loading. II. Fluid volume and tissue pressure changes. *Am. J. Physiol.* 207, 669–671.

Fagard, R. H., Cowley, A. W., Jr., Navar, L. G., Langford, H. G., and Guyton, A. C. (1978). Renal responses to slight elevations of renal arterial plasma angiotensin II concentration in dogs. *Clin. Exp. Pharmacol. Physiol.* 3, 531–538.

Guyton, A. C. (1980). "Circulatory Physiology III: Arterial Pressure and Hypertension," Chapter 10, pp. 139–155. Saunders, Philadelphia, Pennsylvania.

Hall, J. E., Guyton, A. C., Trippodo, N. C., Lohmeier, T. E., McCaa, R. E., and Cowley, A. W., Jr. (1977). Intrarenal control of electrolyte excretion by angiotensin II. *Am. J. Physiol.* 233, F538–F544.

Hall, J. E., Guyton, A. C., Salgado, H. C., McCaa, R. E., and Balfe, J. W. (1978). Renal hemodynamics in acute and chronic angiotensin II hypertension. *Am. J. Physiol.* 235, F174–F179.

Lohmeier, T. E., and Cowley, A. W., Jr. (1979). Hypertensive and renal effects of chronic low level intrarenal angiotensin infusion in the dog. *Circ. Res.* 44, 154–160.

Lohmeier, T. E., Cowley, A. W., Jr., Trippodo, N. C., Hall, J. E., and Guyton, A. C. (1977). Effects of endogenous angiotensin II on renal sodium excretion and renal hemodynamics. *Am. J. Physiol,* 233, F388–F395.

McCaa, R. E. (1977). Role of the renin-angiotensin system in the regulation of aldosterone biosynthesis and arterial pressure during sodium deficiency. *Circ. Res.* 40, I-157-I-162.

Pan, Y. J., and Young, D. B. (1978). Experimental aldosterone hypertension. *Fed. Proc., Fed. Am. Soc. Exp. Biol.* 31, 634.

Pan, Y. J., Young, D. B., and Guyton, A. C. (1978). Effects of renal perfusion pressure on renal function. *Physiologist* 21, 89.

Selkurt, E. E., Hall, P. W., and Spencer, M.P. (1949). Influence of graded arterial pressure decrement on renal clearance of creatinine, *p*-amino-hippurate and sodium. *Am. J. Physiol.* 159, 369–378.

Shipley, R. E., and Study, R. S. (1951). Changes in renal blood flow, extraction of insulin, glomerular filtration rate, tissue pressure and urine flow with acute alterations of renal artery blood pressure. *Am. J. Physiol.* 167, 676–688.

Thompson, D. D., and Pitts, R. F. (1952). Effects of alterations of renal arterial pressure on sodium and water excretion. *Am. J. Physiol.* 168, 490–499.

Thompson, J. M. A., and Dickinson, C. J. (1976). The relationship between the excretion of sodium and water and the perfusion pressure in the isolated, blood-perfused, rabbit kidney, with special reference to changes occurring in clip-hypertension. *Clin. Sic. Mol. Med.* 50, 223–236.

Waugh, W. H. (1972). Angiotensin II: Local renal effects of physiological increments in concentration. *Can. J. Physiol. Pharmacol.* **50,** 711–716.

Young, D. B., and Guyton, A. C. (1977). Steady-state aldosterone dose-response relationships. *Circ. Res.* **40,** 138–142.

Young, D. B., Murray, R. H., Bengis, R. G., and Markov, A. K. (1980). Experimental angiotensin II hypertension. *Am. J. Physiol.* **239,** H391–H398.

18

Sodium and the Effects of Norepinephrine

FRIEDRICH C. LUFT, LAURA I. RANKIN,
DAVID P. HENRY, AND MYRON H. WEINBERGER

I. INTRODUCTION

The kidneys and the regulatory systems that influence their control over sodium and choride homeostasis play a primary role in the regulation of arterial blood pressure (Guyton, 1980). Two renal regulatory systems, which have received considerable attention, are the renin–angiotensin–aldosterone system and the sympathetic nervous system (Guyton *et al.*, 1972). The activities of both systems are in turn modulated by dietary sodium intake (Henry *et al.*, 1980; Luft *et al.*, 1979a,b). We have previously examined the effects of extremes in sodium intake on the interrelationships among the renin–angiotensin–aldosterone system, sympathetic nervous system, renal hemodynamics, and arterial blood pressure (Henry *et al.*, 1980; Luft *et al.*, 1979a,b; Pratt and Luft, 1979). In addition, we have recently studied the effect of low and high sodium intake on the pressor responses and vascular compartmentalization of administered norepinephrine

267

(Rankin *et al.*, 1981a). In these experiments the responses of the renin–angiotensin system and renal hemodynamics were monitored as well (Rankin *et al.*, 1981b). Our studies provide new information about the adaptive changes that occur in response to sodium restriction or loading. Furthermore, they provide additional insight into mechanisms by which excessive salt intake may facilitate the development of arterial hypertension.

II. METHODS

The initial sodium loading studies were conducted in 14 healthy male volunteers who denied a family history of hypertension. Observations were made after at least 3 days of six levels of sodium intake, namely, 10, 300, 600, 800, 1200, and 1500 mEq/24 hr. All 14 subjects were studied at the 10 and 300 mEq/24 hr levels. Eight subjects then received 800 and 1500 mEq/24 hr sodium, while six subjects received 600 and 1200 mEq/24 hr sodium. The subjects were given a constant diet containing 10 mEq sodium, 80 mEq potassium, 65 g protein, 50 g fat, 279 g carbohydrate, 400 mg calcium, and 1000 mg phosphorus daily. All meals were eaten at the Clinical Research Center. Dietary sodium intake was maintained at 10 mEq/24 hr for 7 days. For 3 days 290 mEq sodium, in the form of sodium chloride was added to the diet (300 mEq sodium diet). Either 590 or 790 mEq sodium (600 and 800 mEq sodium diet) was added to the 10 mEq diet for the next 3 days. In order to achieve these high levels of intake, sodium was given with bouillon between meals and at bedtime. For the final 3 days, the subjects were hospitalized and received the 600 mEq or 800 mEq sodium diet. Throughout the night they received 400 or 700 mEq sodium, respectively (1200 and 1500 mEq/24 hr sodium intake) in the form of i.v. normal saline. Fluid intake (distilled water) was allowed *ad libitum*.

The subjects were weighed every morning before breakfast after voiding. Blood pressure was obtained daily before meals by the indirect ausculatory technique. The same mercury manometers (Baum, Inc., New York, N.Y.) and cuffs were employed throughout the study. The subjects rested supine in a darkened room for 5 min after which blood pressure and measurements of heart rate were obtained in the nondominant arm each minute for 5 min. The same observers were responsible for these measurements throughout the study.

Daily 24-hr urine specimens were obtained for the determination of sodium, potassium, creatinine, and norepinephrine concentrations. Acetic acid, which protects against urinary norepinephrine loss during storage, was used as a preservative. At 8:00 A.M. on the morning of the final day at each level of sodium intake, venous blood specimens were obtained from the basilic vein, following 2 hr of ambulation for hematocrit, creatinine, sodium, potassium, plasma renin activity, plasma aldosterone, and plasma norepinephrine concentrations.

On the morning of the final day at each level of sodium intake, blood pressure responses to isometric handgrip were determined as outlined elsewhere (Luft *et al.*, 1979a). In addition, cardiac index, stroke index, end-systolic left vetricular volume, and end-diastolic left ventricular volume were measured noninvasively by means of echocardiography (Luft *et al.*, 1979a,b).

To examine the effect of sodium intake on the responses to administered norepinephrine 8 subjects were recruited. These subjects received either 10 or 800 mEq Na daily for 7 and 5 days, respectively, following random assignment. The previously described diet was used. Sodium homeostasis was documented by determination of 24-hr urinary Na excretion.

On the study day, the subject ate breakfast and lunch as usual. Liberal fluid intake was provided to ensure rapid urine flow rates during the study. After lunch a venous catheter was placed in the dominant arm and priming doses of inulin and p-aminohippurate were infused. Subjects were recumbent during the study. A solution of 5% dextrose in water (D_5W) with sustaining amounts of inulin and PAH was then administered at a rate of 45 ml/hr throughout the study. After 1 hr, a catheter was placed in the radial artery of the nondominant arm. A venous catheter for blood sampling was also placed in the nondominant arm.

Eight consecutive 30-min clearance periods were then conducted. The first two periods provide baseline data. L-Norepinephrine bitartrate (Levophed, Winthrop Laboratories, New York, N.Y.) was infused in D_5W delivered by a Harvard infusion pump into the venous catheter in the dominant arm at rates of 1, 2, 4, 8, and 16 μg/min during consecutive 30-min periods. A final recovery period was also conducted. If mean arterial blood pressure increased more than 25 mm Hg from control, no subsequent increase in norepinephrine infusion rate was performed and the recovery period was conducted during the next 30 min.

At 5, 15, and 25 min of each clearance period, blood pressure was recorded using a P23GB transducer (Statham Gould, Oxnard, Calif.) and an Electronic for Medicine recorder (model VR 12, White Plains, N.Y.). At the midpoint of each period, venous blood was sampled for determination of plasma renin activity, sodium, potassium, inulin, PAH, venous norepinephrine, and aldosterone concentrations. Arterial blood was obtained simultaneously for determination of norepinephrine concentration. Urine was obtained at the end of each period for determination of sodium, potassium, inulin, PAH, and norepinephrine excretion. Diuresis was maintained throughout the study by intravenous D_5W infusion.

Sodium and potassium determinations were made using a flame photometer (Instrumentation Laboratories, Boston, Mass.). Inulin and PAH concentrations were determined by an automated method (AutoAnalyzer, Technicon, Chauncey, N.Y.). Plasma renin activity and aldosterone concentrations were measured by previously reported radioimmunoassay methods (Weinberger *et al.*, 1975b). The concentration of norepinephrine in plasma and urine was measured by a radioenzymatic assay (Henry *et al.*, 1975). Clearances were calculated using the general formula $C_X = (U_X V)P_X$, where U_X is the primary concentration, V is the urinary flow rate (ml/min), and P_X is the plasma concentration. Fractional excretion (FE_X) was calculated using the general formula $FE_X = (U_X P_{In}/P_X U_{In})100$, where U_X and P_X are the urinary concentrations of inulin.

The data were analyzed using repeated measures analysis of variance, two-way analysis of variance, linear regression analysis, Student's t test, or nonparametric approaches as appropriate. The 95% confidence limits were accepted as significant. Results are expressed as mean and standard error of the mean (SEM).

All studies were approved by the Indiana Human Use Committee and informed consent was obtained from all subjects. The protocols were well tolerated in all instances and no deleterious effects were encountered.

III. RESULTS

Table I displays the effects of progressive sodium loading on weight, sodium, and potassium excretion at each level of sodium intake. Sodium excretion approximated sodium intake at each level. A significant kaliuresis occurred at sodium intakes in excess of 300 mEq/day. Figure 1 illustrates the effects of sodium loading on mean blood pressure, response to isometric handgrip, cardiac index, and heart rate. There was a significant progressive increase in mean blood pressure ($p < 0.05$), increase in cardiac index ($p < 0.05$), and decrease in heart rate ($p < 0.05$). No interaction between sodium intake and response to isometric handgrip was identified. Figure 2 illustrates the effects of sodium loading on plasma and urinary norepinephrine values as well as on plasma renin activity (PRA) and plasma aldosterone (PA) concentrations. A significant interaction between sodium intake and each of these substances was identified ($p < 0.05$).

TABLE I

Weight, Urinary, Sodium, and Potassium on the Final Day at Each Level of Sodium Intake

	Sodium intake (mEq/24 hr)					
	10	300	600	800	1200	1500
Subjects (N)	14	14	6	8	6	8
ΔWeight (kg)[a]	—	0.8 ± 0.2[b]	0.7 ± 0.3	2.5 ± 0.4	2.5 ± 0.5	5.5 ± 0.6
$U_{Na}V$ (mEq/24 hr)[a]	15 ± 4	278 ± 18	543 ± 61	706 ± 24	1122 ± 68	1443 ± 36
$U_K V$ (mEq/24 hr)[a]	63 ± 5	71 ± 4	132 ± 13	142 ± 7	150 ± 11	189 ± 14

[a] Significant interaction between variable and sodium intake ($p < 0.05$).
[b] Mean $\pm$ SEM.

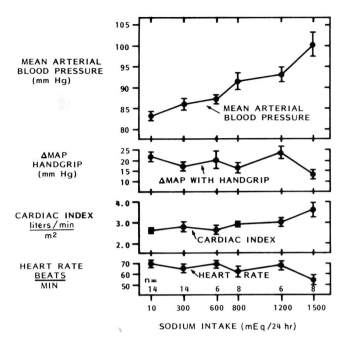

Fig. 1. Hemodynamic effects of increasing sodium intake. Significant changes ($p < 0.05$) in mean blood pressure, cardiac index, and heart rate were observed.

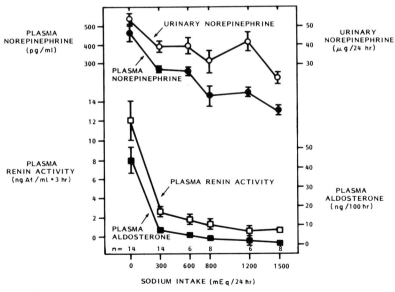

Fig. 2. Humoral effects of increasing sodium intake. Significant changes ($p < 0.05$) in mean blood pressure, cardiac index, and heart rate were observed.

Plasma and urinary norepinephrine values progressively decreased as did PRA and PA concentrations.

A multiple regression analysis was performed with mean blood pressure as the dependent variable and cardiac index, renin, aldosterone, norepinephrine values in plasma, and urinary norepinephrine excretion as independent variables. Plasma norepinephrine concentration and urinary norepinephrine excretion entered the equation. The addition of the remaining independent variables failed to improve the correlation. The expression defining the relationship among mean blood pressure, plasma norepinephrine concentration, and urinary norepinephrine excretion was as followed: MABP $= 105.1 - 0.03\,(P_{Ne}) - 0.24\,(U_{Ne})$ (multiple correlation coefficient $= 0.72$, $p < 0.001$).

Table II illustrates the mean blood pressure values in the norepinephrine infusion experiments. All subjects participating in these studies received all five infusion rates of norepinephrine (1, 2, 4, 8, 16 μg/min) when studied during the low Na phase. However, during the high Na period, six subjects developed an increase of >25 mm Hg mean arterial pressure with infusion of 8 μg norepinephrine/min. Thus, only two subjects received 16 μg/min norepinephrine during the high Na regimen. At the 800 mEq/day level of Na intake the basal blood pressure was modestly but significantly ($p < 0.05$) greater than at the 10 mEq/day level of Na intake. As the infusion rate was increased, the blood pressure was greater for a given norepinephrine infusion rate after the high Na than the low Na diet ($p < 0.05$). In addition, the incremental increase in blood pressure at each of the four lower infusion rates (excluding 16 μg/min) was greater after the high sodium diet ($p < 0.05$) than during the low sodium intake when compared by paired-t test.

Table III outlines both arterial and venous plasma norepinephrine values. During the basal state arterial and venous values were not different. With infu-

TABLE II

Mean Arterial Blood Pressure Values (mm Hg during Norepinephrine Infusion)

Period (infusion rate)	10 mEq Na intake	800 mEq Na intake
Basal	92.2 ± 2.8^a	94.5 ± 3.6
1 μg/min	94.1 ± 2.7	101.2 ± 3.9
2 μg/min	95.5 ± 2.3	104.6 ± 4.6
4 μg/min	99.0 ± 2.2	108.4 ± 4.6
8 μg/min	106.8 ± 1.5	123.2 ± 5.1
16 μg/min	117.2 ± 2.0	$118.1 \pm 4.9\ (N = 2)$

[a] Mean ± SEM.

TABLE III

Arterial and Venous Plasma Norepinephrine Concentrations (pg/ml) during Norepinephrine Infusion

Period (infusion rate)	Plasma	10 mEq Na intake	800 mEq Na intake
Basal	Arterial	192 ± 35[a]	86 ± 17
	Venous	264 ± 63	107 ± 16
1 μg/min	Arterial	592 ± 79	381 ± 47
	Venous	612 ± 181	272 ± 27
2 μg/min	Arterial	957 ± 79	773 ± 104
	Venous	643 ± 69	482 ± 60
4 μg/min	Arterial	1946 ± 124	1786 ± 229
	Venous	953 ± 95	899 ± 101
8 μg/min	Arterial	3133 ± 275	3512 ± 375
	Venous	1684 ± 226	1634 ± 318
16 μg/min	Arterial	8872 ± 592	5896 ± 947 ($N = 2$)
	Venous	3889 ± 351	3436 ± 1662 ($N = 2$)

[a] Mean ± SEM.

sion there was an incremental increase. The arterial levels were greater ($p <$ 0.01) than the venous levels after the infusion of exogenous norepinephrine. The arterial norepinephrine concentration and its urinary excretion rate were highly correlated during both studies ($r = 0.86$, $r = 0.89$, $p < 0.001$). The slopes of this relationship were not different in the two studies. The infusion of norepinephrine affected renal hemodynamics. The clearances of inulin and PAH decreased ($p < 0.01$) in a stepwise fashion as the dose of norepinephrine was increased (Table IV), and this relationship was not altered by the sodium intake. A rapid return to control levels was observed in the recovery period. As shown in Table V, the basal fractional excretion of NA (FE_{Na}) was higher after the high Na diet than the low Na diet ($p < 0.001$). With increasing doses of NE, the FE_{Na} decreased ($p < 0.05$) when the subjects were on the high Na diet. No effect was detected on the low Na diet. No change in the fractional potassium excretion was observed during the norepinephrine infusions. In addition, the plasma concentrations of sodium and potassium were unaltered by sodium intake or norepinephrine infusion.

The effect of increasing doses of exogenous norepinephrine on plasma renin activity (PRA) is displayed in Table VI. The stimulated PRA noted in control periods during the low Na diet increased further with infusion of 16 μg/min ($p <$ 0.01). In contrast, the high Na diet suppressed control renin levels ($p < 0.01$) and the subsequent infusion of norepinephrine did not result in a detectable change in PRA. A correlation between A_{NE} and PRA was seen only during the low NA intake ($r = 0.25$, $p < 0.05$). However, urinary norepinephrine excre-

TABLE IV

The Effect of Administered Norepinephrine on Glomerular Filtration Rate and Renal Blood Flow (ml/min)

Period (infusion rate)	Clearance	10 mEq Na + intake	800 mEq Na + intake
Basal	CI	106 ± 5[a]	126 ± 6
	CPAH	630 ± 28	651 ± 44
1 μg/min	CI	102 ± 5	105 ± 6
	CPAH	574 ± 37	540 ± 43
2 μg/min	CI	103 ± 4	106 ± 8
	CPAH	539 ± 19	505 ± 21
4 μg/min	CI	98 ± 6	96 ± 7
	CPAH	493 ± 22	450 ± 34
8 μg/min	CI	93 ± 5	95 ± 6
	CPAH	425 ± 22	422 ± 26
16 μg/min	CI	84 ± 9	84 ± 9
	CPAH	392 ± 62	$379 \pm 0 \ (N = 2)$

[a] Mean $\pm$ SEM.

TABLE V

The Fractional Excretions of Sodium (FE_{Na}) and Potassium (FE_K) Expressed as Percent during Norepinephrine Administration

Period (infusion rate)	Excretion	10 mEq Na + intake	800 mEq Na + intake
Basal	FE_{Na}	0.346 ± 0.095[a]	3.328 ± 0.406
	FE_K	14.78 ± 3.93	22.36 ± 2.12
1 μg/min	FE_{Na}	0.256 ± 0.065	2.804 ± 0.343
	FE_K	9.28 ± 0.79	19.88 ± 2.08
2 μg/min	FE_{Na}	0.250 ± 0.056	2.627 ± 0.244
	FE_K	8.29 ± 0.74	13.88 ± 0.99
4 μg/min	FE_{Na}	0.298 ± 0.059	2.346 ± 0.201
	FE_K	15.30 ± 7.60	11.56 ± 1.26
8 μg/min	FE_{Na}	0.232 ± 0.058	2.220 ± 0.269
	FE_K	7.41 ± 0.92	10.25 ± 1.74
16 μg/min	FE_{Na}	0.214 ± 0.060	$1.035 \pm 0.45 \ (n = 2)$
	FE_K	7.06 ± 0.77	$8.14 \pm 4.72 \ (n = 2)$

[a] Mean $\pm$ SEM.

TABLE VI

The Effect of Norepinephrine Administration on Renin (PRA; ng AI/ml/3 hr) and Aldosterone (PA; μg/dl)

Period (infusion rate)	Renin aldosterone	10 mEq Na + intake	800 mEq Na + intake
Basal	PRA	6.36 ± 1.21^a	0.68 ± 0.17
	PA	11.94 ± 2.18	4.33 ± 0.45
1 μg/min	PRA	5.00 ± 0.93	0.73 ± 0.16
	PA	10.24 ± 1.03	4.24 ± 0.44
2 μg/min	PRA	5.39 ± 0.93	0.62 ± 0.11
	PA	11.72 ± 1.93	4.69 ± 0.64
4 μg/min	PRA	5.45 ± 1.13	0.57 ± 0.05
	PA	10.78 ± 1.55	4.40 ± 0.61
8 μg/min	PRA	8.14 ± 2.10	0.86 ± 0.24
	PA	12.89 ± 2.26	3.51 ± 0.49
16 μg/min	PRA	12.74 ± 3.46	1.34 ± 0.84 ($n = 2$)
	PA	21.24 ± 4.97	6.05 ± 0.75 ($n = 2$)

[a] Mean $\pm$ SEM.

tion and PRA were correlated at both levels of Na intake ($r = 0.31$, $r = 0.25$, $p < 0.05$). The effect of norepinephrine on plasma aldosterone concentration (PA) is also seen in Table VI. Similarly to PRA, the control PA was higher on the 10 mEq Na diet ($p < 0.05$). During the 800 mEq intake, control PA was suppressed and did not change with NE infusion.

V. DISCUSSION

It is well recognized that both the state of sodium balance and the sympathetic nervous system are important in the control of arterial blood pressure. Both of these influences have direct and indirect actions. Moreover, both are intimately related. For example, our data show that dietary sodium loading increased blood pressure in normotensive men associated with an increase in cardiac output. The upright plasma norepinephrine concentration, which provided a means for assessing sympathoadrenal medullary function (Fitzgerald et al., 1980), decreased with sodium loading. Urinary norepinephrine excretion decreased in a similar fashion. Multiple regression analysis revealed a significant, albeit inverse, relationship between blood pressure and plasma and urinary norepinephrine values, which was not improved by the addition of other variables. This regression, which in no way implies cause and effect, provides an obvious demonstration of the close relationship between mean blood pressure following sodium loading and norepinephrine in plasma and urine of normal subjects.

The relationships identified in the sodium loading studies underscored the possibility that sodium intake may influence the response of both the cardiovascular system and the kidneys to circulating norepinephrine. In addition it became apparent that subtle aberrations in sympathetically mediated sodium excretory mechanisms may contribute to elevation of blood pressure in some individuals when they indulge in the high salt intake characteristic of our society. We therefore administered norepinephrine to normotensive men consuming either low or high sodium intakes.

The data obtained from the norepinephrine administration studies clearly show that sodium intake influences the blood pressure response to norepinephrine, a characteristic that has been previously attributed to angiotensin II (Brunner and Gavras, 1980; Weinberger *et al.*, 1972). Several factors could account for this increased sensitivity induced by a high salt diet. The reciprocal relationships observed between changes in blood pressure and pulse rate seen during norepineprhine infusion at both sodium intakes documents the intact nature of the baroreceptor reflex. An increase in the number, affinity or type ($\alpha 1$, $\alpha 2$) of sympathetic receptor sites could have altered the sensitivity to norepinephrine, but these aspects were not evaluated in the current study. However, we did examine another aspect of sympathetic function which also could have influenced the vascular response, namely, arterial and venous norepinephrine concentrations. High dietary sodium intake was associated with a decrease in both basal arterial and venous norepinephrine concentrations when compared to those seen after the low sodium diet (Table II). These observations are in accord with a substantial body of evidence indicating that sodium loading decreases sympathetic tone. Efferent renal nerve activity has been reported to decrease with volume expnasion (Colindres and Gottschalk, 1978). It has been suggested that this effect is mediated by an increase in pressure sensed in the atria, carotid body, or aorta (Colindres and Gottschalk, 1978; Prosnitz and DiBona, 1978).

Tissue norepinephrine content (de Champlain *et al.*, 1967), as well as the concentration in plasma and urine (Henry *et al.*, 1980; Luft *et al.*, 1979b), have been shown to vary inversely with the sodium balance and volume status. Some investigators have identified changes in catecholamine metabolism induced by potassium loss (Krakoff, 1972) which can be seen with large sodium loads (Luft *et al.*, 1979a). Thus, alterations in the rate of norepinephrine metabolism induced by the changes in sodium and/or potassium balance may be responsible for the differences in blood pressure response following norepinephrine administration at low and high sodium intake.

The sympathetic nervous system is known to be involved in renal sodium homeostasis. However, the mechanism by which sympathetic stimulation induces sodium reabsorption is not completely clear. In the present studies we were only able to detect a change in fractional excretion of sodium after the high sodium diet, perhaps because the basal level of sodium excretion after the low sodium inake period was too low to permit detection of a further decrease. Nonetheless, during the high salt period a dose-related decrease in fractional excretion of sodium, similar to observations in previous studies (Bello-Reuss *et al.*, 1976; Besarab *et al.*, 1977; DiBona, 1978; Gill, 1979; Gill and Casper, 1972), was observed. The second component responsible for renal sodium handling, the renin–aldosterone system, demonstrated virtually complete suppression by the high sodium intake and was not detectably increased by norepinephrine infusion. We cannot, of course, exclude the participation of unexamined factors also thought to influence renal sodium handling. Thus, it would appear that the observed decrease in sodium excretion during high sodium (Gill, 1979) intake was due to a direct effect of norepinephrine on the renal tubule or to decreases in renal blood flow and filtration rate. During sodium depletion, apparent maximal sodium reabsorption prevented the detection of an increase in reabsorption induced by norepinephrine infusion, despite similar decreases in renal blood flow and glomerular filtration rate. To our knowledge, this dependence or norepinephrine-induced sodium reabsorption on the state of sodium balance in man is a unique observation.

The effect of norepinephrine on plasma renin activity was also influenced by the state of sodium balance. We detected a significant increase in PRA with norepinephrine infusion after the low sodium period but not while on a high sodium intake. This observation suggests that when renin release is suppressed by high sodium intake sympathetic stimulation of renin release cannot be achieved. It is of interest to note, however, that urinary norepinephrine excretion correlated with plasma renin activity at both levels of sodium intake. This relationship implies that urinary norepinephrine excretion may be a better indicator of renal sympathetic nerve activity than plasma concentrations, a concept that we have previously suggested (Bello-Reuss *et al.*, 1976; Boren *et al.*, 1980; Henry *et al.*, 1979; Luft *et al.*, 1980). Additional evidence is provided by a recent study which identified a correlation between basal PRA and norepinephrine-stimulated PRA in diuretic-treated humans (Beretta-Piccoli *et al.*, 1980). In that study sodium intake was not controlled and thus the relative contributions of sodium and sympathetic stimuli on renin release cannot be assessed. The differential effect of sodium intake on renin release has also been noted with angiotensin II by Williams and colleagues who observed that they could only detect suppression of PRA by angiotensin II infusion when subjects were receiving a low sodium diet, but not after a more liberal (200 mEq/day) sodium intake (Williams *et al.*, 1978).

Renin release is thought to be mediated by decreases in renal blood flow or pressure (baroreceptor), changes in sodium concentration delivered by the tubule (macula densa), or direct adrenergic stimulation. Studies utilizing α-adrenergic blockade (Veda *et al.*, 1970) or the denervated, nonfiltering kidney (Johnson *et al.*, 1971) have demonstrated sympathetic influences on renin release without alterations in flow, pressure, or sodium handling. The infusion of epinephrine has also been shown to cause dose-related degrees of renin release even though norepinephrine plasma concentrations did not change (Fitzgerald *et al.*, 1980). In that study sodium intake was not determined. In the present studies, blood pressure increased with norepinephrine infusion, which would be expected to reduce renin release by the baroreceptor mechanism. In addition, we have previously demonstrated β-adrenergic stimulation of renin release as well as the potential of juxtaglomerular nerves to stimulate renin release in isolated kidney slices devoid of hemodynamic and metabolic influences (Aoi *et al.*, 1976; Weinberger *et al.*, 1975a). The failure to detect a significant increase in renin activity during the high sodium phase of the study may have resulted from the technical limitations of assay measurements at low levels or to an interaction between the state of sodium balance and sympathetic-mediated renin release.

It is likely that the physiological role of the renin system has undergone drastic revision with the ever-increasing sodium ingestion of acculturated man (Freis, 1976) Brunner and Gavras (1980) have recently raised the question whether, under conditions of our present salt-eating habits, the renin system is even necessary for the welfare of the organism. They point out that considerable attention has been paid to pharmacologic blockade of this system in order to evoke a desirable therapeutic effect, e.g., lowering blood pressure. From that standpoint our studies conducted at the 10 mEq/day level of sodium intake are particularly relevant since they confirm an important interrelationship of the renin system and sympathetic nervous system during sodium depletion. Hyperactivity of the sympathetic nervous system during periods of high sodium intake may be especially deleterious because of the greater impact of that system on arterial blood pressure during the sodium repleted state and possibly an even greater tendency toward sympathetic-mediated sodium retention. In addition suppression of the sympathetic nervous system may be necessary to facilitate the excretion of large sodium loads.

V. SUMMARY

To identify interactions between sodium intake and the sympathetic nervous system (SNS) as reflected by plasma and urinary norepinephrine (NE) values, we performed sodium loading studies across a very wide sodium intake (10–1500 mEq/day), as well as NE administration studies at different levels of sodium intake in normotensive subjects. Sodium intakes > 600 mEq/day increased arterial blood pressure and cardiac index. Plasma and urinary NE decreased and were inversely related to mean blood pressure. The pressor responses to administered NE were enhanced by high sodium intake as was renal sodium retention. NE administration stimulated the renin system at low sodium intake. These observations reveal qualitative and quantitative interactions between sodium homeostasis and the SNS which may influence blood pressure in man in several ways. High sodium intake may increase the vascular sensitivity to the SNS. SNS activity may influence sodium homeostasis in an adverse fashion at high sodium intake. SNS suppression may be necessary to facilitate the excretion of sodium at high intakes.

ACKNOWLEDGMENT

Supported in part by USPHS Grant HL 14159, Specialized Center of Research (SCOR) in Hypertension and RR 00750 (General Clinical Research Center).

REFERENCES

Aoi, W., Henry, D. P., and Weinberger, M. H. (1976). Evidence for a physiological role of renal sympathetic nerves in adrenergic stimulation of renin release in the rat. *Circ. Res.* **38**, 123–126.

Bello-Reuss, E., Trevino, D. L., and Gottschalk, C. W. (1976). Effect of renal sympathetic nerve stimulation on proximal water and sodium reabsorption. *J. Clin. Invest.* **57**, 1104–1108.

Beretta-Piccoli, C., Weidman, P., Meier, A., Grimm, M., Keusch, G., and Gluck, Z. (1980). Effect of short term norepinephrine infusion on plasma catecholamines, renin and aldosterone in normal and hypertensive man. *Hypertension* **2**, 623–630.

Besarab, A., Silva, P., Landsberg, L., and Epstein, F. H. (1977). Effect of catechlolamines on tubular function in the isolated perfused rate kidney. *Am. J. Physiol.* **233**, F34–F45.

Boren, K. R., Henry, D. P., Selkurt, E. E., and Weinberger, M. H. (1980). Renal modulation of urinary cathecholamine excretion during volume expansion in the dog. *Hypertension* **2**, 383–389.

Brunner, H. R., and Gavras, H. (1980). Is the renin system really necessary? *Am. J. Med.* **69**, 739–745.

Colindres, R. E., and Gottschalk, C. W. (1978). Neural control of renal tubular sodium reabsorption in the rat: Single nephron analysis. *Fed. Proc., Fed. Am. Soc. Exp. Biol.* **37**, 1218–1220.

de Champlain, J., Krakoff, C. R., and Axelrod, J. (1967). Cathecholamine metabolism in experimental hypertension in the rat. *Circ. Res.* **20**, 136–140.

DiBona, G. F. (1978). Neural control of renal tubular sodium reabsorption in the dog. *Fed. Proc., Fed. Am. Soc. Exp. Biol.* **37**, 1214–1217.

Fitzgerald, G. A., Barnes, P., Hamilton, C. A., and Dollery, C. T. (1980). Circulating adrenaline and blood pressure: The metabolic effects and kinetics of infused adrenaline in man. *Eur. J. Clin. Invest.* **10**, 401–406.

Freis, E. D. (1976). Salt, volume and the prevention of hypertension. *Circulation* **53**, 589–595.

Gill, J. R. (1979). Neural control of renal tubular sodium reabsorption. *Nephron* **23**, 116–118.

Gill, J. R., and Casper, A. G. T. (1972). Effect of renal alpha-adrenergic stimulation on proximal tubular sodium reabsorption. *Am. J. Physiol.* **223**, 1201–1205.

Guyton, A. C. (1980). "Arterial Pressure and Hypertension," p. 352. Saunders, Philadelphia, Pennsylvania.

Guyton, A. C., Coleman, T. G., Cowley, A. W., Scheel, K. W., Manning, R. D., and Norman, R. A. (1972). Arterial pressure regulation. *Am. J. Med.* **52**, 584–594.

Henry, D. P., Starman, B. T., Johnson, D. G., and Williams, R. H. (1975). A sensitive radioenzymatic assay for norepinephrine in tissue and plasma. *Life Sci.* **16,** 375–385.

Henry, D. P., Dentino, M., Gibbs, P. S., and Weinberger, M. H. (1979). Vascular compartmentalization of plasma norepinephrine in normal man. *J. Lab. Clin. Med.* **94,** 429–437.

Henry, D. P., Luft, F. C., Weinberger, M. H., Fineberg, N. S., and Grim, C. E. (1980). Norepinephrine in urine and plasma following provocative maneuvers in normal and hypertensive subjects. *Hypertension* **2,** 20–28.

Johnson, J. A., Davis, J. O., and Witty, R. T. (1971). Effects of catecholamines and renal nerve stimulation on renin release in the nonfiltering kidney. *Circ. Res.* **29,** 646–653.

Krakoff, L. R. (1972). Potassium deficiency and cardiac metabolism in the rat. *Circ. Res.* **30,** 608–613.

Luft, F. C., Rankin, L. I., Bloch, R., Weyman, A. E., Willis, L. R., Murray, R. H., Grim, C. E., and Weinberger, M. H. (1979a). Cardiovascular and humoral responses to extremes of sodium intake in normal black and white men. *Circulation* **60,** 697–706.

Luft, F. C., Rankin, L. I., Henry, D. P., Bloch, R., Grim, C. E., Weyman, A. E., Murray, R. H., and Weinberger, M. H. (1979b). Plasma and urinary norephinephrine values at extremes of sodium intake in normal man. *Hypertension* **1,** 261–266.

Luft, F. C., Weinberger, M. H., Grim, C. E., Henry, D. P., and Fineberg, N. S. (1980). Nocturnal electrolyte excretion and its relationship to the renin system and sympathetic activity in normal and hypertensive man. *J. Lab. Clin. Med.* **95,** 395–406.

Pratt, J. H., and Luft, F. C. (1979). The effect of extremely high sodium intake on plasma renin activity, plasma aldosterone concentration and urinary excretion of aldosterone metabolites. *J. Lab. Clin. Med.* **93,** 724–729.

Prosnitz, E. H., and DiBona, G. F. (1978). Effect of decreased renal sympathetic nerve activity on renal tubular sodium reabsorption. *Am. J. Physiol.* **235,** F557–F651.

Rankin, L. I., Henry, D. P., Weinberger, M. H., Gibbs, P. S., and Luft, F. C. (1981a). Sodium intake alters the effects of norepinephrine on the renin system and the kidney. *Am. J. Kidney Dis.* **1,** 177–184.

Rankin, L. I., Luft, F. C., Henry, D. P., Gibbs, P. S., and Weinberger, M. H. (1981a). Sodium intake alters the blood pressure effects of norepinephrine. *Hypertension* **3,** 650–656.

Ueda, H., Yasuda, H., Takabatake, Y., Iizuke, M., Iizuke, T., Ihori, M., and Sakamoto, Y. (1970). Observations on the mechanism of renin release by cathecholamine. *Circ. Res.* **26–27,** Suppl. II, II-195–II-200.

Weinberger, M. H., Ramsdell, J. W., Rosner, D. R., and Geddes, J. J. L. (1972). Effect of chlorothiazide and sodium on vascular responsiveness to angiotensin II. *Am. J. Physiol.* **223,** 1049–1052.

Weinberger, M. H., Aoi, W., and Henry, D. P. (1975a). The direct effect of beta-adrenergic stimulation on renin release by rat kidney slices in vitro. *Circ. Res.* **37,** 318–324.

Weinberger, M. H., Kem, D. C., Gomez-Sanchez, C., Kramer, N. J., Martin, B. T., and Nugent, C. A. (1975b). The effect of dexamethasone on the control of plasma aldosterone concentration in normal recumbent man. *J. Lab. Clin. Med.* **85,** 957–967.

Williams, G. H., Hollenberg, N. K., Moore, T. J., Dluhy, R. G., Bavli, S. Z., Solomon, H. S., and Mersey, J. H. (1978). Failure of renin suppression by angiotensin II in hypertension. *Circ. Res.* **42,** 46–52.

19

The Role of the Sympathetic Nervous System in the Modulation of Sodium Excretion

MYRON H. WEINBERGER, FRIEDRICH C. LUFT,
AND DAVID P. HENRY

I. INTRODUCTION

The sympathetic nervous system is known to influence sodium excretion by the kidney in a variety of ways. An increase in sympathetic activity can increase renal blood flow and pressure and thus alter sodium handling by such indirect hemodynamic effects. More recently it has been demonstrated that phar-

281

THE ROLE OF SALT IN
CARDIOVASCULAR HYPERTENSION

macologic agonists or antagonists of sympathetic activity, renal nerve stimulation, or denervation can alter renal sodium handling directly (DiBona, 1977). At present it appears that α-adrenergic activity results in an increase in renal tubular sodium reabsorption (DiBona, 1977; Gill and Casper, 1972; Morgunov and Baines, 1981; Strandhoy et al., 1974; Zambraski et al., 1976) and that dopamine is a natriuretic agent (Alexander et al., 1974; Davis et al., 1968; Goldberg, 1972; Kuchel et al., 1978; McDonald et al., 1964), and that both effects can occur independent of changes in renal hemodynamics. Most of this information has been obtained under contrived experimental conditions.

However, recent studies in humans have suggested a link between urinary dopamine and sodium excretion or balance (Adam, 1980; Alexander et al., 1974; Kuchel et al., 1979a,b; Oates et al., 1979). Other studies have demonstrated a relationship between the state of sodium balance and sympathetic nerve activity measured by direct nerve recordings or by the level of norepinephrine in tissue, plasma, or urine (Boren et al., 1980; Clement et al., 1972; deChamplain, 1972; Faucheux et al., 1977; Giachette et al., 1979; Henry et al., 1980; Krakoff et al., 1967; Luft et al., 1979a,b; Miller et al., 1980; Romoff et al., 1979). These studies have been interpreted as evidence that sodium loading suppresses sympathetic nerve activity and sodium depletion activates it. Thus, a feedback system for noradrenergic activity and sodium balance can be envisioned with an opposing relationship between dopaminergic activity and sodium balance. This has led us to hypothesize that there are separable noradrenergic and dopaminergic systems operating in the kidney to modulate renal handling of sodium.

Previous studies by our group and others provide convincing support for the use of the urinary excretion of norepinephrine (Boren et al., 1980; Henry et al., 1979b; Morgunov and Bains, 1981; Unger et al., 1978) and dopamine (Adam, 1980; Boren et al., 1980; Unger et al.,1978) as markers, primarily, of renal noradrenergic and dopaminergic activity, respectively. The recent development of a sensitive and specific method for measuring free dopamine in urine as well as its major nondietary metabolite, dihydroxyphenylacetic acid (DOPAC) (Boren et al., 1980; Henry, 1979a) has provided us with an opportunity to explore this hypothesis further. The present study was designed to examine relative renal noradrenergic and dopaminergic activities after equilibration at two extremes of dietary sodium intake in normal men and to compare the effects of a more vigorous method of volume expansion and contraction in normal and hypertensive men.

II. METHODS

The studies to be described have been approved by the Indiana University Medical Center Human Use Committee and informed consent was obtained from all subjects prior to study. All studies were conducted in the Clinical Research Center. Two protocols were used: (1) dietary sodium loading and restriction; (2) rapid sodium and intravascular volume expansion and contraction. For the dietary study, eight normotensive men (24–38 years) were studied in equilibrium after low and high levels of sodium intake. The basic diet was constant throughout and consisted of 10 mEq Na, 80 mEq potassium, 65 g protein, 50 g fat, 280 g carbohydrate, 400 mg calcium, and 1000 mg phosphorus daily. The high Na diet was identical with the exception that 290 mEq Na was added to the diet in the form of NaCl. An additional 500 mEq NaCl was given in bouillon between and with meals to attain a total Na intake of 800 mEq/day. The high sodium was given for 5 days and the low sodium diet for 7 days. Each subject was randomly assigned to enter the study on either low or high Na intake. The second phase was performed after 3–7 days of an intervening normal diet. Sodium homeostasis was documented by determination of 24 hr urinary Na excretion. The second study utilized a protocol developed by us for the evaluation of hypertension and applied to over 1500 normotensive and hypertensive subjects (Grim *et al.*, 1977; Luft *et al.*, 1977a,b). On the evening of admission a basal nocturnal (Luft *et al.*, 1980) urine specimen was collected from 10 P.M. to 6 A.M. the following morning. This urine collection and all subsequent ones were analyzed for concentrations of sodium (Na), potassium (K), creatinine, norepinephrine (NE), dopamine (DA), and the major dopamine metabolite of nondietary origin, dihydroxyphenylacetic acid (DOPAC) by methods to be described. At 6 A.M. the subjects were awakened, asked to void, and then were ambulatory for 2 hr. At 8 A.M. they again voided and blood samples were obtained for Na, K, creatinine, plasma renin activity (PRA), and aldosterone (PA). The subjects then assumed the recumbent position and received a 4-hr intravenous infusion of 2 liters of isotonic (0.9%) saline (500 ml/hr). At 12 noon the 4-hr urine collection was terminated and blood was obtained for PRA, PA, Na, K, and creatinine. This procedure was designed to evaluate the suppressibility of the renin–aldosterone axis by inducing rapid volume expansion (Kem *et al.*, 1971). We have subsequently recognized that it also induces suppression of components of the sympathetic nervous system (Henry *et al.*, 1980; Miller *et al.*, 1980) and the fractional excretion of sodium (Luft *et al.*, 1977a, 1980). After completion of the infusion the subjects were permitted to move about and received a diet containing 150 mEq Na and 70 mEq K. At 10 P.M. the 10-hr ("day") urine collection was terminated. At 8 A.M. the next morning, a 10-hr nocturnal urine collection was completed. The total Na intake on this "saline" day was 458 mEq.

At 6 A.M. on the following morning, while recumbent, and again at 8 A.M. following 2 hr of ambulation, blood samples were obtained. The diet on this day was restricted to 10 mEq Na, 70 mEq K, and 25 ml water/kg body wt. Furosemide (40 mg) was given orally at 10 A.M., 2 P.M., and 6 P.M. A day urine collection was terminated at 10 P.M. and a night specimen completed at 8 A.M. on the morning following sodium and volume depletion. This "Lasix day" was utilized to evaluate the stimulability of the renin system to sodium and volume depletion (Grim *et al.*, 1977). Subsequent studies have indicated that it also stimulated the sympathetic nervous system (Henry *et al.*, 1980) and that the nocturnal or basal sodium excretion approached zero (Luft *et al.*, 1980).

Concentrations of Na and K in plasma and urine were measured by flame photometry (Instrumentation Laboratories, Boston, Mass.) and creatinine by an automated technique (Technicon, Chauncy, N.Y.). The concentrations of NE in plasma and urine were measured by a radioenzymatic assay (Henry *et al.*, 1979b). The data were analyzed statistically by analysis of variance, *t* test, nonparametric techniques (Walsh, Wilcoxon, Mann-Whitney *U*), where appropriate, and linear regression. The 95% limits of probability were accepted as significant. The data are expressed as mean ± SEM.

III. RESULTS

In study 1, after equilibration on 10 and 800 mEq of dietary Na intake, the urinary excretion rates of NE, DA, and DOPAC were measured as shown in Fig. 1. With dietary sodium loading a significant ($p < 0.03$) decrease in NE excretion

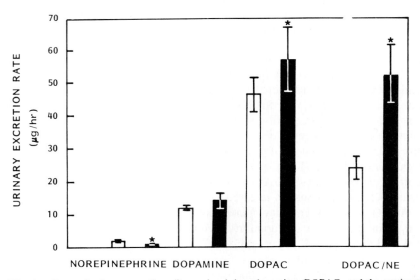

Fig. 1.   Rates of urinary excretion of norepinephrine, dopamine, DOPAC, and the natriuretic index (DOPAC/NE) in normotensive men after ingestion of sodium at either 10 mEq/day (open bars) or 800 mEq/day (closed bars). Asterisks denote values significantly ($p < 0.05$) different from 10 mEq/day levels.

rate and increase ($p < 0.03$) in DOPAC excretion rate were seen. DA excretion was not significantly influenced by the level of sodium intake. In an attempt to utilize a single measurement to reflect the relative renal noradrenergic and dopaminergic activities as influenced by sodium intake we calculated the ratio of DOPAC to NE excretion rates as a potentially useful "natriuretic" index. This ratio, also shown in Fig. 1, increased significantly ($p < 0.03$) with dietary sodium loading.

To examine these relationships further we made similar measurements in the second, rapid volume expansion–volume contraction study. In this study we utilized the nocturnal excretion rate as a measure of "basal" sympathetic activity. We measured the urinary excretion rates of NE, DA, and DOPAC during the sleep period the evening before (control) and after intravenous volume expansion with 2 liters of normal saline which was given between 8 A.M. and noon (saline) and during the sleep period following sodium and volume depletion induced by the low salt diet and three doses of furosemide (depletion). The nocturnal excretion rates of sodium, potassium and the catecholamines measured are tabulated in Table I for the normal and hypertensive subjects. During the sleep period following saline infusion, normal subjects demonstrated a significant increase in urinary sodium excretion rate and in the natriuretic ratio (DOPAC/NE) when compared to control observations but not in the other measurements. During the night following sodium and volume depletion, normal subjects evinced a significant decrease in sodium, DA, and DOPAC excretion rates and a significant increase in NE; the natriuretic index also decreased significantly. In the hypertensive group similar significant changes in urinary sodium excretion were seen in response to the saline loading and depletion protocol. This group also demonstrated a significant increase in NE excretion after sodium and volume depletion and a significant decrease in the natriuretic index. The hypertensives did not have changes in DOPAC excretion that were as marked as those observed in the normal subjects. Significant ($p < 0.05$) differences between the normal and hypertensive subjects were seen on several occasions. Normal subjects had significantly higher values for DOPAC and the DOPAC/NE ratio during the control night as well as both nights after the saline load. The hypertensives had significantly higher urinary excretion rates of NE on both the night following the saline load and following volume contraction. Nocturnal dopamine excretion was not significantly different between the two groups on any night.

To examine the relationship between the urinary excretion rates of NE, DA, and DOPAC and the excretion of sodium and potassium during these different states of sodium loading and depletion, we calculated the correlation coefficients among these measures during the study. As shown in Table II, several consistent and significant relationships were observed. In the normal subjects significant direct correlations between sodium excretion and DA ($p < 0.05$), DOPAC ($p < 0.001$), and the natriuretic ratio, DOPAC/NE, ($p < 0.001$) were seen, with an

TABLE I

Nocturnal Responses to Saline Loading and Volume Depletion in Normal and Hypertensive Subjects (Mean ± SEM)

Response	Normals			Hypertensives		
	Control	Saline	Depletion	Control	Saline	Depletion
Sodium excretion (mEq/hr)	5.14 ± 1.0^a	10.81 ± 1.4^b	0.50 ± 0.1^b	3.97 ± 1.1	10.53 ± 1.4^b	0.65 ± 0.4^b
Potassium excretion (mEq/hr)	1.07 ± 0.1	1.12 ± 0.2	1.86 ± 0.2	1.40 ± 0.3	1.68 ± 0.4	1.98 ± 0.2
NE (μg/hr)	0.86 ± 0.1	0.74 ± 0.1^c	1.15 ± 0.2	1.34 ± 0.3	1.20 ± 0.2^c	1.70 ± 0.2
DA (μg/hr)	9.40 ± 2.0	9.22 ± 1.5^a	5.41 ± 1.4	12.94 ± 1.7	18.45 ± 5.4	8.02 ± 1.6
DOPAC (μg/hr)	49.36 ± 2.8	58.81 ± 5.9^c	32.27 ± 4.4^d	38.31 ± 3.8	41.90 ± 1.5	32.74 ± 4.6
DOPAC/NE	59.5 ± 6.5^c	82.6 ± 11.1^a	30.1 ± 3.6^b	34.8 ± 7.0	39.8 ± 6.5	20.3 ± 3.7

[a] $p < 0.01$ compared to saline.
[b] $p < 0.01$ compared to control.
[c] $p < 0.05$ compared to saline.
[d] $p < 0.05$ compared to control.

TABLE II

Coefficients of Correlation between Nocturnal Catecholamine and Electrolyte Excretion Rates in Normal and Hypertensive Subjects

Rates	Normals	Hypertensives
DA and Na	0.40[a]	0.44[a]
DA and K	−0.22	0.50[b]
DOPAC and Na	0.70[c]	0.42[a]
DOPAC and K	−0.41[a]	0.17
NE and Na	−0.49[b]	0.21
NE and K	0.33	0.02
DOPAC/NE and Na	0.75[c]	0.37
DOPAC/NE and K	−0.46[a]	−0.06

[a] $p < 0.05$
[b] $p < 0.01$.
[c] $p < 0.001$.

inverse correlation with NE ($p < 0.05$). Reciprocal (inverse) correlations between potassium excretion and DOPAC ($p < 0.05$) and the natriuretic ratio ($p < 0.05$) were also seen in the normal subjects. In the hypertensives these significant correlations were less consistently observed, being limited to direct correlations between sodium excretion and DA ($p < 0.05$) and DOPAC ($p < 0.05$). Specifically, no significant correlations between either sodium or potassium excretion and the natriuretic ratio (DOPAC/NE) were seen in the hypertensive group, in marked contrast to the observations in the normotensive group.

IV. DISCUSSION

Several recent developments have permitted us to utilize rates of urinary excretion of norepinephrine, DA, and DOPAC to estimate relative noradrenergic and dopaminergic activities in the kidney. Previous studies in humans have demonstrated an increase in the rate of urinary excretion of NE with assumption of upright posture, a stimulus to sympathetic activity (Henry *et al.*, 1979b). Furthermore, this increase in urinary norepinephrine excretion rate occurred in the face of a decrease in glomerular filtration rate and was associated with a norepinephrine clearance rate that exceeded that of creatinine. Thus, the kidney contributes NE to urine during stimulation of the sympathetic nervous system. Using the canine model, a more specific documentation of the role of the kidney in modulating catecholamine excretion was performed (Boren *et al.*, 1980; Morgunov and Baines, 1981). These studies also demonstrated net production of NE and DA by the kidney in the control state. With volume expansion a marked increase in DA excretion was observed. Since almost all of the DA appearing in the circulation is conjugated (and biologically inactive), free urinary dopamine must be derived from: (1) deconjugation, (2) synthesis by renal dopaminergic neurons or, (3) synthesized from circulating DOPA by renal decarboxylases. Thus, urinary DA excretion, and presumably that of its major nondietary metabolite, DOPAC, should reflect intrarenal dopaminergic activity. Our ability to measure NE, DA, and DOPAC with high sensitivity and specificity was facilitated by the development of new modifications of radioenzymatic methodology by one of us (DPH) (Henry, 1979a).

Our previous studies in humans utilizing the rapid volume expansion–volume contraction protocol have observed inverse responses of NE excretion to the state of sodium balance (Henry *et al.*, 1980). Other investigators have also observed an effect of sodium loading or depletion on excretion of NE (Alexander *et al.*, 1974; Boren *et al.*, 1980; Faucheux *et al.*, 1977; Luft *et al.*, 1979a,b; Miller *et al.*, 1980; Romoff *et al.*, 1979). A substantial body of experimental evidence suggests that sodium balance influences sympathetic nerve activity (Alexander *et al.*, 1974; Boren *et al.*, 1980; Clement *et al.*, 1972; Giachette *et al.*, 1979; Krakoff *et al.*, 1967; Morgunov and Baines, 1981) and that noradrenergic factors influence renal tubular handling of sodium with α-adrenergic stimulation favoring sodium reabsorption (DiBona, 1977; Gill and Casper, 1972; Morgunov and Baines, 1981; Strandhoy *et al.*, 1974; Zambraski *et al.*, 1976). Thus, the experimental evidence favoring the concept of a feedback loop between sympathetic nerve activity and sodium reabsorption is impressive. In addition, while the opposing, natriuretic effect of dopamine has been clearly demonstrated in experimental animals, only recently has a possible relationship between the state of sodium balance and urinary dopamine excretion in humans been explored (Alexander *et al.*, 1974; Kuchel *et al.*, 1978, 1979a,b; Oates *et al.*, 1979). For these reasons the present studies, testing the existence of a reciprocal renal modulatory system in the kidney for handling sodium under varying conditions of sodium balance in normotensive and hypertensive men, are particularly timely, feasible, and appropriate.

As evidenced in the study utilizing equilibration on low or high dietary sodium intake in normotensive men, reciprocal changes in rates of excretion of NE and DOPAC were observed consistently (Fig. 1). These changes, reproduced by the more rapid volume expansion volume contraction protocol, are compatible with the hypothesis that the renal noradrenergic and dopaminergic systems may be reciprocally related to renal sodium handling. From our knowledge of the actions of norepinephrine and dopamine on renal tubular sodium excretion, such a reciprocal physiological mechanism makes teleological sense. Further support for these relationships in the normal subjects is obtained from the highly significant and consistent correlations between NE, DA, DOPAC, and the natriuretic index and the urinary excretion of sodium and, frequently, potassium.

In hypertensive humans a variety of alterations in sympathetic activity have been reported. While most reports have focused on elevated levels of NE in plasma or urine of hypertensive subjects (DeChamplain, 1972; DeQuattro and Chan, 1972; Esler *et al.*, 1977; Henry *et al.*, 1980; Kuchel, 1977; Luft *et al.*, 1980), abnormalities of dopamine excretion have also been reported in some forms of hypertension (Kuchel, 1977; Kuchel *et al.*, 1979a,b), particularly those manifesting an "exaggerated natriuresis" (Luft *et al.*, 1979b). In the present study, hypertensive subjects demonstrated only the increase in NE in response to volume contraction and failed to show significant changes in DA and DOPAC with volume expansion and contraction as did the normal subjects, providing additional points of contrast. None of the hypertensives had received antihypertensive agents for several weeks prior to study so that pharmacologic interference is not a likely explanation. In addition, significant correlations between urinary sodium and potassium excretion and the other parameters measured were less consistently observed in the hypertensive subjects.

These studies provide new evidence in support of a dual noradrenergic-dopaminergic modulatory influence on renal sodium handling in man. They provide a new concept of a natriuretic index expressing these reciprocal influences and identify unique and potentially important differences between normal and hypertensive men. Additional studies confirming and extending these new findings are indicated.

V. SUMMARY

To investigate the existence of opposing renal noradrenergic and dopaminergic modulation of renal sodium excretion, rates of urinary excretion of NE, DA, and DOPAC were measured in different states of sodium balance. A natriuretic index, DOPAC/NE, was found to correlate closely with the state of sodium balance in normal men subjects to either very low (10 mEq/day) or very high (800 mEq/day) sodium intakes. Additional studies utilizing rapid sodium and volume expansion and contraction confirmed the utility of this natriuretic index. Hypertensive men had significantly lower values for this index than did normotensive subjects under similar conditions. These studies provide new evidence of abnormalities in the adrenergic–dopaminergic system in human hypertension and support a link between these systems and renal handling of sodium.

ACKNOWLEDGMENTS

These studies were supported in part by USPHS grants HL 14159, Specialized Center of Research (SCOR) Hypertension, HL 27294 and RR 00750 (General Clinical Research Center).

The authors wish to acknowledge the expert statistical assistance provided by Dr. Naomi Fineberg and the help of Ms. Toni Moore in the preparation of the manuscript.

REFERENCES

Adam, W. R. (1980). Aldosterone and dopamine receptors in the kidney: Sites for pharmacologic manipulation of renal function. *Kidney Int.* **18**, 623–635.

Alexander, R. W., Gill, J. R., Yamabe, H., Lovenberg, W., and Keiser, H. R. (1974). Effects of dietary sodium and of acute saline infusion on the interrelationship between dopamine excretion and adrenergic activity in man. *J. Clin. Invest.* **54**, 194–200.

Boren, K. R., Henry, D. P., Selkurt, E. E., and Weinberger, M. H. (1980). Renal modulation of urinary catecholamine excretion during volume expansion in the dog. *Hypertension* **2**, 383–389.

Clement, D. L., Pelletier, C. L., and Shepherd, J. T. (1972). Role of vagal afferents in the control of renal sympathetic nerve activity in the rabbit. *Circ. Res.* **31**, 824–830.

Davis, B. B., Walter, M. J., and Murdaugh, H. V. (1968). The mechanism of the increase in sodium excretion following dopamine infusion. *Proc. Soc. Exp. Biol. Med.* **129**, 210–213.

DeChamplain, J. (1972). Hypertension and the sympathetic nervous system. *In* "Perspectives in Neuropharmacology" (S. H. Snider, ed., pp. 215–265. Oxford Univ. Press, London and New York.

DeQuattro, V., and Chan, S. (1972). Raised plasma catecholamines in some patients with primary hypertension. *Lancet* **1**, 806–809.

DiBona, G. F. (1977). Neurogenic regulation of renal tubular sodium reabsorption. *Am. J. Physiol.* **233**, F73–F81.

Esler, M., Julius, S., Zweifler, A., Randall, O., Harburg, E., Gardiner, H., and DeQuattro, V. (1977). Mild high-renin essential hypertension: Neurogenic human hypertension? *N. Engl. J. Med.* **296**, 405–411.

Faucheux, B., Buu, N. T., and Kuchel, O. (1977). Effects of saline and albumin on plasma and urinary catecholamines in dogs. *Am. J. Physiol.* **232**, F123–F127.

Giachette, A., Rubenstein, R., and Clark, T. L. (1979). Noradrenaline storage in deoxycorticosterone-saline hypertensive rats. *Eur. J. Pharmacol.* **57**, 99–106.

Gill, J. R., Jr., and Casper, A. G. T. (1972). Effect of renal alpha adrenergic stimulation on proximal tubular sodium reabsorption. *Am. J. Physiol.* **223**, 1201–1207.

Goldberg, L. I. (1972). Cardiovascular and renal actions of dopamine: Potential clinical applications. *Pharmacol. Rev.* **24**, 1–29.

Grim, C. E., Weinberger, M. H., Higgins, J. T., and Kramer, N. J. (1977). Diagnosis of secondary forms of hypertension: A comprehensive protocol *JAMA, J. Am. Med. Assoc.* **237**, 1331–1337.

Henry, D. P. (1979). Radioenzymatic assays for catecholamines and related compounds. *In* "Catecholamines: Basic and Clinical Frontiers" (E. Usden, I. J. Kopin, and J. Barkas, eds.), pp. 859–876. Pergamon, Oxford.

Henry, D. P., Dentino, M., Gibbs, P. S., and Weinberger, M. H. (1979). Vascular compartmentalization of plasma norepinephrine in normal man: The relationship between venous and arterial NE concentration and the urinary excretion of NE. *J. Lab. Clin. Med.* **94**, 429–437.

Henry, D. P., Luft, F. C., Weinberger, M. H., Fineberg, N. S., and Grim, C. E. (1980). Norepinephrine in urine and plasma following provocative maneuvers in normal and hypertensive subjects. *Hypertension* **2**, 20–28.

Kem, D. C., Weinberger, M. H., Mayes, D. M., and Nugent, C. A. (1971). Saline suppression of plasma aldosterone in hypertension. *Arch. Intern. Med.* **128**, 380–384.

Krakoff, L. R., DeChamplain, J., and Axelrod, J. (1967). Abnormal storage of norepinephrine in experimental hypertension in the rat. *Circ. Res.* **21**, 583–588.

Kuchel, O. (1977). Autonomic nervous system in hypertension: Clinical aspects. *In* "Hypertension" (J. Genest, E. Koiw, and O. Kuchel, eds.), pp. 93–113. McGraw-Hill, New York.

Kuchel, O., Buu, N. T., and Unger, T. (1978). Dopamine-sodium relationship: Is dopamine a part of the endogenous natriuretic system? *Contr. Nephrol.* **13**, 27–35.

Kuchel, O., Buu, N. T., Hamet, P., Nowaczynski, W., and Genest, J. (1979a). Free and conjugated dopamine in pheochromocytomas, primary aldosteronism and essential hypertension. *Hypertension* **1**, 267–273.

Kuchel O, Buu, N. T., Unger, T., Lis, M., and Genest, J. (1979b). Free and conjugated plasma and urinary dopamine in human hypertension. *J. Clin. Endocrinol. Metab.* **48**, 425–429.

Luft, F. C., Grim, C. E., Higgins, J. T., and Weinberger, M. H. (1972a). Differences in response to sodium administration in normotensive white and black subjects. *J. Lab. Clin. Med.* **90**, 555–562.

Luft, F. C., Grim, C. E., Willis, L. R., Higgins, J. T., and Weinberger, M. H. (1977b). Natriuretic response to saline infusion in normotensive and hypertensive man. The role of renin suppression in exaggerated natriuresis. *Circulation* **55**, 779–784.

Luft, F. C., Rankin, L. I., Bloch, R., Weyman, A. E., Willis, L. R., Murray, R. H., Grim, C. E., and Weinberger, M. H. (1979a). Cardiovascular and humoral responses to extremes of sodium intake in normal black and white men. *Circulation* **60**, 697–706.

Luft, F. C., Rankin, L. I., Henry, D. P., Bloch, R., Grim, C. E., Weyman, A. E., and Weinberger, M. H. (1979). Plasma and urinary norepinephrine values at extremes of sodium intake in normal men. *Hypertension* **1**, 261–266.

Luft, F. C., Weinberger, M. H., Grim, C. E., Henry, D. P., and Fineberg, N. S. (1980). Nocturnal electrolyte excretion and its relationship to the renin system and sympathetic activity in normal and hypertensive man. *J. Lab. Clin. Med.* **95**, 395–406.

McDonald, R. H., Goldberg, L. I., and McNay, J. L. (1964). Effects of dopamine in man: Augmentation of sodium excretion, glomerular filtration rate and renal plasma flow. *J. Clin. Invest.* **43**, 1116–1121.

Miller, J. Z., Luft, F. C., Grim, C. E., Henry, D. P., Christian, J. C., and Weinberger, M. H. (1980). Genetic influences on plasma and urinary norepinephrine after volume expansion and contraction in normal men. *J. Clin. Endocrinol. Metab.* **50**, 219–222.

Morgunov, N., and Baines, A. D. (1981). Renal nerves and catecholamine excretion. *Am. J. Physiol.* **240**, F75–F81.

Oates, N. S., Ball, S. G., Perkins, C. M., and Lee, M. R. (1979). Plasma and urine dopamine in man given sodium chloride in the diet. *Clin. Sci.* **56**, 261–264.

Romoff, M. S., Keusch, Campese, V. M., Wang, M. S., Friedler, R. M., Weidmann, P., and Massry, S. G. (1979). Effect of sodium intake on plasma catecholamines in normal subjects. *J. Clin. Endocrinol. Metab.* **48**, 26–31.

Strandhoy, J. W., Schneider, E. G., Willis, L. R., and Knox, F. G. (1974). Intrarenal effects of phenoxybenzamine on sodium reabsorption. *J. Lab. Clin. Med.* **83**, 263–270.

Unger, T., Buu, N. T., and Kuchel, O. (1978). Renal handling of free and conjugated catecholamines following surgical stress in the dog. *Am. J. Physiol.* **235**, F542–F547.

Zambraski, E. J., DiBona, G. F., and Koloyanides, G. J. (1976). Effect of sympathetic blocking agents on the antinatriuresis of reflex renal nerve stimulation. *J. Pharmacol. Exp. Ther.* **198**, 464–472.

20

β-Adrenergic Responsiveness in Deoxycorticosterone-Salt-Induced Hypertension in Rats

MICHAEL J. KATOVICH AND MELVIN J. FREGLY

I. INTRODUCTION

Chronic administration of mineralocorticoid hormones is accompanied by hypertension in both intact (Tobian and Redleaf, 1957) and uninephrectomized

293

rats drinking saline (Dusting *et al.*, 1973; Selye *et al.*, 1943). The mechanism(s) responsible for the induction of hypertension is not yet clear but may be related to several factors including an increased concentration of catecholamines in blood (Reid *et al.*, 1975), enhanced sympathetic nervous activity (Reid *et al.*, 1975), enhanced vascular reactivity (Dusting *et al.*, 1973; Berecek and Bohr, 1977, 1978; Berecek *et al.*, 1980b), sodium retention and expansion of extracellular volume (Haack *et al.*, 1977; Tarazi, 1969), alterations in the concentration of electrolytes in the arterial wall (Tobian and Redleaf, 1957), and an increased concentration of vasopressin in blood (Haack *et al.*, 1977; Mohring *et al.*, 1977). Regardless of the ultimate pathogenic mechanism, the development of deoxycorticosterone (DOC)-induced hypertension seems to depend on the presence of sodium (de Champlain, 1973; Tobian and Redleaf, 1957).

A significant cardiovascular change related to the development of DOC-salt-induced hypertension is that of an enhanced vascular reactivity to norepinephrine (Dusting *et al.*, 1973; Berecek and Bohr, 1977, 1978) which was observed prior to a rise in arterial pressure in both rats (Berecek *et al.*, 1980a) and pigs (Berecek and Bohr, 1978). This suggests that a change in vascular reactivity, per se, may be a primary pathogenic factor in the development of DOC-salt hypertension. Of particular interest is the fact that sodium deficiency prevented the occurrence of an increased vascular reactivity (Berecek *et al.*, 1980b) and the changes in electrolyte concentration of the arterial wall (Tobian and Redleaf, 1957) in the DOC-salt-treated rat. This lends support to the potential role of sodium in the enhanced responsiveness of vascular smooth muscle to α-adrenergic agonists.

Since the development of DOC-salt-induced hypertension is accompanied by an increased cardiovascular responsiveness to α-adrenergic agonists, a question arises as to the responsiveness of the β-adrenergic system of the DOC-salt-treated rat. Administration of β-adrenergic antagonists has produced inconsistent results. Similar doses (10–20 mg/kg/day) of propranolol have been shown both to increase (Dusting and Rand, 1974), and to decrease (Conway *et al.*, 1975) systolic blood pressure in DOC-hypertensive rats. It has also been shown that administration of isoproterenol, a β-adrenergic agonist, to DOC-salt-treated rats elicits cardiac arrhythmias in doses that are well tolerated by control rats (Guideri *et al.*, 1978). This myocardial sensitization to isoproterenol is characteristic of both gluco- and mineralocorticoid-treated rats and a high sodium diet is not an absolute requirement for development of this phenomenon in either case (Guideri *et al.*, 1978). These results suggest the possibility that β-adrenergic responsiveness may be increased in DOC-salt-treated rats. It is therefore an objective of these studies to determine whether the metabolic responsiveness to β-adrenergic stimulation was altered in DOC-salt-treated rats. In addition, an attempt was made to determine whether chronic treatment with NaCl, in the absence of DOC, can affect β-adrenergic responsiveness.

II. METHODS

A. Experiment 1: Effect of Deoxycorticosterone (DOC)-Salt-Induced Hypertension on β-Adrenergic Responsiveness

Twenty-five male rats of the Blue Spruce Farms (Sprague–Dawley) strain weighing from 236 to 294 g were used. The rats were housed in groups of three in hanging stainless steel cages that were kept in a windowless room maintained at 25 ± 1°C and illuminated from 0700 to 1900 hours. All rats were given Purina Laboratory Chow and 0.15 M NaCl solution to drink *ad libitum*.

The animals were divided into two groups. The experimental group (14 rats) was administered deoxycorticosterone pivalate (DOC) (Percorten pivalate, CIBA-Geigy, N.J.) intramuscularly (i.m.), at a dose of 5 mg/rat/week. The control group (11 rats) was administered saline, i.m. in the same volume (0.2 ml). At weekly intervals throughout the study the systolic blood pressure of each rat was measured indirectly from the tail by means of a Narco Bio Systems transducer and physiograph. Body weight was also measured weekly.

During the fourth through sixth weeks of the study, the response of heart rate to administration of the β-adrenergic agonist, isoproterenol, was studied. Heart rates were measured at an ambient temperature of 25° ± 1°C. Each rat was lightly anesthetized with ether and electrode paste was applied to the chest above the heart. Discs for recording the EKG were secured to the chest with adhesive tape and heart rate was recorded on a Narco Bio Systems physiograph. Each rat was placed in a restraining cage consisting of a wire mesh tunnel with a wooden floor similar to that described by Adolph *et al.* (1954). After a 1-hr equilibration period, the control or resting (0 time) heart rate was measured. On completion of control measurement *dl*-isoproterenol (Isuprel, Wintrop Laboratories) was administered s.c., at doses of either 2.5, 5, or 10 μg/kg body wt. Heart rate was then recorded every 5 min for the first 30 min and every 10 min for the next 30 min. Both groups were tested simultaneously and the experiments were designed to randomize the dose of isoproterenol as well as to ensure that there were at least 5 days between tests for each rat. At least six animals from each group were administered the three doses of isoproterenol.

During the ninth week of the study, 11 animals from each group were placed in individual stainless steel metabolic cages equipped with funnels for collection of urine. Finely ground Purina Laboratory Chow and 0.15 M NaCl solution were provided *ad libitum*. Two days after the animals were placed in individual cages, a 24-hr measurement of intakes of food and NaCl solution was made. Each animal was also weighed. The water containers were infant nursing bottles with cast bronze spouts as described by Lazarow (1954). The food cups were spillproof and have been described by Fregly (1960). Urine volume was also collected under light mineral oil to prevent evaporation.

Temperatures of the skin of the tail and colon were measured prior to and following s.c. administration of dl-isoproterenol (5 to 10 μg/kg) during the tenth and twelfth weeks of treatment with DOC. The rats were lightly restrained in tunnel-type cages as described in the study above in which heart rate was measured. Colonic temperature was measured with a copper–constantan thermocouple inserted 5 cm into the colon and taped to the tail. The temperature of the dorsal surface of the tail was also measured by means of a second thermocouple placed on the skin of the tail approximately 2 cm from its base. This thermocouple was held in place by weaving it into a single layer of gauze sponge 3 cm long, the ends of which were bound to the tail with adhesive tape. The temperatures were measured at 1-min intervals by a recording potentiometer.

After being placed in the restraining cages, an adjustment period of 1 hr was allowed before temperatures were recorded. Thirty minutes later all animals were administered isoproterenol (5 or 10 μg/kg body wt, s.c.) and measurements were continued for 2 hr. The doses of isoproterenol administered to the rats were randomized and there were at least 5 days between treatments for each rat. The data were analyzed by calculating the mean colonic and tail-skin temperatures for each group during every 10 min of the experiment.

During the sixteenth week of treatment with DOC, the rate of oxygen consumption was measured in the same six animals from each group that were used previously to study the effect of administration of 5 μg isoproterenol/kg on tail-skin temperature. Rate of oxygen consumption was measured with an open circuit system and a Beckman DM-11 oxygen analyzer. Each rat was restrained in a wire mesh cage which was sealed in a cylindrical, water-jacketed, Lucite chamber. Water temperature was adjusted to maintain the temperature inside the chamber at 25 $\pm$ 1°C. Room air was drawn through the chamber at a rate of 350 ml/min. The concentration of oxygen in effluent air was measured by the oxygen analyzer. Rate of oxygen consumption was calculated as ml of oxygen consumed (STPD) per min per kg body $wt^{0.75}$. At the beginning of each trial animals were placed in the Lucite chambers for 1 hr prior to initiation of the study. Thirty minutes after the initial measurements were completed, the wire mesh cages were quickly removed from the chamber and 5 μg isoproterenol/kg were administered s.c. to each rat. The animals were returned immediately to the chamber and rate of oxygen consumption measured every 5 min for the next hour.

During the twenty-third to twenty-fifth week of the study, the left carotid artery of each animal was cannulated with PE 50 tubing after anesthesia with sodium pentobarbitol (35 mg/kg body wt). The cannula was filled with heparinized saline and threaded subcutaneously to an area behind the neck where it was exteriorized and plugged with a solid stainless steel stylette. Each rat was allowed to recover from surgery and was kept in an individual stainless steel cage. Five days after implantation of the cannula, it was connected to a Narco Bio Systems transducer (Model P-1000B) and direct blood pressures of the unanesthetized rats were recorded on a Narco Bio Systems physiograph. Each animal was allowed to move freely in its home cage during the entire experiment. One hour after the initial blood pressure was recorded, 10 μg isoproterenol/kg body wt were administered s.c. Blood pressure was then measured for the next 60 min.

All data were analyzed and compared by means of Student's t test with significance set at the 95% confidence limit (Daniel, 1974).

B. Experiment 2: Effect of Ingestion of 0.15 M NaCl Solution on β-Adrenergic Responsiveness

Twelve male rats of the Blue Spruce Farms (Sprague–Dawley) strain weighing from 254 to 296 g were used. The animals were divided into two groups of six each. One group received 0.15 M NaCl solution as the sole drinking fluid, while the second group was given tap water. Food (Purina Laboratory Chow) was available to both groups *ad libitum*. The animals were maintained under the same experimental conditions as those described in experiment 1.

Seven weeks after initiation of 0.15 M NaCl solution as the sole drinking fluid, the response of heart rate to administration of 5 μg isoproterenol/kg s.c. was studied. During the ninth week of the study, the response of tail-skin temperature to a s.c. administration of 10 μg isoproterenol/kg also was studied. Saline intake and systolic blood pressures were measured during the tenth week of the study. Protocols for both studies were identical to those described in experiment 1.

III. RESULTS

A. Experiment 1

The effects of graded doses of isoproterenol on heart rate of the DOC-salt-treated and control-salt-treated rats are shown in Figs. 1–3. In Fig. 1A resting heart rates of both groups were nearly identical. Following administration of 2.5 μg isoproterenol/kg both groups responded with an increase in heart rate. Mean heart rate of the control-salt-treated group was elevated significantly above that of the DOC-salt-treated group for the first 20 min after administration of isoproterenol. By 60 min after administration of isoproterenol, mean heart rates of both groups approached pretreatment values. Figure 1B summarizes the mean change in heart rate of both groups. The control-salt-treated group responded with an increase in heart rate of about 150 beats/min for the first 20 min. This

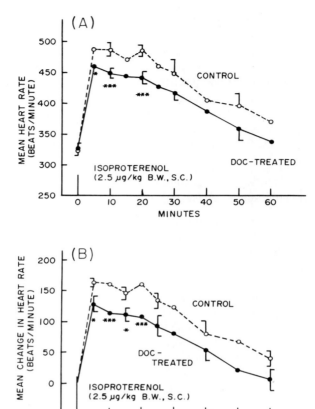

Fig. 1. Effect of administration of isoproterenol (2.5 μg/kg body wt, s.c.) on mean heart rate (A) in DOC-salt-treated (solid circle) and control-salt-treated (open circle) groups. The mean increase in heart rate (B) during 1 hr after administration of isoproterenol is also shown. One standard error is set off at each mean. Significance of the difference from control is expressed as *$p < 0.05$; ***$p < 0.01$.

was elevated significantly ($p < 0.05$) above that of the DOC-salt-treated group (115 beats/min). Figures 2 and 3 summarize the responses of heart rate after administration of 5 and 10 μg isoproterenol/kg, respectively. In both studies a similar pattern was observed, that is, the DOC-salt-treated group was less responsive to isoproterenol than the control-saline-treated group. In all three trials, heart rates measured prior to treatment were comparable for both groups (325–350 beats/min). The control-salt-treated group had a mean maximal heart rate approximating 500 beats/min compared to about 450 beats/min for the DOC-salt-treated group following administration of isoproterenol. The major effect of increasing the dose of isoproterenol was an increase in the duration of the maximal response of heart rate to the β-adrenergic agonist.

The effect of the weekly injection of DOC on intakes of food and 0.15 M NaCl solution, urine output, blood pressure, and body weight are summarized in Fig. 4. DOC-salt-treatment had no effect on food intake (Fig. 4A) whereas there was at least a threefold increase in the volume of 0.15 M NaCl solution consumed during the 24 hr period (Fig. 4B). The increase in fluid intake, however, did not result in an increase in body weight gain (Fig. 4E). A threefold increase

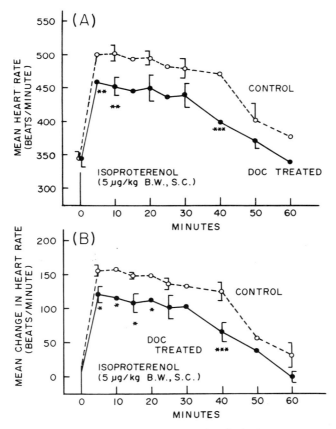

Fig. 2. Effect of administration of isoproterenol (5.0 μg/kg body wt, s.c.) on mean heart rate (A) in DOC-salt-treated (solid circle) and control-salt-treated (open circle) groups. The mean increase in heart rate (B) during 1 hr after administration of isoproterenol is shown. One standard error is set off at each mean. Significance of the difference from control is expressed as *$p < 0.05$; **$p < 0.02$, ***$p < 0.01$.

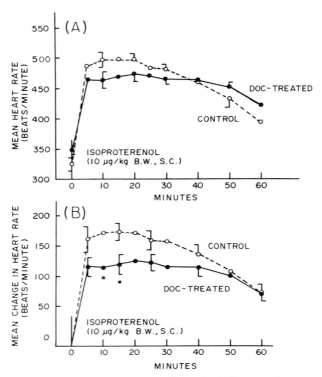

Fig. 3. Effect of administration of isoproterenol (10.0 μg/kg body wt, s.c.) on mean heart rate (A) in DOC-salt-treated (solid circle) and control-salt-treated (open circle) groups. The mean increase in heart rate (B) during 1 hr after administration of isoproterenol is shown. One standard error is set off at each mean. Significance of the differences from control is expressed as described in Fig. 2.

in urine output above control level was observed in the DOC-salt-treated group (Fig. 4C). Systolic blood pressure was elevated significantly in the DOC-salt-treated group compared to the control-salt-treated group (Fig. 4D). The mean systolic blood pressure of the DOC-salt-treated group was significantly elevated above that of the control-salt-treated group by the sixth week of treatment with DOC.

Following administration of 5 μg isoproterenol/kg (Fig. 5A), both groups responded with an increase in mean tail-skin temperature. At this dose the mean maximal increase in tail-skin temperature was reached by both groups within 40–50 min postinjection. However, the mean tail-skin temperature of the DOC-salt-treated group was elevated significantly above that of the control-salt-treated group from 30 to 80 min postinjection. The tail-skin temperatures of both groups returned toward pretreatment values by the end of the 120-min experiment. Simultaneous measurements of colonic temperature after treatment with iso-

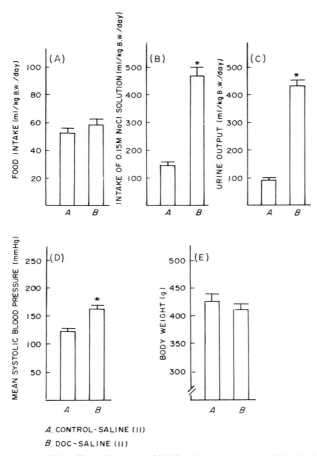

Fig. 4.   Summary of the effect of 9 weeks of DOC-salt-treatment on (A) 24 hr food intake; (B) 24 hr intake of 0.15 *M* NaCl solution; (C) 24 hr urinary volume; (D) indirect systolic blood pressure; and (E) mean body weight. One standard error set off at each mean. Number of rats is shown in parentheses. Significance of the difference from control is expressed as $*p < 0.01$.

proterenol (Fig. 5B) revealed nearly identical responses in both groups. At the higher dose of isoproterenol (10 μg/kg) similar results were observed. A difference between studies was that the mean response of tail-skin temperature in both groups was higher and more prolonged at a dose of 10 μg of isoproterenol/kg than at a dose of 5 μg/kg (Fig. 6A). Mean colonic temperatures of both groups were similar (Fig. 6B).

Resting rates of oxygen consumption were similar in both groups (Fig. 7). Within 5–10 min following administration of 5 μg isoproterenol/kg, an elevation

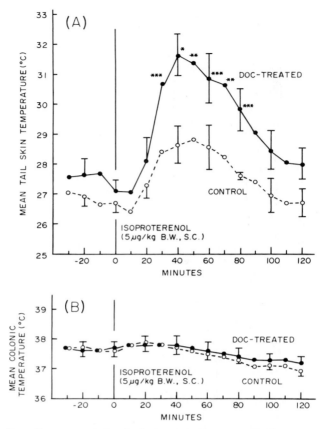

Fig. 5. Effect of isoproterenol (5 μg/kg body wt, s.c.) on mean tail-skin (A) and mean colonic (B) temperatures of DOC-salt-treated (solid circle) and control-salt-treated (open circle) groups. One standard error is set off at each mean. Significance of the difference from control is expressed as *p < 0.01; **p < 0.02; ***p < 0.05.

in the rate of oxygen consumption was observed. Both groups responded in a similar manner. The rate of oxygen consumption returned to pretreatment values by 40 min postinjection, the time at which mean tail-skin temperatures reached maximal levels in the studies described above.

Direct measurement of both systolic (Fig. 8) and diastolic blood (Fig. 9) pressures in awake, unrestrained animals demonstrated an enhanced responsiveness to administration of isoproterenol in the DOC-salt-treated group compared to the control-saline-treated group. Pretreatment systolic and diastolic blood pressures were elevated significantly (p < 0.01) in the DOC-salt-treated group compared to the control-saline-treated group. Administration of 10 μg isoproterenol/kg was accompanied by a decrease in systolic blood pressure (Fig. 8A) in both groups. The change in blood pressure (Fig. 8B) of the control group was between 10 and 15 mm Hg during the first 5 min following administration of isoproterenol compared to a decrease of 30 mm Hg in the DOC-treated group. Within less than 30 min after administration of isoproterenol, systolic blood pressure was near pretreatment value in the control group while it was still reduced 10–15 mm Hg in the DOC-treated group. This same decrease in pressure

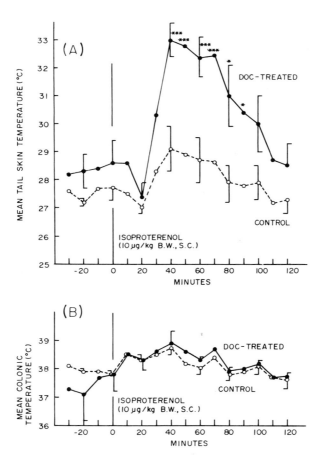

Fig. 6.   Effect of isoproterenol (10 μg/kg body wt, s.c.) on mean tail-skin (A) and mean colonic (B) temperatures of DOC-salt-treated (solid circle) and control-salt-treated (open circle) groups. One standard error is set off at each mean. Significance of the difference from control is the same as that described in Fig. 5.

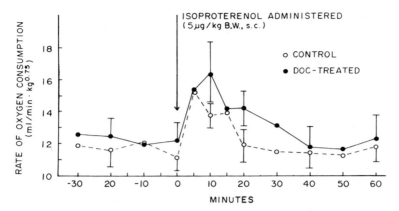

Fig. 7.   Effect of isoproterenol (5 μg/kg body wt, s.c.) on the rate of oxygen consumption of DOC-salt-treated (closed circle) and control-salt-treated (open-circle) groups. One standard error is set off at each mean.

was maintained throughout the 50 min period in the DOC-treated group. Similar results were observed for the response of diastolic blood pressure to administration of 10 μg isoproterenol/kg (Fig. 9).

B. Experiment 2

Maintenance of rats on 0.15 M NaCl solution as their sole drinking fluid did not alter the responsiveness of heart rate to the β-adrenergic agonist, isoproterenol. At a dose of 5 μg isoproterenol/kg the increase in heart rate of the group receiving 0.15 M NaCl solution was virtually identical to that of the control group (Fig. 10). Both groups started at comparable resting values (320–340 beats/min), and following treatment with isoproterenol, mean heart rates of both groups approached 475 beats/min (Fig. 10A). The mean changes in heart rate of both groups were similar and were approximately 150 beats/min (Fig. 10B).

Resting mean tail-skin temperatures of both the 0.15 M NaCl-treated and control groups were about 28°C (Fig. 11A). Following administration of 10 μg isoproterenol/kg, both groups responded with a similar increase in tail-skin temperature which was maximal at 50–70 min after treatment. Within 80 min after injection, tail-skin temperatures of both groups returned to pretreatment values. There was no effect of isoproterenol on colonic temperatures (Fig. 11B).

Systolic blood pressure was not affected during the 10-week study. Both the 0.15 M NaCl-treated and control groups had similar systolic blood pressures of 125 $\pm$ 3 and 121 $\pm$ 6 mm Hg, respectively. Food intake was 45.6 $\pm$ 3.2

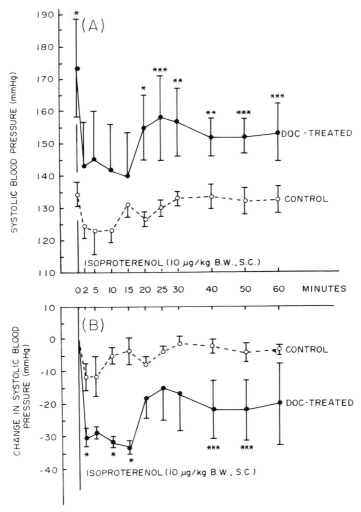

Fig. 8. Effect of administration of 10 μg isoproterenol/kg s.c. on direct mean systolic blood pressure (A) and change in mean systolic blood pressure (B) in unanesthetized DOC-salt-treated (solid circle) and the control-salt-treated (open circle) groups. One standard error is set off at each mean. Significance of the difference from control is expressed as *$p < 0.01$; **$p < 0.02$; ***$p < 0.05$.

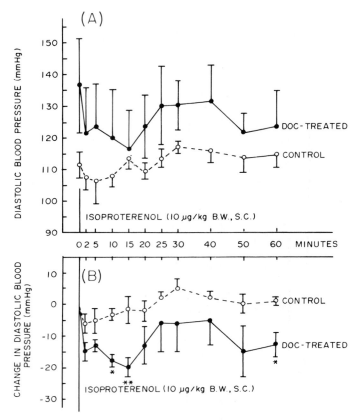

Fig. 9. Effect of administration of 10 μg isoproterenol/kg s.c. on direct mean diastolic blood pressure (A) and change in mean diastolic blood pressure (B) in unanesthetized DOC-salt-treated (solid circle) and the control-salt-treated (open circle) groups. One standard error is set off at each mean. Significance of the difference from control is expressed as **$p < 0.02$; *$p < 0.01$.

g/kg/day and 42.7 ± 2.9 g/kg/day, respectively. Intake of 0.15 M NaCl solution by the experimental group was 87.4 ± 8.9 ml/kg/day while water intake by the control group was 54.8 ± 6.1 ml/kg/day.

IV. DISCUSSION

Chronic treatment of rats with deoxycorticosterone and saline was accompanied by an increase in blood pressure, and an altered responsiveness to administration of a β-adrenergic agonist. The latter is particularly interesting since the responses of blood pressure and tail-skin temperature to administration of iso-proterenol were increased in DOC-treated rats compared to those of controls while the responsiveness of heart rate to administration of isoproterenol was attenuated. The difference in responsiveness may be related to differences in receptor types mediating the responses. Thus, changes in heart rate following administration of isoproterenol have been attributed to activation of β_1 adrenoreceptors while changes in diastolic blood pressure and peripheral resistance have been as-sociated with activation of β_2 adrenoreceptors (Lands *et al.*, 1967). The results of these studies suggest, but do not prove, that chronic treatment with DOC may increase responsiveness of β_2 adrenoreceptors while reducing the responsiveness of β_1 adrenoreceptors.

The increase in tail-skin temperature accompanying administration of iso-proterenol to rats is a reliable test of β-adrenergic responsiveness. It is inhibited

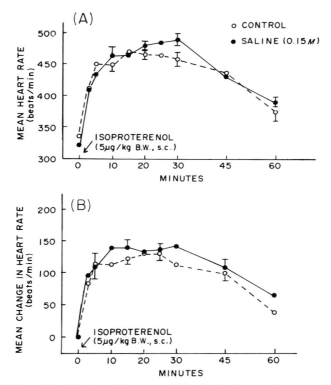

Fig. 10. Effect of administration of isoproterenol (5 μg/kg body wt, s.c.) on mean heart rates of the group ingesting 0.15 *M* NaCl solution as its sole drinking fluid (solid circle) as well as the group ingesting water (open circle) is shown in (A). The mean increases in heart rate during one hour after administration of isoproterenol are shown in (B). One standard error is set off at each mean.

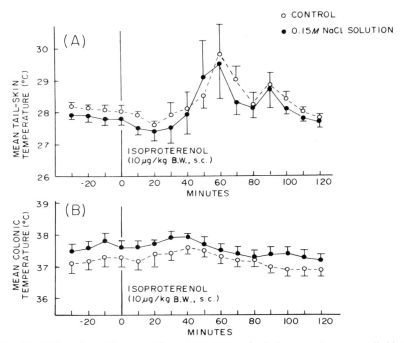

Fig. 11.   Effect of administration of isoproterenol (10 μg/kg body wt, s.c.) on mean tail-skin (A) and mean colonic (B) temperatures of the group ingesting 0.15 M NaCl solution as its sole drinking fluid (solid circle) as well as the group ingesting tap water (open circle). One standard error is set off at each mean.

by a prior administration of the β-adrenergic antagonist, propranolol (Fregly *et al.*, 1980), and cannot be induced by administration of graded doses of the α-adrenergic agonist, phenylephrine (Fregly *et al.*, 1975). The tail of the rat serves an important function in temperature regulation (Rand *et al.*, 1965). When body temperature is elevated and the rat is threatened with overheating, the tail vasculature dilates and tail-skin temperature increases to facilitate heat loss. The mechanism by which administration of isoproterenol induces an increase in tail-skin temperature is not known with certainty and could result from a direct effect on the vasculature or it could occur secondarily to an increase in heat production and body temperature induced by isoproterenol (Fregly *et al.*, 1980). The present study attempted to determine whether the greater increase in tail-skin temperature observed in the DOC-treated rats following administration of iso-proterenol was related to an increased metabolic responsiveness. The increase in rate of oxygen consumption (and metabolic rate) in response to administration of isoproterenol at a dose of 5 μg/kg was not different when DOC-treated rats were compared to controls (Fig. 7). This suggests that the enhanced responsiveness of the DOC-treated group may be related to direct effects of isoproterenol on the vasculature rather than to an indirect effect on metabolic rate and body temperature. This explanation is consistent with the enhanced responsiveness of blood pressure to administration of isoproterenol which was also observed in DOC-treated rats (Fig. 9).

Administration of isoproterenol to DOC-treated rats resulted in a twofold greater decrease in the blood pressure (systolic and diastolic) of DOC-treated rats than in controls (Figs. 8 and 9). The greater reduction in diastolic pressure in DOC-treated rats may be attributed to a greater dilatory responsiveness of peripheral vasculature to administration of a β-adrenergic agonist. The reduced responsiveness of heart rate, which accompanies administration of isoproterenol to DOC-treated rats, also suggests that isoproterenol may have affected the vasculature directly. The large increase in heart rate accompanying administration of isoproterenol to the control group most likely decreased stroke volume and cardiac output because of the reduced cardiac filling time at the very fast heart rates accompanying administration of the β-adrenergic agonist. The expected response, a reflex increase in peripheral vasoconstriction, was antagonized, in part at least, by the direct effect of isoproterenol on peripheral vasculature. In the case of the DOC-treated rat, heart rate did not increase to the same high level as that observed in the control animals (Figs. 1–3) and presumably cardiac output was less affected. Despite the latter, a greater decrease in diastolic blood pressure occurred in this group (Fig. 9). This would appear to reflect a greater direct vasodilatory effect of isoproterenol on the vascular smooth muscle.

The reduced responsiveness of heart rate to administration of isoproterenol observed in DOC-treated rats may be related to a reduction in the number of β-adrenergic receptors in cardiac tissue (Woodcock et al., 1978, 1979). The decrease in receptor number would appear to be specific to cardiac tissue since no decrease in the number of β-adrenergic receptors in renal cellular membranes was observed by these investigators (Woodcock et al., 1978). Both the increased vascular responsiveness and the increased responsiveness of tail-skin temperature to administration of isoproterenol suggest that either the number of β-adrenergic receptors or their affinity for β-adrenergic agonists or both may actually be increased in the tissues associated with these responses. An explanation for these differences in regional responsiveness to β-adrenergic stimulation is not available.

It was reported by others (Dusting et al., 1973; Bereck and Bohr, 1977, 1978; Berecek et al., 1980a) that an enhanced vascular reactivity to administration of an α-adrenergic agonist accompanied chronic administration of DOC and NaCl to rats. The enhanced responsiveness could be prevented if the DOC-treated rats were administered a sodium-deficient diet (Berecek et al., 1980b). This lends support to a role for sodium in the increased α-adrenergic responsiveness of DOC-treated rats. The question of the individual contributions of DOC and NaCl to the changes in β-adrenergic responsiveness observed here remains to be answered. Animals ingesting saline solution are not an adequate control group for the DOC-saline-treated group since the latter ingested nearly three times more saline solution than the former. However, they also excreted nearly three times as much urine. Additional experiments will be required to determine whether intakes of NaCl alone at levels accompanying administration of the dose of DOC used here affect responsiveness to isoproterenol in a similar fashion.

The study in which the β-adrenergic responsiveness of rats given 0.15 M NaCl solution to drink was compared with that of controls ingesting tap water suggests that at least at this level of intake (0.8 g NaCl/kg/day) NaCl has no significant effect. Additional studies, not described here, were carried out in which rats received only 0.25 M NaCl solution to drink. Intake of NaCl by these animals was 1.3 g NaCl/kg/day. The results of these studies also failed to reveal differences in β-adrenergic responsiveness from the control group.

It is of interest that chronic administration of DOC to rats is accompanied by an increased vascular responsiveness to both α- and β-adrenergic agonists. The increased α-adrenergic responsiveness was observed prior to an elevation of blood pressure in DOC-treated rats (Berecek et $al.$, 1980a). Similar studies have not been carried out to determine when an increased β-adrenergic responsiveness occurs in relation to the elevation of blood pressure. Such a study would be of obvious interest since the effect on blood pressure of the increased α-adrenergic responsiveness could be at least partially antagonized by an increased β-adrenergic responsiveness. Information regarding the time of development of the increased β-adrenergic responsiveness in rats administered DOC, as well as the participation of the ingestion of excessive amounts of sodium chloride on it, awaits additional experimentation.

V. SUMMARY

Chronic administration of 5 mg of deoxycorticosterone (DOC) pivalate/rat/week to male rats resulted in a significant increase in systemic blood pressure, intake of 0.15 M NaCl solution, and urinary volume without significant changes in body weight and food intake. Stimulation of a β-adrenergic receptor-mediated response was accompanied by an attenuated response of heart rate in DOC-salt-treated rats administered isoproterenol (2.5, 5.0, and 10.0 μg/kg) compared to salt-treated controls. In contrast, the DOC-salt-treated group had a twofold increase in the response of blood pressure to acute administration of isoproterenol when compared to the control-salt-treated group. This enhanced response may be mediated by β_2-adrenergic receptors on peripheral vasculature. The response of tail-skin temperature to administration of isoproterenol was greater in the DOC-salt-treated group than the control-salt-treated group. This enhanced response apparently was not due to an enhanced rate of oxygen consumption in the DOC-salt-treated group and may be attributed to the enhanced vasodilatory response accompanying administration of isoproterenol in the DOC-salt-treated group. Animals maintained on 0.15 M NaCl solution as their sole drinking fluid showed no alteration in either β_1- or β_2-adrenergic responsiveness compared to those given tap water to drink. The results of this study suggest that chronic treatment with DOC in combination with NaCl may alter β-adrenergic responsiveness by increasing β_2-adrenergic responsiveness while decreasing β_1-adrenergic responsiveness.

ACKNOWLEDGMENTS

Supported by a grant from the American Heart Association, Florida Affiliate, Suncoast Chapter and by Grant HL 14526-09 from the National Heart, Lung, and Blood Institute.

The authors thank Mr. Bill Kelly, Ms. June Senff, and Mrs. Charlotte Edelstein for technical assistance and graphic illustrations, and Mrs. Gail Storin for preparation of manuscript.

REFERENCES

Adolph, E. F., Barker, J. P., and Hoy, P. A. (1954). Multiple factors in thirst. *Am. J. Physiol.* **178,** 538–562.

Berecek, K. H., and Bohr, D. J. (1977). Structural and functional changes in vascular resistance and reactivity in the deoxycorticosterone acetate (DOCA)-hypertensive pig. *Circ. Res.* **40,** 146–152.

Berecek, K. H., and Bohr, D. J. (1978). Whole body reactivity during the development of deoxycorticosterone acetate hypertension in the pig. *Circ. Res.* **42,** 764–771.

Berecek, K. H., Stocker, M., and Gross, F. (1980a). Changes in renal vascular reactivity at various stages of deoxycorticosterone hypertension in rats. *Circ. Res.* **46,** 619–624.

Berecek, K. H., Murray, R. D., and Gross, F. (1980b). Significance of sodium, sympathetic innervation, and central adrenergic structures on renal vascular responsiveness in DOCA-treated rats. *Circ. Res.* **47,** 675–683.

Conway, J., Darwin, K., Hilditch, A., Loveday, B., and Reeves, M. (1975). Effect of propranolol on blood pressure in normal and hypertensive rats. *Clin. Sci. Mol. Med.* **48,** 101S–103S.

Daniel, W. W. (1974). "Biostatistics: A Foundation for Analysis in the Health Sciences," pp. 224–268. Wiley, New York.

de Champlain, J. (1973). The influence of sodium on the sympathetic system in relation to experimental hypertension. *In* "Hypertension: Mechanisms and Management" (G. Onesti, K. E. Kim, and J. H. Moyer, eds.), pp. 147–164. Grune & Stratton, New York.

Dusting, G., and Rand, M. (1974). An antihypertensive action of propranolol in DOCA/salt-treated rats. *Clin. Exp. Pharmacol. Physiol.* **1,** 87–98.

Dusting, G. J., Harris, G. S., and Rand, M. J. (1973). A specific increase in cardiovascular reactivity to sodium retention in DOCA-salt-treated rats. *Clin. Sci. Mol. Med.* **45,** 571–581.

Fregly, M. J. (1960). A simple and accurate feeding device for rats. *J. Appl. Physiol.* **15,** 539.

Fregly, M. J., Nelson, E. L., Resch, G. E., Field, F. P., and Lutherer, L.O. (1975). Reduced beta-adrenergic responsiveness in hypothyroid rats. *Am. J. Physiol.* **229,** 916–924.

Fregly, M. J., Barney, C. C., Kelleher, D. L., Katovich, M. J., and Tyler, P. E. (1980). Temporal relationship between the increase in metabolic rate and tail-skin temperature following administration of isoproterenol to rats. *In* "Thermoregulatory Mechanisms and Their Therapeutic Implications" (B. Cox, P. Lomax, A. S. Milton, and E. Schonbaum, eds.), pp. 12–18. Karger, Basel.

Guideri, G., Greer, M., and Lehr, D. (1978). Potentiation of isoproterenol cardiotoxicity by corticoids. *Res. Commun. Chem. Pathol. Pharmacol.* **21,** 197–212.

Haack, D., Mohring, J., Mohring, B., Petri, M., and Hackenthal, E. (1977). Comparative study on development of corticosterone and DOCA hypertension in rats. *Am. J. Physiol.* **323,** F403–F411.

Lands, A. M., Arnold, A., McAuliff, J. P., Luduena, F. P., and Brown, T. G., Jr. (1967). Differentiation of receptors activated by sympathomimetic amines. *Nature (London)* **214,** 597–598.

Lazarow, A. (1954). Methods for quantitative measurement of water intake. *Methods Med. Res.* **6,** 225–229.

Mohring, J., Mohring, B., Petri, M., and Haack, D. (1977). Vasopressor role of ADH in the pathogenesis of malignant DOC hypertension. *Am. J. Physiol.* **232,** F260–269.

Rand, R. P., Burton, A. C., and Ing, T. (1965). The tail of the rat in temperature regulation and acclimatization. *Can. J. Physiol. Pharmacol.* **43,** 257–267.

Reid, J. L., Zivin, J. A., and Kopin, I. J. (1975). Central and peripheral adrenergic mechanisms in the development of deoxycorticosterone-saline hypertension in the rat. *Circ. Res.* **37,** 569–579.

Selye, H., Hall, C. E., and Rowley, E. M. (1943). Malignant hypertension produced by treatment with deoxycorticosterone acetate and sodium chloride. *Can. Med. Assoc. J.* **49,** 88–92.

Tarazi, R. C., Dustan, H. P., Frohlich, E. D. (1969). Relation of plasma to interstitial fluid volume in essential hypertension. *Circulation* **40,** 357–365.

Tobian, L., and Redleaf, P. D. (1957). Effect of hypertension on arterial wall electrolytes during deoxycorticosterone administration. *Am. J. Physiol.* **189,** 451–454.

Woodcock, E. A., Funder, J. W., and Johnston, C. I. (1978). Decreased beta-adrenoceptors in hypertensive rats. *Clin. Exp. Pharmacol. Physiol.* **5,** 545–550.

Woodcock, E. A., Funder, J. W., and Johnston, C. I. (1979). Decreased cardiac beta-adrenergic receptors in deoxycorticosterone-salt and renal hypertensive rats. *Circ. Res.* **45,** 560–565.

21

Mild Hypertension and Obesity in Salt-Loaded and Non-Salt-Loaded Ventromedial Hypothalamic Lesioned Rats

EFRAIN REISIN, DANIEL H. SUAREZ,
ALLAN A. MACPHEE, AND EDWARD D. FROHLICH

THE ROLE OF SALT IN
CARDIOVASCULAR HYPERTENSION

I. INTRODUCTION

Since the first description of experimental bilateral electrolytic lesions of the ventral medial hypothalamic nuclei (VMH) (Hetherington and Ranson, 1939), the development of obesity associated with other anatomic, metabolic and endocrinologic changes has become well established (Bray and York, 1979). However, the arterial pressure changes in these VHM lesioned animals have remained controversial (Bernardis and Skelton, 1965; Nosaka, 1966; Bernardis *et al.*, 1967; Bernardis, 1972) despite the rather strong clinical association of obesity and hypertension (Short and Johnson, 1939; Levy *et al.*, 1946; Epstein *et al.*, 1965; Kannel *et al.*, 1967). Additionally, a naturally developing experimental model of genetically induced obesity-hypertension has been introduced (Koletsky, 1973, 1975).

In a preliminary study we have shown increased *l*-norepinephrine responsiveness in female VMH-lesioned rats (Reisin and Wilson, 1981). The present study was designed to find out more about the pathophysiological alterations associated with the increased arterial pressure of obesity induced (VMH) hypertension and their relationship to changes in plasma and total blood volumes and systemic hemodynamics in Wistar rats receiving either a normal or a high salt intake.

II. METHODS

A. Bilateral VMH Lesions

Thirty-six Wistar rats (Hilltop Laboratory Animals, Inc., Chetsworth, California) with repeated tail systolic plethysmographic arterial pressures under 140 mm Hg (Pfeffer *et al.*, 1971) were used in this study.

Bilateral sterotaxic lesions of the VMH areas (David Kopf stereotaxic apparatus) were made electrolytically in rats weighing between 260 and 300 g under sodium pentobarbital (50 mg/kg intraperitoneally) anesthesia. The tooth bar was positioned 2.5 mm below the level of the intraaural line. A stainless steel monopolar anodal electrode was positioned 2.5 mm posterior to the bregma, 0.5 mm to both sides of the midline, and then lowered 9 mm deep. Lesions were made by passing a constant anodal current (1.5 mA) for 15 sec through the electrode (epoxilite 6001) which was insulated except for a 0.5-mm area at the tip. The cathode was attached to the temporalis muscle. In sham animals the electrode was similarly positioned using the same coordinates, but in these rats no lesioning current was passed. After the lesions were made, all rats were housed in individual cages with *ad libitum* access to water and mashed wet food; one-half of the rats received tap water and the other half received 1.5% NaCl solution. Over the ensuing 8 weeks following the VMH lesions 24-hr urinary collections were obtained in each rat for two consecutive days in order to determine sodium and potassium excretion.

B. Plasma and Total Blood Volume Determinations

On the sixtieth day following lesion placement, cannulas (PE 50) were inserted, under light ether anesthesia, into the lower abdominal aorta and left ventricle through the right femoral and carotid arteries, respectively. Confirmation of the catheter tip locations was made by pressure tracings, both cannulas having been filled with heparinized saline. These catheters were then passed subcutaneously for exteriorization at the dorsal neck area. When the rats had fully recovered from anesthesia (after at least 3 hr) they were placed in a plastic chamber ($20 \times 9 \times 9$ cm) where they remained unrestrained. Arterial pressure and heart rate were recorded on a Grass polygraph (model 79 D) connected to a Statham P23Db strain gauge. Approximately 0.74 μCi/g (about 10^6 cpm/kg R^{125}ISA in a 0.2–0.3 ml saline gravimetrically determined volume) was injected through the left ventricular catheter that was immediately followed by a 0.1-ml 0.9% NaCl flush. Blood (0.2 ml) was withdrawn from the femoral catheter after 10 min for determination of hematocrit and plasma volume. Plasma and R^{125}ISA standard samples were placed in a deep-well gamma Packard scintillation counter and counted for 10 and 1 min, respectively. Plasma volume (PV) was calculated using the following formula:

$$PV \text{ (ml)} = \frac{\text{(ml injected)} - \text{(counts/min ml}^{-1}\text{ RISA stock solution)}}{\text{(counts/min ml}^{-1}\text{ plasma)}}$$

Total blood volume (BV) was calculated using the following formula:

$$BV = \frac{PV \text{ (ml)}}{1 - \left(0.8 \times \dfrac{\text{hematocrit}}{100} \right)}$$

where 0.8 is the F cells ratio as previously determined in our laboratory for Wistar rats (Trippodo, 1981).

C. Hemodynamic Measurement

Systemic hemodynamic indices were determined with approximately 40,000 radioactive microspheres (15 μm diameter)(3M Company, St. Paul, Minn.) that were placed in a 5 cm length silastic tubing (i.d. 0.040 mm $\times$ o.d. 0.085 mm, Dow Chemical Co., Midland, MI), labeled with either ^{85}Sr or ^{141}Ce, using the reference sample method and calculation described previously (Ishise et al., 1980).

Nine rats were used in each experimental group. At the termination of the study each rat was killed by exsanguination. The brains were removed, and localization of lesions was confirmed from paraffin-embedded material. The sliced sections were cut at 7μm mounted on glass slides and stained with hematoxylin and eosine.

D. Statistical Methods

All values presented in the text, tables, and figures are means ± 1 SEM. The effects of the VMH lesion and salt intake were determined by one way analyses of variance (ANOVA). In all cases, when a significant ($p < 0.05$) F ratio was obtained, the Duncan test was used to determine which of the groups differed significantly from the others (Duncan, 1955).

III. RESULTS

A. Weight, Mean Arterial Pressure, and Heart Rate

Total body weight of the VMH-lesioned rats was greater than that of the sham control animals ($p < 0.01$); and the non-salt-loaded rats were heavier than the

TABLE I

Body Weight, Mean Arterial Pressure, Heart Rate, and Systemic Hemodynamics in Bilateral Ventromedial Hypothalamic Lesioned (VMH) and Sham-Treated Rats (Non-Salt-Loaded and Salt-Loaded)[a]

Property	Non-salt-loaded		Salt-loaded		p^{1b}	p^{2b}
	VMH	Sham	VMH	Sham		
Weight (g)	567 ± 19	462 ± 12	505 ± 4	415 ± 16	**	**
Heart rate (beats/min)	389 ± 16	401 ± 13	401 ± 19	387 ± 9	NS	NS
Mean arterial pressure (mm Hg)	128 ± 3	118 ± 3	133 ± 4	120 ± 3	**	NS
Cardiac output (ml/min)	115 ± 7	112 ± 5	105 ± 4	106 ± 5	NS	NS
Total peripheral resistance index (mm Hg/ml/min/kg)	0.6 ± .03	0.5 ± .02	0.6 ± .02	0.5 ± .03	***	NS

[a] Each group presents the mean ($\pm$ SEM) for nine rats.
[b] p^1, lesion versus sham; p^2, Non-salt-loaded versus salt-loaded; NS, not significant; *$p < 0.05$; **$p < 0.01$; ***$p < 0.001$.

salt-loaded rats ($p < 0.01$). Mean arterial pressure (MAP) was higher in rats with VMH lesions than in the sham operated controls ($p < 0.05$) (Table I). The salt-loaded animals had a slightly higher (but insignificantly so) mean arterial pressure as compared to the rats with normal salt intake. Heart rates were similar in all four groups (Table I).

B. Systemic Hemodynamics

Cardiac output (CO) was similar in all four groups studied (Table I). However, cardiac index (output per kg body wt) was reduced in the VMH-lesioned rats with high salt intake as compared with their sham controls (211 ± 12 versus 256 ± 12 ml/min/kg, $p < 0.05$) and reduced (but not significantly so) in the VMH-lesioned rats receiving normal salt intake as compared with their sham controls (205 ± 33 versus 231 ± 22 ml/min/kg). The VMH-lesioned rats had a higher total peripheral resistance index (TPRI) than their sham controls ($p < 0.001$) whether salt-loaded or not (Table I). However, the difference in diet did not produce any significant change in TPRI.

C. Urinary Volume and Electrolyte Excretion

The 24-hr urinary volume and sodium excretion were significantly greater in the VMH-lesioned rats than in their sham controls ($p < 0.01$) (Table II), as expected; urinary sodium excretion was greater in the groups with high salt intake than in the groups with regular salt intake ($p < 0.001$), but more so in the VMH lesioned rats than in the sham control rats ($p < 0.01$). Potassium excretions were similar in all four experimental groups (Table II).

D. Intravascular Volume

Plasma and total blood volumes were not expanded in the VMH-lesioned rats. In fact, when blood volume was expressed in terms of body weight it was actually contracted in the obese rats as compared with their sham controls ($p < 0.001$) (Table II). The VMH-lesioned and sham control animals with high salt intake had shown an expanded blood volume/kg body wt when compared with their regular salt intake control rats ($p < 0.001$ and $p < 0.001$, respectively) (Table II).

E. Brain Histology

Brain histological studies revealed extensive bilateral damage to the ventromedial hypothalamic nuclei of all VMH-lesioned rats. Additionally, in both groups of animals with VMH lesions, some rats had bilateral destruction of the

TABLE II

Urinary Volume Collection (24 Hr) for Sodium and Potassium Excretion, and Intravascular Volume Measurements in Bilateral Ventromedial Hypothalamic Lesioned (VMH) and Sham-Treated Rats (Non-Salt-Loaded and Salt-Loaded)[a]

| | Non-salt-loaded | | Salt-loaded | | | |
	VMH	Sham	VMH	Sham	p^{1b}	p^{2b}
Urinary volume (ml/24 hr)	44 ± 11	17 ± 1	87 ± 15	56 ± 8	**	***
U_{Na} (mEq/24 hr)	22 ± 4	13 ± 3	91 ± 7	59 ± 7	**	***
U_K (mEq/24 hr)	25 ± 5	24 ± 4	21 ± 4	22 ± 2	NS	NS
Plasma volume (ml)	13 ± 2	12 ± 1	13 ± 1	14 ± 1	NS	NS
Total blood volume (ml/kg)	34 ± 1	46 ± 2	38 ± 1	54 ± 2	***	***

[a] Each group presents the mean (± SEM) for nine rats.
[b] p^1, VMH versus sham; p^2, non-salt-loaded versus salt-loaded; NS, not significant; *$p < 0.5$; **$p < 0.01$; ***$p < 0.001$.

nuclei arcustus, dorsomedialis, and periventricularis or unilateral lesions of the columme fornicus and fasciculo mamillothalamicus.

IV. DISCUSSION

Previous reports have been contradictory with respect to the effect of VMH destruction on arterial pressure. In one earlier study bilateral VMH lesions prevented the rise of arterial pressure that normally was observed in weanling rats but similar lesions in adult rats did not change arterial pressure (Bernardis and Skelton, 1965). Another study demonstrated an increased arterial pressure which was related to an extensive bilateral medioanteromedial lesion in the hypothalamus (Nosaka, 1966).

Increased salt intake has been implicated in the development of hypertension in both animals and humans (Selye *et al.,* 1943; Meneely *et al.,* 1953, 1957; Dahl *et al.,* 1958). A salt load has been reported to aggravate the hypertension of spontaneously hypertensive rats by further elevating total peripheral resistance (Chrysant *et al.,* 1979); a similar effect was reported for the salt-sensitive rat (Dahl strain) (Tobian *et al.,* 1974). By contrast, high salt intake did not increase arterial pressure in the salt-resistant rat of the Dahl strain (Tobian *et al.,* 1974) or in WKY rats. Hemodynamic studies in the normotensive WKY rats revealed an increased cardiac output and fall in total peripheral resistance when the WKY rats were salt loaded (Chrysant *et al.,* 1979).

The Wistar rats used in the present experiments were initially normotensive; but bilateral VMH lesions produced obesity and mild hypertension in them. A recent study in mice indicated that bilateral VMH destruction (with gold thioglucose) increased cardiac norepinephrine turnover in the fasting and feeding states and strongly suggested enhanced sympathetic activity (Young and Landsberg, 1981). This sympathetic hyperactivity associated with bilateral VMH lesions could explain the increased arterial pressure, but further studies are necessary to verify this hypothesis in rats.

The responses to salt loading in VMH-lesioned and sham rats were similar. These results are somewhat surprising for this is one of the few forms of chronic hypertension that is associated with no further rise in arterial pressure with salt loading. Perhaps this is because the kidneys were undisturbed. Nevertheless, VMH-lesioned rats and sham-treated rats that received salt excess demonstrated an expanded blood volume.

In conclusion, bilateral VMH lesions in male Wistar rats were associated with obesity and mild hypertension. The hypertension was related to an increased total peripheral resistance and contracted blood volume (per kg body wt). Increased salt intake expanded the blood volume (per kg body wt) in both VMH-lesioned and sham-treated rats, but did not amplify the increased arterial pressure in either.

V. SUMMARY

Clinical and experimental studies report a positive correlation between obesity, high salt intake, and arterial pressure. In order to study this relationship in an animal model, obesity was produced in male Wistar rats by bilateral electrolytic lesion of the ventromedial hypothalamic nuclei (VMH). Age- and sex-matched rats served as controls. After the lesions were made, all rats had *ad libitum* access to water and mashed wet food; one-half of the rats received tap water and the other half received 1.5% NaCl. After 60 days, intraarterial pressure was recorded when the animals were conscious and without an anesthetic effect. Plasma volume was determined with R^{125} ISA and systemic hemodynamics were determined in each rat with radioactive (^{85}Sr or ^{141}Ce) microspheres (15 μm). Lesioned rats had a higher body weight, increased mean arterial pressure, increased total peripheral resistance, and contracted blood volume(per kg body wt). Increased salt intake expanded the blood volume (per kg body weight) in both VMH-lesioned and sham-treated rats but did not amplify the increased arterial pressure in either. The sympathetic hyperactivity associated with bilateral VMH lesions previously described in mice could explain the increased arterial pressure but further studies are necessary to verify these hypothesis in rats.

ACKNOWLEDGMENT

Supported, in part, by a grant-in-aid from the American Heart Association, Louisiana, Inc.

REFERENCES

Bernardis, L. L. (1972). Delayed ventricular changes in the hypothalamics of weanling rat following electrolytic lesions of the ventromedial nucleus. *J. Neuro-Visc. Relat.* **32,** 347–354.

Bernardis, L. L., and Skelton, F. R. (1965). Blood pressure in female and male rats following ventromedial hypothalamic lesions placed at four different ages. *Proc. Soc. Exp. Biol. Med.* **120,** 756–760.

Bernardis, L. L., Phil, D., Brownie, A. C., Molteni, A., and Skelton, F. R. (1967). Effect of ventromedial hypothalamic lesions on adrenal regeneration hypertension in young adult rats. *Lab. Invest.* **16,** 516–525.

Bray, G. A., and York, D. A. (1979). Hypothalamic and genetic obesity in experimental animals: An autonomic and endocrine hypothesis. *Physiol. Rev.* **59,** 719–809.

Chrysant, S. G., Walsh, G. M., Kern, D. C., and Frohlich, E. D. (1979). Hemodynamic and metabolic evidence of salt sensitivity in spontaneously hypertensive rats. *Kidney Int.* **15,** 33–37.

Dahl, L. J., Silver, L., and Christie, R. W. (1958). The role of salt in the fall of blood pressure accompanying reduction in obesity. *N. Engl. J. Med.* **258,** 1186–1192.

Duncan, D. B. (1955). Multiple range and multiple F tests. *Biometrics* **11,** 1–42.

Epstein, F. H. (1965). Prevalence of chronic disease and distribution of selected physiological variably in a total community of Tecumseh, Washington. *Am. J. Epidemiol.* **81,** 307–322.

Hetherington, A. W., and Ranson, S. W. (1939). Experimental hypothalamics-hypophyseal obesity in the rat. *Proc. Soc. Exp. Biol. Med.* **41,** 465–466.

Ishise, S., Pegram, B. L., Yamamoto, J., Kitomura, Y., and Frohlich, E. D. (1980). Reference sample microsphere method cardiac output and blood flows in conscious rat. *Am. J. Physiol.* **239,** H443–H449.

Kannel, W. B., Brand, N., Skinner, J. J., Dawber, T. R., and McNamara, P. M. (1967). The relation of adiposity to blood pressure and development of hypertension. The Framingham study. *Ann. Intern. Med.* **67,** 48–59.

Koletsky, S. (1973). Obese spontaneously hypertensive rats. A model for study of atherosclerosis. *Exp. Mol. Pathol.* **19,** 53–60.

Koletsky, S. (1975). Pathologic findings and laboratory data in a new strain of obese hypertensive rats. *Am. J. Pathol.* **80,** 129–140.

Levy, R. L., White, P. D., Stroud, W. D., and Hillman, C. C. (1946). Overweight: Its prognostic significance in relation to hypertension and cardiovascular renal disease. *JAMA, J. Am. Med. Assoc.* **131,** 951–953.

Meneely, G. R., Tucker, R. G., Darby, W. J., and Auerbach, S. H. (1953). Chronic sodium chloride toxicity in albino rat. II. Occurrence of hypertension and syndrome of edema and renal failure. *J. Exp. Med.* **98,** 71–79.

Meneely, G. R., Ball, C. O. T., and Youmans, J. B. (1957). Chronic sodium chloride toxicity: Protective effect of added potassium chloride. *Ann. Intern. Med.* **47,** 263–213.

Nosaka, S. (1966). Hypertension induced by extensive medial anteromedian hypothalamic destruction in the rat. *Jpn. Circ. J.* **30,** 509–523.

Pfeffer, J. M., Pfeffer, M. A., and Frohlich, E. D. (1971). Validity of an indirect tail-cuff method for determining systolic arterial pressure in unanesthetized normotensive and spontaneously hypertensive rats. *J. Lab. Clin. Med.* **78,** 957–962.

Reisin, E., and Wilson, J. R. (1981). Increased pressor reactivity in ventromedial hypothalamic lesion-induced obesity. *Life Sci.* **29,** 53–60.

Selye H., Hall, C. E., and Rowley, E. M. (1943). Malignant hypertension produced by treatment with deoxycorticosterone acetate and sodium chloride. *Can. Med. Assoc. J.* **49,** 88–92.

Short, J. J., and Johnson, H. J. (1939). An evaluation of the influence of overweight and blood pressure of healthy men. *Am. J. Med. Sci.* **198,** 220–224.

Tobian, L., Ganguli, M., and Dahl, L. (1974). Cardiac output in strains of rats sensitive or resistant to NaCl hypertension. *Circulation* **50,** 31 (abstr.)

Trippodo, N. C. (1981). Total circulatory capacity in the rat. Effects of epinephrine and vasopressin on compliance and unstressed volume. *Circ. Res.* **49,** 923–931.

Young, J. B., and Landsberg, L. (1981). Impaired suppression of sympathetic activity during fasting in the gold thioglucose-treated mouse. *J. Clin. Invest.* **65,** 1086–1094.

22

The Loop of Henle Is the Nephron Site Responsible for Escape from the Sodium-Retaining Effects of Mineralocorticoids

JOHN A. HAAS AND FRANKLYN G. KNOX

I. INTRODUCTION

The prolonged administration of mineralocorticoids concurrent with an abundance of sodium in the diet results in retention of the dietary intake of sodium for

323

Copyright © 1982 by Academic Press, Inc.
All rights of reproduction in any form reserved.
ISBN 0-12-267280-1

a few days. After this period of sodium retention, sodium balance is restored despite the continued administration of mineralocorticoids. This return to sodium balance is termed the "escape" from the salt-retaining effects of mineralocorticoids (Davis and Howell, 1953).

The nephron site of enhanced sodium reabsorption and those involved in escape may not be the same. Previous studies with isolated cortical collecting tubules have shown that mineralocorticoids enhance sodium reabsorption in this nephron segment (Gross et al., 1975; O'Neil and Helman, 1977). However, because no diminution of the enhanced sodium reabsorption in the cortical collecting tubule has been demonstrated, it seems likely that the return to sodium balance, i.e., "escape," is accomplished when increased sodium delivery from another nephron segment overcomes cortical collecting duct sodium reabsorption.

The present studies were undertaken, therefore, to ascertain by free-flow micropuncture the effect of chronic mineralocorticoid treatment on sodium reabsorption along the nephron. In the first series, Groups 1 and 2, the effect of chronic DOCA treatment on collecting duct sodium reabsorption was evaluated in rats by comparing fractional sodium delivery out of the superficial late distal tuuble with the fraction of sodium remaining at the base and tip of the papillary collecting duct (Haas et al., 1979). The second series, Groups 3, 4, 5, and 6, was undertaken to evaluate the effect of chronic DOCA treatment on loop of Henle sodium reabsorption in both superficial and deep nephrons (Kohan and Knox, 1980).

II. METHODS

Six groups of Munich–Wistar rats were studied. The different groups and protocols employed are outlined below.

Group	Treatment	Micropuncture protocol
1	Normal salt diet; isotonic saline; controls for Group 2	Superficial late distal tubules and base and tip of papillary collecting duct
2	Normal salt diet; isotonic saline; DOCA-treated	Same as Group 1
3	Normal salt diet; isotonic saline; controls for Group 4	Superficial proximal and distal tubules
4	Normal salt diet; isotonic saline; DOCA-treated	Same as Group 3

Group	Treatment	Micropuncture protocol
5	Normal salt diet; isotonic saline; controls for Group 6	Superficial proximal tubule and descending and ascending limbs of deep nephrons
6	Normal salt diet; isotonic saline; DOCA-treated	Same as Group 5

In Groups 1–6, male Munich–Wistar rats (100–225 g) were given normal Purina rat chow (sodium concentration 0.1 mEq/g) up to 15 hr before experimentation and had free access to isotonic saline for 3 days prior to the experiment. DOCA (15 mg/kg) was administered subcutaneously for 3 days prior to experimentation to Groups 2, 4, and 6. This was sufficient time for the rats to escape from the sodium retaining effects of mineralocorticoids (Mohring and Mohring, 1972). On the day of the acute experiment, the rats were anesthetized with Inactin and a tracheostomy was performed. Body temperature was maintained between 36° and 38°C with a heated micropuncture table. Catheters were inserted into a jugular vein for infusions, a carotid artery for blood sampling and blood pressure monitoring, and the dome of the bladder for contralateral kidney urine collection. Through a left subcostal incision, the left kidney was immobilized and placed in a holder and bathed in mineral oil. The papilla was exposed by excision of the ureter. The rats were primed with 0.5 ml of a 7% inulin in a 0.9% saline solution, and the rate of inulin infusion was kept at 1.2 ml/hr for the duration of the experiment. Simultaneously, a 10% body weight volume expansion with 0.9% saline was given over 1 hr, after which the infusion was altered to match urine volume in Groups 1 and 2, or in Groups 3–6, followed by a 4% body weight saline infusion for the remainder of the experiment. Following completion of the 10% body weight expansion, micropuncture samples were collected and 2–4 clearance periods were obtained from the right kidney via the bladder catheter.

Superficial proximal and distal tubule segments were identified by lissamine green injection and punctured with pipettes 4–12 μm o.d. as previously described (Knox and Gasser, 1974). Papillary collecting duct samples were taken at the base of the papilla (base collections) and from the tip of the papilla by the axial introduction of the pipette into a duct of Bellini (tip collection). Descending and ascending limb collections were punctured with pipettes 5–7 μm o.d. and papillary collecting ducts with pipettes of 10–15 μm. Inulin concentrations in tubule fluid, plasma, and urine were determined by the microflurormetric method of Vurek and Pegram (1966). The volume of tubule fluid was measured with micropipettes calibrated with a radioactive tracer. Sodium concentrations in tubular fluid were measured with a helium-glow photometer. Sodium concentrations in plasma and urine were measured by flame photometry. Comparison of the data within groups was determined by the paired t test and between groups by the group t test.

III. RESULTS

A summary of the clearances from the contralateral kidney and micropuncture data for Groups 1 and 2 is shown in Table I. Glomerular filtration rate (GFR) and fractional sodium excretion ($FE_{Na}\%$) were not significantly different in the two groups. In Group 1, rats which received saline drinking water alone, the tubule fluid:plasma concentration ratio of Na divided by that of inulin (TF/P) Na/In $\times$ 100 or fractional delivery of sodium ($FD_{Na}\%$) at the superficial distal tubule was 8.3 $\pm$ 0.8%, whereas $FD_{Na}\%$ to the base of the papilla was 10.4 $\pm$ 1.1%. $FD_{Na}\%$ at the tip of the papilla was significantly less than at the base of the papilla, $\Delta4.6 \pm 1.0\%$, $p < 0.005$. In Group 2, rats that received DOCA and saline drinking water, $FD_{Na}\%$ at the superficial distal tubule was significantly greater than at the base of the papillary collecting duct, $\Delta6.6 \pm 1.7\%$, $p <$ 0.005. $FD_{Na}\%$ at the tip of the papilla was also significantly less than at the base, $\Delta3.6 \pm 1.1\%$, $p < 0.01$. Single nephron glomerular filtration ($SNGFR$) rate was not significantly different between the two groups.

A summary of the clearances from the contralateral kidney and the micropuncture data for Groups 3, 4, 5, and 6 is shown in Table II. In Groups 3 and 4, GFR, $FE_{Na}\%$, and $SNGFR$ were not different in the two groups. $FD_{Na}\%$ to the late proximal tubule was similar in control (60.1 $\pm$ 1.8%) and DOCA-treated rats

TABLE I

Summary of Clearance and Micropuncture Data for Groups 1 and 2

	Contralateral kidney		(TF/P) Na/In $\times$ 100[b]			
	GFR (nl/min)	$FE_{Na}\%$[a]	Superficial distal tubule	Base papilla	Tip papilla	Distal $SNGFR$ (nl/min)
Group 1 ($n = 9$) control rats receiving isotonic saline drinking water						
Mean	0.8	6.5	8.3	10.4[c]	5.9	49
$\pm$ 1 SEM	0.1	0.9	0.8	1.1	0.6	6
Group 2 ($n = 10$): DOCA-treated rats receiving isotonic saline drinking water						
Mean	1.2	6.5	16.1[c,d]	9.5[c]	5.9	49
$\pm$ 1 SEM	0.2	1.6	2.6	1.9	1.2	5

[a] Fractional sodium excretion.

[b] Tubule fluid: plasma concentration ratio of Na divided by that of inulin or fractional delivery of sodium ($FE_{Na}\%$).

[c] Statistically significant; paired t test.

[d] Statistically significant; group t test.

TABLE II

Summary of Clearance and Micropuncture Data for Groups 3–6

	Contralateral kidney		(TF/P) Na/In × 100 Superficial		$SNGFR^b$ (nl/min)	
	GFR^a	$FE_{Na}\%$	Late proximal	Early distal	LP	ED
Group 3 ($n = 12$): Control rats receiving isotonic saline drinking water						
Mean	0.58	8.9	60.1	13.3	18.2	19.4
± 1 SEM	0.04	0.5	1.8	1.0	1.6	1.2
Group 4 ($n = 12$): DOCA-treated rats receiving isotonic saline drinking water						
Mean	0.63	8.0	61.0	19.9^c	17.1	16.7
± 1 SEM	0.04	0.7	1.9	1.6	1.4	1.2

	GFR^a	$FE_{Na}\%$	Superficial late proximal	Deep loop of Henle	LP	LH
Group 5 ($n = 9$): Control rats receiving isotonic saline drinking water						
Mean	0.51	8.5	53.6	41.8	19.0	21.9
± 1 SEM	0.06	0.6	3.1	3.3	1.7	2.8
Group 6 ($n = 9$): DOCA-treated rats receiving isotonic saline drinking water						
Mean	0.48	7.8	49.3	51.8^c	18.6	25.3
± 1 SEM	0.04	0.8	3.3	3.9	1.8	3.2

[a] Values are expressed as $ml \cdot min^{-1} \cdot 100$ g body wt^{-1}.

[b] Values are expressed as $nl \cdot min^{-1} \cdot 100$ g body wt^{-1}.

[c] Statistically significant; group t test.

(61.0 ± 1.9%), but $FD_{Na}\%$ to the superficial early distal tubule was significantly increased in DOCA-treated rats (19.9 ± 1.6%) compared to control rats (13.3 ± 1.0%). $FD_{Na}\%$ to the superficial early distal tubule was also evaluated by subtracting $FD_{Na}\%$ to the superficial early distal tubule from $FD_{Na}\%$ in the superficial late proximal tubule in each rat. $FD_{Na}\%$ (late proximal minus early distal) was significantly lower in DOCA-treated rats (41.1 ± 2.0%) than in controls (46.8 ± 2.3%), $p < 0.05$.

In Groups 5 and 6, GFR, $FE_{Na}\%$, and $SNGFR$ were not different in the two groups. As in Groups 3 and 4, $FD_{Na}\%$ in the superficial late proximal tubule was similar in DOCA-treated and control animals. However, $FD_{Na}\%$ to the loop of Henle in the deep nephrons was increased in DOCA-treated (51.8 ± 3.9%) compared to control rats (41.8 ± 3.3%, $p < 0.05$). Again, $FD_{Na}\%$ between the deep loop of Henle and superficial late proximal tubule (late proximal minus deep loop of Henle) was significantly lower in DOCA-treated rats (−4.4 ± 3.7%) compared to controls (11.5 ± 3.1%, $p < 0.005$). These data provide additional evidence that $FD_{Na}\%$ to the loops of Henle in the deep nephrons is significantly greater in DOCA-treated than control rats. Sodium delivery out of the proximal tubule is not different between the control and DOCA-escape rats. In contrast, sodium delivery in the superficial early distal tubule as well as the loop of Henle in deep nephrons is markedly enhanced. However, this difference is abolished at the base of the papillary collecting duct, $10.4 \pm 1.1\%$ versus $9.5 \pm 1.9\%$, $\Delta 2.26 \pm 0.4\%$, NS. Finally, sodium reabsorption by the papillary collecting duct is similar in control and DOCA-escaped rats.

IV. DISCUSSION

In contrast to controls, fractional delivery of sodium between the late proximal and early distal tubule of superficial nephrons was greater in the DOCA-escaped rats. Additionally, $FD_{Na}\%$ to the bend of the deep loop of Henle was increased. Other studies have been unable to detect an effect of DOCA treatment on pars recta and/or loop of Henle sodium transport (Schnermann et al., 1975; Sonnenberg, 1973). However, these studies were conducted during hydropenia, which, without volume replacement for surgical losses, may have masked differences between DOCA-treated and control animals (Maddox et al., 1977). Thus, superimposed volume expansion in the present studies (Haas et al., 1979; Kohan and Knox, 1980) may have unmasked the contribution of the loop of Henle in escape. Therefore, based on these studies, the loop of Henle in both superficial and deep nephrons appears likely to be the nephron segment responsible for the increase in sodium delivery in mineralocorticoid escape.

As shown in Table I, $FD_{Na}\%$ was greater in the papillary collecting duct base than in the superficial late distal tubule in control rats, whereas $FD_{Na}\%$ decreased between the superficial late distal tubule and papillary collecting duct base in the DOCA-escaped rats. This difference in $FD_{Na}\%$ is consistent with the in vitro observation in the rabbit of enhanced sodium reabsorption by cortical collecting tubules after chronic mineralocorticoid treatment (Gross et al., 1975; O'Neil and Helman, 1977). The marked increase in sodium delivery to the distal tubule may be the mechanism that accounts for the return to sodium balance in the presence of an increase in sodium reabsorption by the cortical collecting duct.

Another important aspect of the present studies is that sodium was reabsorbed along the papillary collecting duct in both control and DOCA-escaped rats. This is in contrast to the conclusion drawn in a microcatheterization study that papillary collecting duct sodium reabsorption was completely inhibited after DOCA treatment in the rat (Sonnenberg, 1976). The reason for the failure to detect sodium reabsorption in the papillary collecting duct with microcatheterization may be due to technical difficulties associated with the technique (Stein et al., 1976).

Thus, fractional delivery of sodium is increased from the superficial nephron segment containing the pars recta and loop of Henle. Fractional delivery of sodium is also increased in DOCA escape in deep nephrons at the bend of the loop of Henle. Finally, escape from the sodium-retaining effects of mineralocorticoids occurs when sodium delivery from both superficial and deep nephrons is increased enough to overcome mineralocorticoid-stimulated sodium reabsorption by the cortical collecting tubule.

V. SUMMARY

In vitro studies of isolated perfused cortical collecting tubules from rabbits have demonstrated that prior chronic treatment with deoxycorticosterone acetate (DOCA) increases sodium reabsorption in this nephron segment. On the other hand, it is known that animals return to sodium balance in the presence of mineralocorticoid excess. To evaluate collecting duct sodium reabsorption, *in vivo*, fractional sodium delivery ($FD_{Na}\%$) out of the superficial late distal tubule was compared with the fraction of filtered sodium remaining at the base and tip of the papillary collecting duct in control and DOCA-escaped rats. Additionally, $FD_{Na}\%$ from the superfiical late proximal tubule, early superficial distal tubule, and the loop of Henle in deep nephrons was determined.

Our results indicate that DOCA escape is not due to a greater delivery of sodium from the superficial proximal tubule. However, sodium delivery is increased from the loop of Henle of both superficial and deep nephrons. Consequently, escape from the sodium-retaining effects of mineralocorticoids occurs when this increased sodium delivery overcomes mineralocorticoid-stimulated sodium reabsorption by the cortical collecting tubule.

REFERENCES

Davis, J. O., and Howell, D. S. (1953). Comparative effect of ACTH, cortisone and DOCA on renal function, electrolyte excretion and water exchange in normal dogs. *Endocrinology* **52**, 245–255.

Gross, J. B., Iami, M., and Kokko, J. P. (1975). A functional comparison of the cortical collecting tubule and the distal convoluted tubule. *J. Clin. Invest.* **55**, 1284–1294.

Haas, J. A., Berndt, T. J., Youngberg, S. P., and Knox, F. G. (1979). Collecting duct sodium reabsorption in deoxycorticosterone-treated rats. *J. Clin. Invest.* **63**, 211–214.

Knox, F. G., and Gasser, J. (1974). Altered distal sodium reabsorption in volume expansion. *Mayo Clin. Proc.* **49**, 775–781.

Kohan, D. E., and Knox, F. G. (1980). Localization of the nephron sites responsible for mineralocorticoid escape in rats. *Am. J. Physiol.* **239**, F149–F153.

Maddox, D. A., Price, D. C., and Rector, F. C., Jr. (1977). Effects of surgery on plasma volume and salt and water excretion in rats. *Am. J. Physiol.* **233**, F600–F606.

Mohring, J., and Mohring, M. (1972). Re-evaluation of DOCA escape phenomenon. *Am. J. Physiol.* **223**, 1237–1245.

O'Neil, R. G., and Helman, S. I. (1977). Transport characteristics of renal collecting tubules: Influences of DOCA and diet. *Am. J. Physiol.* **233**, F544–F558.

Schnermann, J., Hermle, M., Schmidmeier, E., and Dahlheim, J. (1975). Impaired potency for feedback regulation of glomerular filtration rate in DOCA-escaped rats. *Pfluegers Arch.* **358,** 325–338.

Sonnenberg, H. (1973). Proximal and distal tubular function in salt-deprived and in salt-loaded deoxycorticosterone acetate-escaped rats. *J. Clin. Invest.* **52,** 263–273.

Sonnenberg, H. (1976). Collecting duct function in deoxycorticosterone acetate-escaped, normal and salt-deprived rats: Response to hypervolemia. *Circ. Res.* **39,** 282–288.

Stein, J. H., Osgood, R. W., and Kunau, R. T. (1976). Direct measurements of papillary collecting duct sodium transport in the rat. *J. Clin. Invest.* **58,** 767–773.

Vurek, G. G., and Pegram, S. E. (1966). Fluorometric method for the determination of inulin. *Anal. Biochem.* **16,** 409–419.

23

Is a Circulating Sodium Transport Inhibitor Involved in the Pathogenesis of Essential Hypertension?

GRAHAM MACGREGOR AND HUGH DE WARDENER

THE ROLE OF SALT IN
CARDIOVASCULAR HYPERTENSION

I. INTRODUCTION

Dahl *et al.* first proposed in 1969 that an explanation of results of experiments they performed in parabiotic rats could be that a saluretic substance was present which also had the capacity to raise blood pressure. This hypothesis was extended by Haddy and Overbeck in 1976 who suggested that the rise in blood pressure which occurs with volume expansion might be due to an increase in a circulating sodium transport inhibitor which, while increasing sodium excretion, would at the same time cause a rise in blood pressure. There was no explanation at this time of how such an inhibitor of sodium transport could cause a rise in blood pressure. Blaustein, one year later, suggested a possible mechanism whereby an inhibitor of sodium transport could cause a rise in intracellular calcium in the smooth muscle cell. Such a rise would cause an increase in the tone and excitability of the smooth muscle cell and an increase in peripheral resistance with the eventual development of high blood pressure. The above hypotheses have recently been extended by de Wardener and MacGregor (1980) to explain the link between sodium intake, the numerous abnormalities of sodium transport, and the development of high blood pressure in essential hypertension. This chapter outlines this hypothesis and presents some of the evidence that supports it.

The hypothesis proposes that the development of essential hypertension in man is due to an inherited defect in the ability of the kidney to excrete sodium (Fig. 1). As sodium intake increases to levels above 50 mmol/day there is a tendency

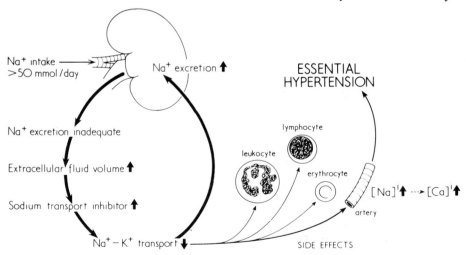

Fig. 1. Hypothesis for the possible role of a circulating sodium transport inhibitor in the etiology of essential hypertension. This figure is reproduced by kind permission of *Kidney International* (de Wardener and MacGregor, 1980).

for sodium retention and an increase in extracellular volume. This gives rise to an increased secretion of a circulating sodium transport inhibitor. This inhibitor of sodium transport reduces tubular reabsorption of sodium and thereby increases sodium excretion. This tends to correct the tendency for an increase in extracellular volume in these patients. As a side effect, this increase in a sodium transport inhibitor will inhibit sodium transport in other cells, in particular, the circulating red and white cells and, more importantly, smooth muscle cell of the arteriole. Inhibition of sodium transport will give rise to an increase in intracellular sodium which by the mechanism Blaustein (1977) has outlined causes a rise in intracellular calcium and an increase in the tone of the smooth muscle cell leading eventually to development of hypertension. This hypothesis necessarily implies that the rate of development and the height of the blood pressure will first depend on sodium intake, and second on the severity of the inherited defect in eliminating sodium from the kidney.

II. SODIUM INTAKE

While there is controversy about the importance of sodium intake in the development of essential hypertension, the prevalence of high blood pressure in different communities is directly related to dietary sodium intake (Gleibermann, 1973) and urinary sodium excretion (Dahl, 1961; Sinnett and Whyte, 1973; Oliver *et al.*, 1975; Fukuda, 1954; Takamatsu, 1955; Sasaki, 1964). Studies in three communities have shown that high blood pressure is unknown when

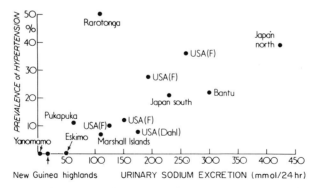

Fig. 2. Georgraphic distribution of the relationship between the prevalence of hypertension and urinary sodium excretion (hypertension defined as diastolic pressure > 90 mm Hg and/or systolic pressure > 140 mm Hg). Data obtained from following references: Yanomamo (Oliver *et al.*, 1975); New Guinea Highlands (Sinnett and Whyte, 1973); Eskimo (Dahl, 1961); Marshall Islands (Dahl, 1961); USA(F) (Table 6: Dawber *et al.*, 1967); Pukapuka and Rarotonga (Prior *et al.*, 1968); Japan south (Sasaki, 1964); Japan north (Fukuda, 1954); Bantu (Isaacson *et al.*, 1963). This figure is reproduced by kind permission of *Nephron*.

sodium intake is less than 50 mmol/day (Dahl, 1961; Sinnett and Whyte, 1973; Oliver *et al.*, 1975; Fig. 2). One objection to the accumulating evidence that sodium intake is important in the development of hypertension has been that within a community there is no relationship between the prevalence of high blood pressure and sodium intake (Miall, 1959; Simpson *et al.*, 1978). However, this relationship could only occur if all individuals in the community were equally liable to develop high blood pressure and there was a very wide range of sodium intake. This does not occur in the western world and it is, therefore, not surprising that within one western community there is no relationship between sodium intake and the prevalence of high blood pressure.

III. DEFECT IN THE KIDNEY'S ABILITY TO EXCRETE SODIUM

The hereditary nature of essential hypertension in man is well known (Pickering, 1968). There is in man for obvious reasons no direct evidence that the genetic fault lies in the kidney. However, in the Dahl salt-sensitive and salt-resistant rats (Tobian *et al.*, 1966; Dahl *et al.*, 1972, 1974) and the Milan spontaneously hypertensive rats (Bianchi *et al.*, 1973, 1974a; Fox and Bianchi, 1976), the kidney cross-transplantation experiments clearly indicate that the blood pressure goes with the kidney. The association between sodium intake and prevalence of high blood pressure in the stock colony rat (Meneely *et al.*, 1953; Smirk and Hall, 1958), the Dahl salt-sensitive rat (Dahl *et al.*, 1962; Dahl and Schackow, 1964), and the retention of sodium that occurs in the Milan spontaneously hypertensive rat during the development of hypertension (Bianchi *et al.*, 1974b, 1975, 1977) suggests that the underlying abnormality in these rats' kidneys is a difficulty in eliminating sodium.

IV. CORRECTED STATE OF VOLUME EXPANSION

If there is a difficulty in excreting sodium by the kidney in patients who are going to develop, or who have, essential hypertension, there will be a tendency for an increase in extracellular volume secondary to the sodium retention. The hypothesis proposes that this tendency for an increase in extracellular volume is corrected by the presence of an increased concentration of a circulating sodium transport inhibitor which, by inhibiting sodium reabsorption in the tubule, will increase sodium excretion. It would be expected therefore that in patients with essential hypertension extracellular fluid volume measurements as well as blood volume would be within the normal limits (Schalekamp *et al.*, 1974). Two lines of evidence, however, suggest that there is a state of continuous correction of a tendency for volume expansion. First, many patients with hypertension have an accelerated natriuresis when challenged with sodium (Baldwin *et al.*, 1958; Lowenstein *et al.*, 1970), which is unrelated to changes in colloid, osmotic, or hydrostatic pressure in the kidney (Willassen and Ofstad, 1978), and is greatest in patients with the lowest plasma renin activity. (Krakoff *et al.*, 1970) An exaggerated natriuresis also occurs in normal subjects who are salt loaded or who have been given mineralocorticoid (Rovner *et al.*, 1965), and in patients with primary aldosteronism (Biglieri and McIllroy, 1966), situations where there is a state of continuous correction of a tendency for volume expansion. Second, it has been found repeatedly that 30–50% of patients with essential hypertension have an abnormally low value of plasma renin activity (Dunn and Tannen, 1974), which is also suggestive of a corrected state of volume expansion. It might also be expected that in low renin patients the increase in the circulating sodium transport inhibitor would be greatest.

V. INHIBITION OF SODIUM TRANSPORT IN THE ARTERIOLES

There is no direct evidence in man that sodium transport is inhibited in the smooth muscle cells of the arterioles of patients with essential hypertension, apart from the original findings of Tobian and Binion (1952) of an increase in the sodium content of renal arteries in patients with hypertension. The mechanism whereby an increase in the concentration of circulating sodium transport inhibitor might cause an increase in the tone of smooth muscle cells has been reviewed by Blaustein (1977). Theoretical calculations by Blaustein of the sensitivity of this system shows a very small rise in intracellular sodium would give a rise in intracellular calcium concentration which, in its turn, would increase the resting tone of vascular smooth muscle by approximately 50%.

VI. EVIDENCE FOR A CIRCULATING SODIUM TRANSPORT INHIBITOR IN NORMAL MAN AND ANIMAL

The existence of a circulating substance other than aldosterone which controls urinary sodium excretion is based on a multiplicity of whole animal experiments (de Wardener, 1977). These initial observations were followed by a number of experiments which demonstrate that the substance in the plasma changes urinary sodium excretion directly by inhibiting Na^+,K^+-ATPase activity.

Lichardus *et al.* (1968), using an extract of plasma, and Nutbourne *et al.* (1970), using whole blood, observed a reduction of the short circuit current in the frog skin with plasma, or blood obtained from a volume-expanded animal. Clarkson *et al.* (1970), using fragments of dog and rabbit renal tubules, demonstrated that plasma from a blood volume-expanded dog inhibits net sodium and

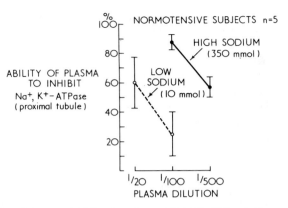

Fig. 3.   Ability of plasma to inhibit guinea pig renal Na^+,K^+-ATPase in five normal subjects on a low sodium (10 mmol/day) and a high sodium diet (350 mmol/day) at different plasma dilutions. This figure is reproduced by kind permission of *Lancet* (de Wardener *et al.*, 1981).

potassium transport in tubular fragments *in vitro* Gonick *et al.* (1977) found that a small molecular weight fraction obtained from rat serum has a significantly greater ability to inhibit renal Na^+,K^+-ATPase when the serum comes from an animal that has received a saline infusion. In man the presence of a circulating Na^+,K^+-ATPase inhibitor was first demonstrated by Poston *et al.* (1980) in normal subjects given fludrocortisone. When leukocytes from a control subjects were incubated in the serum of a person who had been given fludrocortisone, the ouabain sensitive sodium efflux of the leukocytes obtained from the control subject fell to about the same concentration as that of the leukocytes of the person from whom the serum had been obtained. Flier *et al.* (1979) demonstrated that the blood of a toad (*Bufo marinus*) which lives in salt water also contains a Na^+,K^+-ATPase inhibitor. And Gruber *et al.* (1980) obtained an extract from dog blood which inhibits Na^+,K^+-ATPase, the inhibition being greater when the extract is obtained after the dog has been given a large infusion of saline. More recently, de Wardener *et al.* (1981) using a cytochemical technique have demonstrated the presence of a renal Na^+,K^+-ATPase inhibitor in the plasma of man, the circulating concentration of which is related to sodium intake (Fig. 3).

VII. EVIDENCE FOR A RAISED CONCENTRATION OF A CIRCULATING NA^+,K^+-ATPase INHIBITOR IN ESSENTIAL HYPERTENSION

Since the first account by Losse and Wessels (1960) there have been an increasing number of confirmatory reports that sodium transport in the red cells of patients with essential hypertension is abnormal (Gessler, 1962; Wessels *et al.*, 1967; Postnov *et al.*, 1977; Garay and Meyer, 1979; Henningsen *et al.*, 1979; Fadeke Aderounmu and Salako, 1979), Several abnormalities have been reported. More recently, others have demonstrated that there are also abnormalities of sodium transport in the leukocytes (Edmondson *et al.*, 1975; Thomas *et al.*, 1975; Poston *et al.*, 1981) and lymphocytes (Ambrosioni *et al.*, 1979); and some workers have found in both the red and white cells that the Na^+,K^+-ATPase component of sodium transport is abnormal (Fadeke Adernounmu and Salako, 1979; Edmondson *et al.*, 1975; Thomas *et al.*, 1975; Poston *et al.*, 1981).

There is some evidence that suggests that the decreased rate of the Na^+,K^+-ATPase sodium transport is due to a raised concentration of a circulating Na^+,K^+-ATPase inhibitor. Poston *et al.* (1981) incubated leukocytes from normotensive subjects in the plasma of hypertensive patients. As a result these normal leukocytes developed a decrease in Na^+,K^+-ATPase activity of about the same severity as that in the patient's own white cells. This experiment demonstrates that the plasma of patients with essential hypertension contains a substance that increases the plasma's capacity to inhibit Na^+,K^+-ATPase, And suggests that it is this substance that causes the observed abnormality of sodium transport in the patient's own leukocytes (Fig. 4). Similar cross-incubation exper-

White cells from normotensives incubated in :−

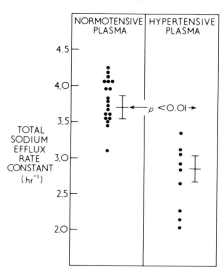

Fig. 4. Total sodium efflux rate constant in white cells from normotensive subjects incubated in either the plasma of other normotensive subjects or patients with high blood pressure. This figure is reproduced by kind permission of Poston *et al.* (1981).

iments of red cells from normotensive subjects in the plasma of patients with essential hypertension did not alter sodium transport of the normal red cells (Poston *et al.*, 1981). This may be due to the necessary differences in the experimental conditions between the two sets of observations.

According to the hypothesis outlined above the abnormalities of sodium transport in the patients' own white cells should be greatest in those hypertensive patients who have the greatest evidence of a tendency to retain sodium. If it is accepted that plasma renin activity is a marker of the state of the extracellular fluid and plasma volume, then the abnormality of white cell sodium transport should be most pronounced in the hypertensive patients who have the lowest PRA. Edmondson and MacGregor (1981) have made observations supporting this prediction. They have found that the extent of the impairment in the Na^+, K^+-ATPase component of the sodium transport of white cells from hypertensive patients is inversely correlated to the rise in PRA induced by a period of sodium deprivation (Fig. 5).

Evidence that the plasma of patients with essential hypertension contains a

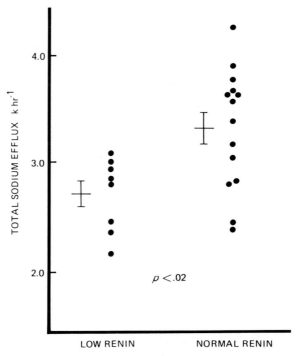

Fig. 5.   Total sodium efflux rate constant in white cells in eight low renin and fourteen normal renin patients with essential hypertension. This figure is reproduced by kind permission of *Br. Med. J.* (Edmondson and MacGregor, 1981).

raised concentration of a Na^+,K^+-ATPase inhibitor has also been obtained with cytochemical techniques. The method used to estimate the plasma's capacity to inhibit Na^+,K^+-ATPase *in vitro* mentioned above is new (de Wardener *et al.*, 1981) and less sensitive than another well-established method that can measure its ability to stimulate glucose-6-phosphate dehydrogenase (G6PD) *in vitro*. But as inhibition of Na^+,K^+-ATPase is associated with stimulation of G6PD it has been found that the plasma's capacity to stimulate G6PD *in vitro* can be used as a marker of its capacity to inhibit Na^+,K^+-ATPase *in vitro*. Using this alternative approach we have found that, as expected, normal plasma stimulated G6PD activity *in vitro,* and that this effect increases with increasing sodium intake (Alaghband-Zadeh *et al.*, 1981a) and with age. We have also found that the ability of plasma from hypertensive patients to stimulate G6PD *in vitro* is greater than in normal subjects (Alaghband-Zadeh *et al.*, 1981), and that it is greatest in patients whose PRA activity is lowest; the latter is in line with the observation of Edmondson and MacGregor (1981) on white cells. As in the normal subjects, changing the sodium intake of the hypertensive patients changed the plasma's capacity to stimulate G6PD *in vitro* but the changes were proportionally much less marked (Alaghband-Zadeh *et al.*, 1981b); after 1 week on a low sodium diet the plasma's ability to increase G6PD *in vitro* was still pronounced. Overall these three sets of observations are consistent with the presence of an increased concentration of a circulating Na^+,K^+-ATPase inhibitor in essential hypertension.

VIII. SUMMARY

There is controversy about the relationship between sodium intake and the prevalence of high blood pressure. Part of this controversy relates to how an increase in sodium intake could cause an increase in peripheral resistance. We have put forward the following hypothesis. In essential hypertension there is an inherited defect of the kidney's ability to excrete sodium which becomes increasingly obvious the greater the sodium intake. This difficulty in sodium excretion by the kidney increases the concentration of a circulating sodium transport inhibitor that affects sodium transport across many cell membranes. In the kidney the inhibitor adjusts urinary sodium excretion back toward normal so that sodium balance is near that of normal subjects on the same intake of sodium. In the arteriolar smooth muscle the inhibition of sodium transport across the cell wall causes a rise in intracellular sodium concentration which, in turn, raises the intracellular calcium concentration and thus increases vascular reactivity. This hypothesis also proposes that the abnormalities of sodium transport in circulating cells *in vivo* are directly due to the increased secretion of the circulating sodium transport inhibitor. Evidence supporting this hypothesis is discussed. First, it is pointed out that there is evidence suggesting that in normal man there is a circulating inhibitor of Na^+,K^+-ATPase, the level of which is related to sodium intake, and that the level of this inhibitor appears to be increased in many hypertensives. Second, the finding that normotsenive white cells incubated in the plasma of hypertensive patients develop the same decrease in the Na^+,K^+-ATPase, dependent sodium transport as the hypertensives' own white cells also suggests that hypertensives have an increase in a circulating Na^+,K^+-ATPase inhibitor.

REFERENCES

Alaghband-Zadeh, J., Clarkson, E. M., Fenton, S., MacGregor, G. A., and de Wardener, H. E. (1981a). The effect of sodium intake on the ability of human plasma to stimulate renal glucose-6-phosphate dehydrogenase (G6PD) in vitro. *Proc. Physiol. Soc., 1981* Abstract C97, p. 53P.

Alaghband-Zadeh, J., Fenton, S., MacGregor, G. A., Markandu, N. D. Roulston, J. E., and de Wardener, H. E. (1981b). An increased ability of plasma from patients with essential hypertension to stimulate renal glucose-6-phosphate dehydrogenase (G6PD) in vitro. *Proc. Physiol. Soc., 1981* Abstract C98, p. 54P.

Ambrosioni, E., Tartagni, F., Montebugnoli, L., and Magnani, B. (1979). Intralymphocytic sodium in hypertensive patients: A significance correlation. *Clin. Sci.* **57**, 325s-327s.

Baldwin, D. S., Biggs, A. W., Goldring, W., Hullet, W. H., and Chasis, H. (1958). Exaggerated natriuresis in essential hypertension. *Am. J. Med.* **24**, 893-902.

Bianchi, G., Fox, U., Di Francesco, G. F., Bardi, U., and Radice, M. (1973). The hypertensive role of the kidney in spontaneously hypertensive rats. *Clin. Sci. Mol. Med.* **45**, 135-139.

Bianchi, G., Fox, U., Di Francesco, G. F., Giovanetti, A. M., and Pagetti, D. (1974a). Blood pressure changes produced by kidney cross-plantation between spontaneously hypertensive rats and normotensive rats. *Clin. Sci. Mol. Med.* **47**, 435-448.

Bianchi, G., Fox, U., and Imbasciati, E. (1974b). The development of a new strain of spontaneously hypertensive rats. *Life Sci.* **14**, 339-347.

Bianchi, G., Baer, P. G., Fox, U., Duzzi, L., Pagetti, D., and Giovanetti, A. M. (1975). Changes in renin, water balance and sodium balance during development of high blood pressure in genetically hypertensive rats. *Circ. Res.,* Suppl. 1, **36/37**, 153-61.

Bianchi, G., Baer, P. G., Fox, U., and Guidi, E. (1977). The role of the kidney in the rat with genetic hypertension. *Postgrad. Med. J.* **53**, Suppl. 2, 123-135.

Biglieri, E. G., and McIllroy, M. B. (1966). Abnormalities of renal function and circulatory reflexes in primary aldosteronism. *Circulation* **33**, 78-86.

Blaustein, M. P. (1977). Sodium ions, calcium ions, blood pressure regulation and hypertension: A reassessment and a hypothesis. *Am. J. Physiol.* **232**(3), C165-C173.

Clarkson, E. M., Talner, L. B., and de Wardener, H. E. (1970). The effect of plasma from blood volume expanded dogs on sodium, potassium and PAH transport of renal tubule fragments. *Clin. Sci.* **38**, 617-627.

Dahl, L. K. (1961). Possible role of chronic excess salt consumption in the pathogenesis of essential hypertension. *Am. J. Cardiol.* **8**, 571-575.

Dahl, L. K., and Schackow, E. (1964). Effects of chronic excess salt ingestion: Experimental hypertension in the rat. *Can. Med. Assoc. J.* **90**, 155-160.

Dahl, L. K., Heine, M., and Tassinar, L. (1962). Effects of chronic excess salt ingestion. Evidence that genetic factors play an important role in susceptibility to experimental hypertension. *J. Exp. Med.* **115**, 1173–1190.

Dahl, L. K., Knusden, K. D., and Iwai, J. (1969). Humoral transmission of hypertension: Evidence from parabiosis, *Circ. Res.* **24**, Suppl. 1, 21–33.

Dahl, L. K., Heine, M., and Thompson, K. (1972). Genetic influences of renal homografts on the blood pressure of rats from different strains. *Proc. Soc. Exp. Biol. Med.* **140**, 852–856.

Dahl, L. K., Heine, M., and Thompson, K. (1974). Genetic influences of the kidneys on blood pressure. Evidence from chronic renal homografts in rats with opposite predisposition to hypertension. *Circ. Res.* **34**, 94–101.

Dawber, T. R., Kannel, W. B., Kagan, A., Donabedian, R. K., McNamara, P. M., and Pearson, G. (1967). Environmental factors in hypertension. *In* "The Epidemiology of Hypertension" (J. Stamler, R. Stamler, and R. B. Pullman, eds.), pp. 255–288. Grune & Stratton, New York.

de Wardener, H. E. (1977). Natriuretic hormone. *Clin. Sci. Mol. Med.* **53**, 1–8.

de Wardener, H. E., and MacGregor, G. A. (1980). Hypothesis: Further observations on Dahl's hypothesis that a saluretic substance may be responsible for a sustained rise in arterial pressure. Its possible role in essential hypertension. *Kidney Int.* **18**, 1–9.

de Wardener, H. E., MacGregor, G. A., Clarkson, E. M., Alaghband-Zadeh, J., Bitensky, L., and Chayen, J. (1981). Effect of sodium intake on ability of human plasma to inhibit renal Na^+-K^+-adenosine triphosphatase in vitro. *Lancet* **1**, 411–412.

Dunn, M. J., and Tannen, R. L. (1974). Low renin hypertension. *Kidney Int.* **5**, 317–325.

Edmondson, P., and MacGregor, G. A. (1981). Leucocyte cation transport in essential hypertension; its relation to the renin-angiotensin system. *Br. Med. J.* (in press).

Edmondson, R. P. S., Thomas, R. D., Hilton, P. J., Patrick, J., and Jones, N. F. (1975). Abnormal leucocyte composition and sodium transport in essential hypertension. *Lancet* **1**, 1003–1005.

Fadeke Aderounmu A., and Salako, L. A. (1979). Abnormal cation composition and transport in erythrocytes from hypertensive patients. *Eur. J. Clin. Invest.* **9**, 364–375.

Flier, J. S., Maretos-Flier, E., Pallotta, J. A., and McIssac, D. (1979). Endogenous digitalis-like activity in the plasma of the toad *Bufo marinus*. *Nature (London)* **279**, 341–343.

Fox, U., and Bianchi, G. (1976). The primary role of the kidney in causing the blood pressure difference between the Milan hypertensive strain (MHS) and normotensive rats. *Clin. Exp. Pharmacol. Physiol., Suppl.* **3**, 71–74.

Fukuda, T. (1954). Investigation on hypertension in farm villages in Akita prefecture. *Chiba Igakkai Zasshi* **29**,490–502.

Garay, R. P., and Meyer, P. (1979). A new test showing abnormal net Na^+ and K^+ fluxes in erythrocytes of essential hypertensive patients. *Lancet* **1**, 349–353.

Gessler, von U. (1962). Intra- und extrazelluläre elektrolytveränderungen bei essentieller hypertonie bor und nach behandlung. *Z. Kreislaufforsch.* **51**, 177–183.

Gleibermann, L. (1973). Blood pressure and dietary salt in human populations. *Ecol. Food Nutr.* **2**, 143.

Gonick, H. C., Kramer, H. J., Paul, W., and Lu, R. (1977). Circulating inhibitor of sodium potassium activated adenosine triphosphate after expansion of extracellular fluid volume in rats. *Clin. Soc. Mol. Med.* **53**, 329–334.

Gruber, K. A., Whitaker, J. M., and Buckalew, V. M., Jr. (1980). Endogenous digitalis-like substance in plasma of volume expanded dogs. *Nature (London)* **287**, 743–745.

Haddy, F. J., and Overbeck, H. W. (1976). The role of humoral agents in volume expanded hypertension. *Life Sci.* **19**, 935–948.

Henningsen, N. C., Mattsson, S., Nosslin, B., Nelson, D., and Ohlsson, O. (1979). Abnormal whole-body and cellular (erythrocytes) turnover of $^{22}Na^+$ in normotensive relatives of probands with established essential hypertension. *Clin. Sci.* **57**, 321s–324s.

Isaacson, L. C., Modlin, M., and Jackson, W. P. U. (1963). Sodium intake and hypertension. *Lancet* **1**, 946.

Krakoff, L. R., Goodwin, F. J., Baer, L., Torres, M., and Laragh, J. H. (1970). The role of renin in the exaggerated natriuresis of hypertension. *Circulation* **42**, 335–345.

Lichardus, B., Pliska, V., Uhrin, V., and Barth, T. (1968). The cow as a model for investigating natriuretic activity. *Lancet* **1**, 127–129.

Losse, H., Wehmeyer, H., and Wessels, F. (1960). The water and electrolyte content of erythrocytes in arterial hypertension. *Klin. Wocheschr.* **38**, 393–395.

Lowenstein, J., Beranbaum, E. R., Chasis, H., and Baldwin, S. D. (1970). Intrarenal pressure and exaggerated natriuresis in essential hypertension. *Clin. Sci.* **38**, 359–374.

Meneely, G. R., Tucker, R. G., Darby, W. J., and Auerbach, S. H. (1953). Chronic sodium chloride toxicity: Hypertension, renal and vascular lesions. *Ann. Intern. Med.* **39**, 991–998.

Miall, W. E. (1959). Follow-up study of arterial pressure in the population of a Welsh mining valley. *Br. Med. J.* **2**, 1204–1210.

Nutbourne, D. M., Howse, J. D., Schrier, R. W., Talner, L. B., Ventom, M. G., Verroust, P. J., and de Wardener, H. E. (1970). The effect of expanding the blood volume of a dog on a short circuit current across an isolated frog skin incorporated in the dog's circulation, *Clin. Sci.* **38**, 629–648.

Oliver, W. J., Cohen, E. L., and Neel, J. V. (1975). Blood pressure, sodium intake and sodium related hormones in the Yanomamo Indians; a no salt culture. *Circulation* **52**, 146–151.

Pickering, G., ed. (1968). "High Blood Pressure," 2nd ed., Vol. 12, pp. 236–290. London.

Postnov, Y. V., Orlov, S. N., Shevchenko, A., and Adler, A. M. (1977). Altered sodium permeability, calcium binding and Na^+-K^+-ATPase activity in the red blood cell membrane in essential hypertension. *Pfluegers Arch.* **371**, 263–269.

Poston, L., Wilkinson, S. P., Sewell, R., and Williams, R. (1980). Inhibition of leucocyte sodium transport during mineralocorticoid "escape." *Clin. Sci.* **58**, 9p.

Poston, L., Sewell, R. B., Wilkinson, S. P., Richardson, P. J., Williams, R., Clarkson, E. M., MacGregor, G. A., and de Wardener, H. E. (1981). Evidence for a circulating sodium transport inhibitor in essential hypertension. *Br. Med. J.* **282**, 847–849.

Rovner, D. R., Conn, J. W., Knopf, R. F., cohen, E. L., and Hsueh, M. T.-Y. (1965). Nature of renal escape from the sodium-retaining effect of aldosterone in primary aldosteronism and in normal subjects. *J. Clin. Endocrinol. Metab.* **25**, 53–64.

Sasaki, N. (1964). The relationship of salt intake to hypertension in the Japanese. *Geriatrics* **19**, 735–744.

Schalekamp, M. A., Beevers, D. G., Kolsters, G., Lebel, M., Fraser, R., and Birkenhager, W. H. (1974). Body-fluid volume in low-renin hypertension. *Lancet* **2**, 310–311.

Simpson, F. O., Waal-Manning, H. J., Bolli, P., Phelan, E. L., and Spears, G. F. S. (1978). Relationship of blood pressure to sodium excretion in a population survey. *Clin. Sci. Mol. Med.* **55**, 373s–375s.

Sinnett, P. F., and Whyte, H. M. (1973). Epidemiological studies in a total highland population, Tukisenta, New Guinea. Cardiovascular disease and relevant clinical, electrocardiographic, radiological and biochemical findings. *J. Chronic Dis.* **26**, 265–290.

Smirk, F. H., and Hall, W. H. (1958). Inherited hypertension in rats. *Nature (London)* **182**, 727–728.

Takamatsu, M. (1955). Figure of body fluid of farmers in the north-eastern districts viewed from angle of water and salt metabolism. *Rodo Kagaku* **31**, 349–370.

Thomas, R. D., Edmondson, R. P. S., Hilton, P. J., and Jones, N. F. (1975). Abnormal sodium transport in leucocytes from patients with essential hypertension and the effect of treatment. *Clin. Sci. Mol. Med.* **48**, 169s–170s.

Tobian, L., Coffee, K., MacCrea, P., and Dahl, L. K. (1966). A comparison of the antihypertensive potency of kidneys from one strain of rats susceptible to salt hypertension and kidneys from another strain resistant to it. *J. Clin. Invest.* **45,** 1080.

Tobian, L., Jr., and Binion, J. T. (1952). Tissue cations and water in arterial hypertension. *Circulation* **5,** 754–758.

Wessels, V. F., Junge-Husling, G., and Losse, H. (1967). Unter suchungen zur natriumpermeabilitat der erythrozyten bei hypertonikern und normotonikern mit familiarer hochdruckbelastung. *Z. Kreislaufforsch.* **56,** 374–380.

Willassen, Y., and Ofstad, J. (1978). Renal sodium excretion and peritubular capillary starling forces (PCSF) in essential hypertension. *Proc. Int. Congr. Nephrol., 7th, Krager, 1978,* B.9.

24

Abnormal Erythrocyte Na$^+$,K$^+$ Cotransport System: A Proposed Genetic Marker of Essential Hypertension

RICARDO P. GARAY, PATRICK HANNAERT,
GEORGES DAGHER, CORINNE NAZARET,
ISABELLE MARIDONNEAU, AND PHILLIPE MEYER

I. INTRODUCTION

Essential hypertension appears to result from a combination of genetic and environmental factors, of which an excess of Na$^+$ intake is the most important (Dahl, 1977).

345

THE ROLE OF SALT IN
CARDIOVASCULAR HYPERTENSION

Recent observations from our laboratory and that of others suggested that in rat (De Mendonca *et al.*, 1980; Jones *et al.*, 1973; Postnov *et al.*, 1976) and man (Canessa *et al.*, 1980; Garay *et al.*, 1979, 1980; Postnov *et al.*, 1976; Wessels *et al.*, 1967), primary hypertension is generally connected with abnormal transmembrane Na^+ transport. The observation of an abnormal Na^+ transport in erythrocytes from some hypertensive offspring indicates that it might follow the genetic trasnmission of hypertension.

The search for a genetic marker of hypertension has been stimulated by two practical interests: (1) to distinguish between secondary and primary hypertension and (2) to determine the inherited tendency to develop high blood pressure in the hypertensive offspring.

We present here some preliminary results suggesting that an abnormally low apparent affinity for intracellular Na^+ of the erythrocyte Na^+,K^+ cotransport system may be a genetic marker of primary hypertension.

II. METHODS AND PATIENTS

The different transmembrane pathways involved in net Na^+ and K^+ transport in erythrocytes were analyzed in the following groups: normotensive and secondary hypertensive subjects devoid of familial hypertension, benign and accelerated essential hypertensive patients, and the offspring of hypertensive patients. Ouabain was used to block the Na^+,K^+ pump and furosemide to inhibit the Na^+,K^+ cotransport (details on methods and and patients are given in Dagher and Garay, 1980).

III. RESULTS

A. Erythrocyte Na^+,K^+ Pump

The addition of ouabain (0.1 mmol/liter) to Na^+ loaded erythrocytes incubated in a physiological Na^+ and K^+ Ringer's solution inhibits to a great extent the net cation movements in both hypertensive and normotensive subjects.

In erythrocytes from six out of eight benign essential hypertensive subjects and from all of six young normotensive subjects with abnormal erythrocyte fluxes, born of hypertensive parents, we observed pump fluxes 20–40% higher than in normal erythrocytes. This observation agrees with the increase in Na^+,K^+-ATPase recently reported for benign essential hypertensive subjects (Wambach *et al.*, 1979).

The increase in Na^+,K^+ pump fluxes are not consequent to a change in the maximal turnover rate in conditions of pump saturation with Na^+ and K^+ (Table I).

TABLE I

Na$^+$,K$^+$ Pump and Na$^+$,K$^+$ Cotransport Kinetics in Hypertension

Transport system	Subject	Half-maximal stimulation by internal Na^{+a} (mmole/liter of cells)	Maximal rate^a μmole (liter of cells $\times$ hr)$^{-1}$	Hill's number^a
Na$^+$,K$^+$ pump	Normotensive	—	6860 $\pm$ 1990 (13)	—
	Hypertensive	—	5580 $\pm$ 1030 (6)	—
Na$^+$,K$^+$ cotransport	Normotensive	12.5 $\pm$ 2.5 (10)	486 $\pm$ 147 (10)	1.72 $\pm$ 0.27 (10)
	Hypertensive	24.2 $\pm$ 7.3^b (12)	412 $\pm$ 278 (12)	1.86 $\pm$ 0.53 (12)

^{a} Values represent means $\pm$ SD; numbers in parentheses denote the number of subjects.
^{b} $p < 0.01$.

TABLE II

Outward Na$^+$,K$^+$ Cotransport in Hypertension

Group	Furosemide-sensitive net Na$^+$ extrusion[a] (μmol hr^{-1} liter^{-1} of cells)	Furosemide-sensitive net K$^+$ extrusion[a] (μmol hr^{-1} liter^{-1} of cells)
Normotensive controls	496 ± 125 ($n = 71$)	521 ± 126 ($n = 71$)
Essential hypertensives	200 ± 110[b] ($n = 80$)	247 ± 110[b] ($n = 80$)
Secondary hypertensives[c]	400 ± 67 ($n = 7$)	464 ± 110 ($n = 7$)

[a] Values represent means ± SD; n denotes the number of subjects in each group.
[b] $p < 0.001$.
[c] Devoid of family history of hypertension.

Some preliminary results indicate that it could be a consequence of increased affinity for external K$^+$.

B. Erythrocyte Na$^+$,K$^+$ Cotransport

As shown in Table II, the furosemide-sensitive net Na$^+$ and K$^+$ extrusion is markedly reduced in erythrocytes from essential hypertensive patients. On the other hand, 53.6% of 97 young normotensive offspring of one hypertensive parent and 73.7% of 19 normotensive offspring of both hypertensive parents had an abnormal cotransport. A normal cotransport was found in secondary hypertensive subjects devoid of familial hypertension.

The abnormal Na$^+$ extrusion by the Na$^+$,K$^+$ cotransport system in essential hypertension seems to be consequent to a decreased apparent affinity for internal Na$^+$ (Table I).

C. Passive Na$^+$ and K$^+$ Permeabilities

No difference could be detected between the Na$^+$ and K$^+$ passive permeabilities of erythrocytes from ten hypertensive patients and those from ten normotensive controls.

IV. DISCUSSION

Most of the explanations so far proposed for the hypertensive properties of an excess Na$^+$ intake only consider extracellular Na$^+$. This is especially the case for Guyton's model where arterial blood pressure is related to extracellular Na$^+$ within a highly nonlinear system (Guyton *et al.*, 1977). Hemodynamics is considered most important in regulation, the ultimate responsibility being attributed to the renal capacity for extracellular Na$^+$ excretion.

A great deal of work has been done on urinary Na$^+$ excretion in essential hypertension. At least in moderate essential hypertension, renal function seems to be normal, and a Na$^+$ load promotes faster natriuresis than in normotensives. In addition, there is no definite evidence for an increase in extracellular Na$^+$, either in moderate essential hypertension (Frohlich *et al.*, 1970) or in malignant hypertension, where, despite frequent impairment of renal function, extracellular volume may diminish (Tarazi *et al.*, 1968).

In the body, the Na$^+$ load resulting from Na$^+$ intake is transitory because it is rapidly corrected by two mechanisms: Na$^+$ entry into cells tends to be compensated by Na$^+$ extrusion into the extracellular compartment, while the excess Na$^+$ of the extracellular fluid is mainly corrected by the kidney.

In order to establish whether or not intracellular Na$^+$ is pathogenic, we developed a simple method for measuring Na$^+$ excretion from Na$^+$-replete red blood cells well adapted to the investigation of hypertensive patients.

The net extrusion of an erythrocyte's Na$^+$ load is accomplished by two different mechanisms: the Na$^+$,K$^+$ pump and Na$^+$,K$^+$ cotransport, which operate against the passive Na$^+$ permeability (Fig. 1). An inherited defect in the Na$^+$,K$^+$ cotransport system seems to be genetically associated with essential hypertension. In avian erythrocytes this transport system participates in the regulation of transmembrane Na$^+$ and K$^+$ electrochemical gradients and is under hormonal control. These observations have led us to formulate the hypothesis that essential hypertension may result from an inefficient hormonal regulation of the extrusion of a cellular Na$^+$ load after an excess Na$^+$ intake, due to a functional disorder of

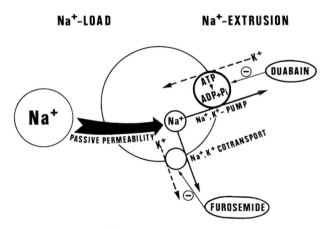

Fig. 1. Schematic diagram of the various factors affecting sodium balance in human red cells. The transport mechanisms on which ouabain and furosemide act are shown.

the Na^+,K^+ cotransport system. Such a process in excitable cells of high surface/volume ratio, such as smooth muscle cells or catecholaminergic neurons, may lead to a temporary or permanent increase in intracellular Na^+, producing critical changes capable of raising blood pressure (Blaustein *et al.*, 1977; De Champlain *et al.*, 1968). The high Na^+,K^+ pump activity seen in some young normotensive offspring of hypertensive parents and benign essential subjects may therefore represent a compensatory mechanism for extruding a cellular Na^+ load and thus preventing severe hypertension in subjects with this genetic abnormality.

The fact that a normal cotransport was found in authentic secondary hypertensive offspring of normotensive parents confirms that this abnormality is not the consequence of high blood pressure per se. Moreover, the familial pattern of the defective cotransport suggests a dominant and an autosomal mode of genetic transmission.

In conclusion, the finding of an abrnomal cotransport in a young normotensive with a family history of hypertension may indicate an inherited tendency to develop high blood pressure and may thus elicit appropriate preventive measures such as a regular medical examination, appropriate Na^+ diet, prevention of excessive weight gain, and clinical follow-up during contraception by estrogens and during pregnancy.

V. SUMMARY

In erythrocytes, the extrusion of a cellular sodium load is accomplished by the ouabain-sensitive Na^+,K^+ pump and by the furosemide-sensitive Na^+,K^+ cotransport, which operate against the passive sodium permeability. All three components of cellular sodium balance were studied in essential hypertension (547 subjects were investigated).

An abnormally low rate of net sodium extrusion by the Na^+,K^+ cotransport system was observed in essential hypertensive patients and in a high proportion of their young normotensive offspring. A normal cotransport system found in secondary hypertensive subjects devoid of familial history of hypertension confirmed that the abnormal cotransport system is not the consequence of high blood pressure per se. At the molecular level, the cotransport abnormality seems to be consecutive to a diminished apparent affinity for intracellular Na^+.

A 20–40% increase in the rate of net sodium extrusion by the Na^+,K^+ pump seems to compensate for the normal cotransport in erythrocytes from some young normotensive subjects born of essential hypertensive parents and from benign essential hypertensive subjects.

No difference could be detected between the passive sodium permeability of erythrocytes from hypertensive subjects and in those from normotensive controls.

Essential hypertension seems to be associated with an inherited defect in the Na$^+$,K$^+$ cotransport system. We propose the use of this system as a tool to distinguish between essential and secondary hypertension and as a diagnostic aid in discovering potential hypertensives among young normotensive subjects born of hypertensive parents.

REFERENCES

Blaustein, M. (1977). Sodium ions, calcium ions, blood pressure regulation and hypertension: A reassessment and a hypothesis. *Am. J. Physiol.* **232**, C165–C172.

Canessa, M., Adragna, N., Solomon, H. S., Connolly, T. M., and Tosteson, D. C. (1980). Sodium-lithium countertransport is increased in red cells of patients with essential hypertension. *N. Engl. J. Med.* **302**, 772–776.

Dagher, G., and Garay, R. P. (1980). A Na$^+$,K$^+$ co-transport assay for essential hypertension. *Can. J. Biochem.* **58**, 1069–1074.

Dahl, L. K. (1977). *In* "Hypertension" (J. Genest, E. Koiw, and O. Kuchel, eds.), pp. 548–559. McGraw-Hill, New York.

De Champlain, J., Krakoff, L., and Axelrod, J. (1968). Relationship between sodium intake and norepinephrine storage during the development of experimental hypertension. *J. Circ. Res.* **23**, 479.

De Mendonca, M., Grichois, M. L., Garay, R. P., Sassard, J., Benishay, D., and Meyer, P. (1980). Abnormal net Na$^+$ and K$^+$ fluxes in erythrocytes of three varieties of genetically hypertensive rats. *Proc. Natl. Acad. Sci. U.S.A.* **77**, 4283.

Frohlich, E. D., Kozul, V. J., Tarazi, R. C., and Dustan, H. P. (1970). Physiological comparison of labile and essential hypertension, *Circ. Res.* **27**, Suppl. 1, 55.

Garay, R. P., and Meyer, P. (1979). A new test showing abnormal net Na$^+$ and K$^+$ fluxes in erythrocytes of essential hypertensive patients. *Lancet* **1**, 349–353.

Garay, R. P., Elghozi, J. L., Dagher, G., and Meyer, P. (1980). Laboratory distinction between essential and secondary hypertension by measurement of erythrocyte cation fluxes. *N. Engl. J. Med.* **302**, 769–771.

Guyton, A. C. (1977). *In* "Hypertension" (J. Genest, E. Koiw, and O. Kuchel, eds.), pp. 566–575. McGraw-Hill, New York.

Jones, A. (1973). Alteration transport in vascular smooth muscle from spontaneously hypertensive rats. Influence of aldosterone, norepinephrine and angiotensin. *Circ. Res.* **563**, 33.

Postnov, Y., Orlov, S., Gulak, P., and Shevchenko, A. (1976). Altered permeability of the erythrocyte membrane for sodium and potassium in spontaneously hypertensive rats. *Pfluegers Arch.* **365**, 257–263.

Postnov, Y., Orlof, V., Shevchenko, A., and Adler, A. (1977). Altered sodium permeability, calcium binding and Na$^+$,K$^+$ ATPase in the red blood cell membrane in essential hypertension. *Pfluegers Arch.* **371**, 263–269.

Tarazi, R. C., Frohlich, E. D., and Dustan, H. P. (1968). *N. Engl. J. Med.* **278**, 762.

Wambach, G., Helber, A., Bonner, C., and Hummerich, W. (1979). Natrium-kalium adenosin triphosphatase-aktivität in Erythrozyten ghost von Patients mit essentieller Hypertonie. *Klin. Wochenschr.* **57**, 169–172.

Wessels, F., Junge-Hulsing, G., and Losse, M. (1967). Untersuchungeer zur Natrium permeabilität der Erytrozyten bei Hypertonitern und Normotonikern mit familäres Hochdruck-belastung. *Z. Kreislaufforsch.* **56**, 374–380.

III

Interaction of Salt with Peripheral Adrenergic Neuroeffector Mechanisms and Regulation of Vascular Smooth Muscle Tone

Introduction

ROSEMARY D. BEVAN

Part III of this volume is derived from a minisymposium on the interaction of salt with peripheral adrenergic neuroeffector mechanisms and its role in the regulation of vascular smooth muscle tone. This was organized in response to a recommendation by the Atherosclerosis, Hypertension and Lipid Metabolism Advisory Committee and supported by the National Heart, Lung, and Blood Institute. The intention of the Symposium was to explore the relationship between salt and blood pressure and the mechanisms whereby salt interacts with those systems involved in blood pressure regulation. There is current interest in genetic variation in the handling of dietary salt in man and laboratory animals, mostly rats. Evidence has accrued which suggests that in hypertension there are both active and passive changes in membrane permeability to cations in circulating blood cells and in vascular smooth muscle and adipocytes. The changes described are not all the same but involve defective handling of sodium that may potentially lead to its accumulation in the cell.

An increase in total peripheral resistance to blood flow is an early feature in human essential hypertension and this has been confirmed in regional vascular beds. In almost all forms of hypertension the increased resistance in the vasculature is associated with functional and structural changes, resulting in a greater effective wall/lumen ratio. The mechanisms by which salt may participate in this process are not clear, although excessive salt intake accelerates and increases the severity of the hypertensive process induced by manipulation of the various systems involved in blood pressure regulation.

The intent of Part III is to focus on the interface of the predominant nerves participating in the regulation of the level of blood vessel contraction or "tone," i.e., the sympathetic nerves and the smooth muscle cells of the vasculature. Due to constraints of time, only those aspects related to the transmembrane Na gradient across the cell and other membrane events that change the permeability of the cell to ions and influence the availability of free intracellular $[Ca^{2+}]$ essential for contraction will be considered. The state of this knowledge in various models of animal hypertension will be reviewed. It must be emphasized that at present

355

THE ROLE OF SALT IN
CARDIOVASCULAR HYPERTENSION

only *in vitro* techniques allow a precise definition of vascular neuroeffector function, so that little information on human blood vessels is available. *In vitro* techniques, however, can assess adrenergic nerve function but not the level of sympathetic nerve traffic.

In the first chapter of Part III, Dr. T. Bolton reviews the mechanisms whereby substances acting on the membrane of the smooth muscle cell influence its permeability to specific ions. Dr. T. Westfall summarizes our present knowledge of the effect of [Na⁺] and salt on the adrenergic neurotransmitter process. Dr. S. Friedman discusses some basic principles underlying the maintenance of the transmembrane Na gradient in vascular smooth muscle. His observations on the role of a change in membrane permeability to ions and the activity of the Na–K pump in a number of experimental models of hypertension are detailed. Dr. F. Haddy reviews the evidence for the role of a circulating ouabain-like factor in certain experimental models of hypertension characterized by low renin levels and gives a cohesive concept concerning its role in hypertension. Dr. M. Blaustein argues for his hypothesis that when sodium metabolism is deranged, leading to elevated intracellular levels, a Na–Ca exchange mechanism plays a critical role in the regulation of free intracellular [Ca^{2+}] in nerve and muscle, leading to increased vascular muscle tone. Dr. C. van Breemen presents experiments indicating a complex relationship between Na and Ca in smooth muscle and an alternative hypothesis for competition for intracellular negatively charged membrane sites.

Excellent as these presentations are, it is evident that detailed knowledge of the generation and control of vascular tone in small resistance vessels is lacking because of the technical difficulties involved. The relative importance of mechanisms leading to contraction and relaxation may differ with the location and size of vessel. Consequently, some observed changes and the hypotheses that they have given rise to await confirmation in resistance vessels and the venous side of the circulation. There is also a lack of knowledge on age-related changes in the mechanisms covered in Part III. It is possible that environmental effects imposed on a genetic factor during the period of growth may have the greatest influence on the function and structure of the vasculature.

Lack of time has precluded a consideration of possible ways that excessive salt intake may participate in effecting structural changes in the vasculature, either secondary to an increase in circulating plasma volume or directly on mechanisms leading to increased components of the wall. In addition, the retention of intra- and/or extracellular water may increase vascular resistance. Although the Na⁺ is the most important osmotically active constituent of the cell, precise measurements of changes in free cell water in hypertension are lacking. Even small changes in resistance vessels could greatly influence blood flow. Other important aspects not covered are the effect of differences in Na/K ratios in the diet on vascular reactivity and the possible role of the chloride ion in vascular smooth muscle tone.

Our understanding of the fundamental processes which are crucial to the function of the normal vascular muscle cell, specifically in relation to sodium and water, are lacking—even more so in cells where there may be altered function due to genetic or environmental causes.

25

Membrane Mechanisms Linking Neurohumoral Receptors to the Effects They Produce in Vascular and Other Smooth Muscles

THOMAS B. BOLTON

THE ROLE OF SALT IN
CARDIOVASCULAR HYPERTENSION

I. INTRODUCTION

The membrane mechanisms that link receptors for neurohumoral substances to the effects they produce in different smooth muscles show a diversity that contributes substantially to the characteristic physiological responses shown by different types of smooth muscles. However, there do appear to be fundamental similarities between the different smooth muscle types, as this chapter will endeavor to describe, and such physiological differences can be viewed as differences in the balance between various fundamental mechanisms which have been shown to exist. Different physiological responses seem to arise, therefore, as variations on a theme resulting from greater or lesser emphasis on a few basic mechanisms.

It is necessary first to describe how contraction and relaxation are controlled in the various smooth muscles before serious discussion of the effects of neurohumoral receptor activation can be attempted. The interaction of the contractile proteins, actin and myosin, in smooth muscle cells results in the development of tension or shortening. It is believed to occur primarily as a result of a rise in intracellular ionized calcium concentration $[Ca^{2+}]_i$ as in other types of muscle. A caveat should be sounded immediately. While $[Ca^{2+}]_i$ may be the primary determinant of the extent of actin–myosin interaction, other processes may exert a significant effect. For example, it is conceivable that the concentrations of other substances may influence the tension achieved at any given $[Ca^{2+}]_i$. The availability of energy in the form of ATP is one such factor. Other substances, by influencing the degree of the actin–myosin interaction, may also exert effects. Cyclic AMP is believed to increase the phosphorylation of the myosin light chain kinase, so weakening its calcium binding and reducing the extent of phosphorylation of the myosin light chain. The net effect is to reduce actin–myosin interaction (Conti and Adelstein, 1980). Activation of β receptors (see Hardman, 1981, for review), PGE_2 receptors (Harbon and Clauser, 1971), and vasoactive intestinal polypeptide receptors (Frandsen et al., 1978) have all been described as increasing cyclic AMP levels in smooth muscle. It is worth emphasizing at this juncture that the complexity of the contractile process is likely to make it susceptible to interference at a number of points. We should not be surprised, therefore, if agents that relax smooth muscle do so by a variety of mechanisms.

II. ACTIONS OF STIMULANTS: PROCESSES RAISING $[Ca^{2+}]_i$

A. Membrane Pores Opened by Depolarization and Admitting Calcium

Most interest in recent years has been focused on the processes and mechanisms that give rise to an increase in $[Ca^{2+}]_i$. These can be divided for convenience into those involved in excitation–contraction coupling and those specific to the activation of receptors for particular neurohumors (for reviews, see Bolton, 1979; Kuriyama, 1981). Excitation–contraction coupling is simply the linking of membrane events to contraction. Smooth muscles, including vascular smooth muscles, generate action potentials to varying degrees. In those smooth muscles that readily generate action potentials, the action potential is probably the most important determinant of tension; modulation of action potential discharge by neurohumoral factors is thus an extremely important, although not necessarily the only, mechanism by which they can vary tension. Other smooth muscles do not readily generate action potentials and it would appear that normally, unless acted on by neurotransmitters or other endogenous substances, their membrane potentials are stable. (Virtually no experiments have been done *in vivo,* but this at present seems a reasonable assumption, from *in vitro* experiments). Neurotransmitters can vary tension in such smooth muscles by changing their membrane potentials. Generally stimulants depolarize the membrane and relaxants hyperpolarize it, but this generalization has important exceptions in vascular muscle (Su and Bevan, 1965; Casteels *et al.,* 1977a; Kuriyama and Suzuki, 1978; Kitamura and Kuriyama, 1979).

Depolarization of the membrane alone, such as may be done by passing continuously an electric current across it, produces considerable tension in some smooth muscles (Ito *et al.,* 1977). This presumably reflects the fact that depolarization of the membrane causes pores, or ion channels, to open in the membrane which admit calcium. We must presume that, where a neurotransmitter also depolarizes a smooth muscle membrane and increases tension, a portion at least of the increase in tension arises because of the opening of more ion channels due to the depolarization.

In smooth muscles that readily generate action potentials, the action potential seems to represent the influx of a substantial amount of calcium into the cell (see Kuriyama, 1981, for references). In other words, the upstroke of the action potential represents a rapid potential change brought about by the opening of ion channels in the membrane which admit calcium ions. The opening of these calcium channels is almost certainly controlled by potential as in the case of virtually all excitable cells.

Thus, in both smooth muscles that readily generate action potentials, and those that do not, the action of stimulant neurotransmitters results in the opening of ion channels that admit calcium into the cell. In both cases, the opening of these channels is a potential-sensitive (or -dependent) phenomenon. That these two types of smooth muscle possess the same fundamental mechanism is supported by the action of tetraethylammonium (TEA). TEA blocks potassium channels and its most striking effect on smooth muscles which do not normally generate action potentials is to convert them into action potential generating cells (see Bolton, 1979). For example, recent papers (Haeusler and Thorens, 1980; Haeusler *et al.,* 1980) describe how the application of TEA to rabbit main pulmonary artery, which is a quiescent smooth muscle not generating action potentials, causes it to discharge action potentials either spontaneously or in response to depolarizing current, and so to contract. Thus, it seems to be true that all smooth muscles possess ion channels that admit calcium when the membrane is depolarized, but their presence need not necessarily result in the ability to generate action potentials.

At this point it is worth mentioning the effects that substances which inhibit the sodium pump, such as the postulated natriuretic hormone, might have in smooth muscle. The sodium pump, besides maintaining both the sodium and potassium gradients across the cell membrane, also may contribute an electrogenic component to the membrane potential. Inhibition of sodium pump activity may result in increased tension development if some reduction of membrane potential occurs. This would have the effect of either increasing the frequency of action potential discharge or of increasing the calcium permeability of the membrane by means of the mechanism described in Section II,A.

B. Pores Admitting Calcium and Operated by Receptors Activated by Neurotransmitters

If the membrane of smooth muscle is depolarized so that the application of neurotransmitters produces no further change in membrane potential, it is known that stimulant substances can still produce contraction (Evans *et al.*, 1958). Under these conditions, as no change in membrane potential occurs, no change in the numbers of open potential-sensitive ion channels can occur. Other mechanisms must presumably exist by which $[Ca^{2+}]_i$ is raised under these conditions.

It can be shown that removal of calcium from the bathing solution will abolish the contractile response to stimulant substances in depolarized smooth muscle (Edman and Schild, 1962). However, in some vascular smooth muscles, contractile responses to norepinephrine have been reported as persisting for an hour or more, even if chelating agents, such as EGTA are incorporated in the bathing solution (Bozler, 1969; Keatinge, 1972; Casteels *et al.*, 1982).

There is abundant evidence that stimulants increase the permeability of the smooth muscle membrane and that this increase in permeability adds to the increase which is caused by the depolarization they produce (Durbin and Jenkinson, 1961; Bolton, 1972). Although it has sometimes been difficult to detect, an increased influx of calcium may occur even in depolarized muscle during the action of the stimulant (Durbin and Jenkinson, 1961; Deth and van Breemen, 1974; Casteels *et al.*, 1977b). It seems plausible that the activation of receptors for stimulant substances opens pores or ion channels that allow the more free movement of inorganic ions across the smooth muscle membrane, i.e., membrane permeability increases. This increase in membrane permeability probably involves calcium ions as well as potassium, sodium, and maybe chloride ions in some cases (Bolton, 1979). The influx of calcium into the cell through receptor-operated ion channels presumably contributes to the rise in $[Ca^{2+}]_i$. Since the calcium entering in this way represents a steady leakage into the cell, tonic changes in tension would be expected to result. It seems likely that influx of calcium through receptor-operated channels may be important in smooth muscles such as the main pulmonary artery of the rabbit (Casteels et al., 1977a,b) which do not readily generate action potentials.

C. Release of Calcium from Bound Sites by Receptor Activation

It has been known for some time that contractile responses to stimulants persist longer in a calcium-free solution than similar responses obtained by depolarizing the membrane with high-potassium solutions (Edman and Schild, 1962; Hinke, 1965). A characteristic of responses to stimulant neurotransmitters is that a single application of the transmitter at high concentrations accelerates the decline of the response to it in calcium-free solution (Edman and Schild, 1962; Ohashi et al., 1974) and generally only a single response can be elicited in calcium-free solution (van Breemen et al., 1972).

If brief exposure to a calcium-containing solution is allowed while in otherwise calcium-free solution, the response to the high concentration of stimulant transmitter is restored. However, the restorative effect of brief exposure to a calcium containing solution can be blocked if calcium "antagonists," such as verapamil, or La^{3+} are present during exposure to calcium (Ohashi et al., 1975; Casteels and Droogmans, 1981). Prior incubation in a calcium-containing, high-potassium solution can potentiate a subsequent response to stimulant neurotransmitter in calcium-free solution (Casteels and Raeymaekers, 1979).

The above results are consistent with there being a store of bound calcium in smooth muscle cells, which is lost slowly to the bathing solution if this is calcium-free. Stimulants such as acetylcholine, norepinephrine, or histamine can act to release calcium from this store, producing contraction of the muscle. Once released in this way, however, the store can only be filled by incubating the muscle for a short period in calcium-containing solution and calcium antagonists will hinder this filling. The calcium content of the store can be increased by certain conditions that increase calcium entry to the cell or accelerate its sequestration within it (Casteels and Raeymaekers, 1979). However, it is worth emphasizing that, at least in action potential generating smooth muscle, the release of calcium is only important in the responsiveness to high concentrations of stimulants. The responses to low concentrations behave quite differently and it would seem that the main physiological mechanism by which transmitters alter tone in action potential generating muscle is by modulation of the frequency of action potential discharge (Brading and Sneddon, 1980).

The role of the releasable calcium stores in the normal physiological response of smooth muscle to stimulants is at present somewhat puzzling. In action potential generating smooth muscle it would not normally seem to be very important *as a contributor to the rise* in $[Ca^{2+}]_i$. It has been suggested (Bolton, 1979) that this releasable calcium store is part of the mechanism linking the activated receptors to the pathways (ion channels) leading to contraction. Thus, it would only be quantitatively important in raising $[Ca^{2+}]_i$ when close to maximal stimulation of receptors is occurring; its main role would be as a link between receptors and the effects they produce and this might be its only role at lower, physiological concentrations of stimulants. However, it may be that in some smooth muscles that do not readily generate action potentials, this releasable calcium can be quantitatively important, even at relatively low concentrations of stimulants, in raising $[Ca^{2+}]_i$. A final point is that where several stimulants are able to produce near maximal or maximal contractions of a smooth muscle, the evidence is that they release calcium from this same store, although their ability to release this stored calcium may vary (van Breemen *et al.*, 1972; Casteels and Raeymaekers, 1979).

D. Summary of Calcium Sources for the Contractile Response

Thus, there seem to be three main mechanisms by which a rise in $[Ca^{2+}]_i$ can be produced in smooth muscle cells (Fig. 1):

1. Ion channels admitting calcium which open when the membrane is depolarized. These are involved in producing action potentials in those smooth muscles generating these; such ion channels are also present, however, in smooth muscles that do not readily generate action potentials.

2. Ion channels which admit calcium into the cell opened by activation of receptors for stimulant substances. These have been called receptor-operated channels (Bolton, 1979) and they also allow ions other than calcium to enter the cell which may cause depolarization of the membrane.

3. Release of calcium from sites where it is stored in the cell on activation of receptors. This calcium may be important for the responses only to high concentrations of stimulant substances.

It should also be remarked that in arterial smooth muscle in calcium-free EGTA-containing solution, small contractions can be produced by norepinephrine or histamine. Such contractions are *not* affected by repeated application of noradrenaline in calcium-free solution, in contradistinction to those responses dependent on calcium stores (see above)(Casteels *et al.*, 1981). It is conceivable that these contractions are independent of $[Ca^{2+}]_i$, as it seems unlikely that the conservation by the cell of calcium releasable from cellular stores by norepinephrine would be so efficient.

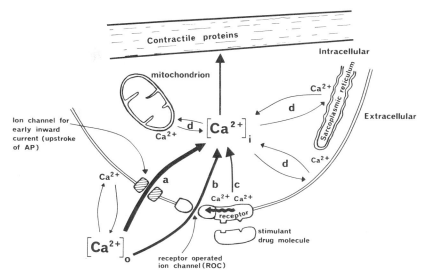

Fig. 1. Schematic representation of postulated calcium sources involved in contraction. In smooth muscles generating action potentials calcium entering through the action potential (AP) channel (a) is of primary importance at lower concentrations of stimulant substances. In smooth muscles that do not generate action potentials, or at higher concentrations of stimulants in those that do, calcium entering through receptor-operated channels (ROCs) (b) is important. Calcium bound within the cell, possibly associated with the receptor, may also be important in some smooth muscles. (Reproduced by permission from Bolton, 1979, in *Physiological Reviews*.)

It has also been suggested that activation of muscarinic, histamine, norepinephrine, or pentagastrin receptors can influence the time and/or potential-dependent behavior of ion channels in smooth muscles, increasing slow potential behavior (Bolton, 1979) and so affecting contractile force (Shuba, 1977; Morgan and Szurszewski, 1980).

III. ACTIONS OF INHIBITORY SUBSTANCES

The mechanisms of action of inhibitory substances, particularly those exogenous to the body, on smooth muscle is, as already remarked, probably diverse because there are many potential sites of interference with the processes of excitation–contraction coupling. Unfortunately, because we know so little with certainty about the details of these processes, the mechanisms of action of vascular relaxants are still obscure. Three types of action are well characterized.

A. Opening of Potassium Channels

The resting potential of most smooth muscles is at least a few millivolts positive to the potassium equilibrium potential so that opening of additional channels allowing potassium to cross the membrane will hyperpolarize it. This type of action has been described for a number of endogenous substances such as ATP (Tomita and Watanabe, 1973) and norepinephrine acting via α receptors (Bülbring and Tomita, 1969). In visceral smooth muscle these effects are blocked by apamin, a toxin from bee venom (Mass et al., 1980). Nonadrenergic, noncholinergic nerve stimulation produces a similar hyperpolarization. In some smooth muscles such as dog descending coronary artery (Mekata, 1980) or gastric fundus (Morgan et al., 1981), which do not readily generate action potentials, there appears to be a leakage of calcium into the cell at the resting membrane potential so that resting tone is present. Hyperpolarization may close ion channels through which calcium is leaking into the cell under these conditions, and relaxation occurs.

B. Effects on Calcium Binding and/or Extrusion

A notable effect of activation of β receptors by catecholamines is the reduction of the tension that is generated in the smooth muscle associated with the discharge of a single action potential. Other effects associated with this are inhibition of spontaneous action potential discharge, and therefore contractions, and hyperpolarization of the membrane. In some smooth muscles, this hyperpolarization is small (Bülbring and den Hertog, 1980) but in others such as the pig coronary artery it can be very substantial (Ito et al., 1979). These effects of β receptor activation have been ascribed to an acceleration of the binding and/or sequestration of calcium within the cell (Edman and Schild, 1963; Casteels and Raeymaekers, 1979; Mueller and van Breemen, 1979; Bülbring and den Hertog, 1980) and may involve inhibition of the actin–myosin interaction via the rise in cyclic AMP that occurs (Conti and Adelstein, 1980).

Another agent that increases cyclic AMP levels is vasoactive intestinal polypeptide (VIP) (Frandsen et al., 1978). VIP relaxes most smooth muscles and in estrogen-dominated guinea pig and rabbit uterus had effects very similar to those of β receptor activation, although it did not produce its effects via β receptors (Bolton et al., 1981). Thus, it reduced the tension response associated with a single action potential and reduced the contractures obtained upon readmitting calcium to a calcium-free, high-potassium solution. Slight hyperpolarization of the membrane was observed and this was probably caused by an increase in potassium permeability.

C. Block of Action Potential Discharge

A number of substances exogenous to the body, loosely called "calcium antagonists," are known to inhibit or block the discharge of action potentials in smooth muscle. These include D600, verapamil, and nifedipine. Such substances will, by inhibiting action potential discharge, reduce or abolish phasic contractions that would normally occur upon application of stimulant substances (e.g., see Golenhofen, 1981). However, no evidence has been obtained that any endogenous substance has a mechanism of action resembling these "calcium antagonists."

D. Summary of Inhibitory Mechanisms

Three mechanisms whereby substances endogenous or exogenous to the body can produce inhibition of smooth muscle contraction are well recognized:

1. Opening of channels allowing potassium ions to escape from the cell, thus hyperpolarizing the membrane. The hyperpolarization will reduce or abolish action potential discharge in those smooth muscles in which this occurs. In smooth muscle not discharging action potentials, the hyperpolarization may close calcium channels already open and reduce resting tension.

2. Increased calcium binding, accompanied by a rise in cyclic AMP, may reduce the tension response associated with an action potential. There are a number of other well recognized phenomena (e.g., hyperpolarization) that are associated with this effect in an, as yet, obscure way.

3. Block of action potential generation.

We must add to the above list a miscellany of inhibitory mechanisms that may underlie the effects of relaxants of vascular and other smooth muscles. Many of these relaxants have been shown to reduce contractures to calcium in high-potassium solution and to reduce calcium influx into the cell. Some increase cyclic AMP levels; others hyperpolarize the membrane and reduce evoked action potential discharge (see Bolton, 1979). Some such as nitroglycerin (Ito *et al.*, 1980) and diltiazem (Ito *et al.*, 1978) have little or no detectable effect on membrane properties of smooth muscle at concentrations that exert an inhibitory effect on tension development. Some investigators (Pöch and Umfahrer, 1976; Gagnon *et al.*, 1980) believe that many vascular relaxants act by increasing cyclic AMP levels (mechanism 2 above?) or cyclic GMP levels (Kukovetz *et al.*, 1979). Intriguing as these suggestions are, as we lack a clear conceptual framework concerning the role of cyclic nucleotides in cell economy (see Hardman, 1981), it is difficult to relate these effects on nucleotide levels to levels of tension.

IV. CONCLUSIONS

In action potential generating smooth muscles, which include the muscle of many small blood vessels, it seems likely that alteration of the frequency of action potential discharge is an important mechanism modulating tension and resistance to blood flow. Effects on permeability of the membrane will depolarize or hyperpolarize, so affecting the readiness with which action potentials and contractions will occur. The opening of receptor-operated ion channels admitting calcium, and the release of bound calcium, may be important in the smooth muscle of larger blood vessels which has less tendency to discharge action potentials. Inhibitory substances, besides acting on the permeability of the cell membrane, also seem to affect the calcium economy of the smooth muscle cell, somehow reducing the tension developed in response to calcium influx or release. Exogenous substances may interfere with contraction at a variety of points as yet incompletely known; endogenous compounds yet to be discovered may act in similar ways.

REFERENCES

Bolton, T. B. (1972). The depolarizing action of acetylcholine or carbachol in intestinal smooth muscle. *J. Physiol.* (*London*) **220,** 647–671.
Bolton, T. B. (1979). Mechanisms of action of transmitters and other substances on smooth muscle. *Physiol. Rev.* **59,** 606–718.
Bolton, T. B., Lang, R. J., and Ottesen, B. (1981). Mechanism of action of vasoactive intestinal polypeptide (VIP) on myometrial smooth muscle of rabbit and guinea-pig. *J. Physiol.* (*London*) **318,** 41–55.
Bozler, E. (1969). Role of calcium in initiation of activity in smooth muscle. *Am. J. Physiol.* **216,** 671–674.
Brading, A. F., and Sneddon, P. (1980). Evidence for multiple sources of calcium for activation of the contractile mechanism of guinea-pig taenia coli on stimulation with carbachol. *Br. J. Pharmacol.* **70,** 229–240.
Bülbring, E., and den Hertog, A. (1980). The action of isoprenaline on the smooth muscle of the guinea-pig taenia coli. *J. Physiol.* (*London*) **304,** 277–296.
Bülbring, E., and Tomita, T. (1969). Increase in membrane conductance by adrenaline in the smooth muscle of guinea-pig taenia coli. *Proc. R. Soc. London, Ser. B* **172,** 89–102.
Casteels, R., and Droogmans, G. (1981). Exchange characteristics of the noradrenaline sensitive Ca store in vascular smooth muscle cells of rabbit ear artery. *J. Physiol.* (*London*) **317,** 263–279.
Casteels, R., and Raeymaekers, L. (1979). The action of acetylcholine and catecholamines on an intra-cellular calcium store in the smooth muscle cells of the guinea-pig taenia coli. *J. Physiol.* (*London*) **294,** 51–68.
Casteels, R., Kitamura, K., Kuriyama, H., and Suzuki, H. (1977a). The membrane properties of the smooth muscle cells of the rabbit main pulmonary artery. *J. Physiol.* (*London*) **271,** 41–61.
Casteels, R., Kitamura, K., Kuriyama, H., and Suzuki, H. (1977b). Excitation-contraction coupling in the smooth muscle cells of the rabbit main pulmonary artery. *J. Physiol.* (*London*) **271,** 63–79.

Casteels, R., Raeymaekers, L., and Suzuki, H. (1981). Calcium-independent contraction of vascular smooth muscle. *J. Physiol. (London)* **313**, 33–34P.

Conti, M. A., and Adelstein, R. S. (1980). Phosphorylation by cyclic adenosine 3′, 5′-monophosphate-dependent protein kinase regulates myosin light chain kinase. *Fed. Proc., Fed. Am. Soc. Exp. Biol.* **39**, 1569–1573.

Deth, R., and van Breemen, C. (1974). Relative contributions of Ca^{2+} influx and cellular Ca^{2+} release during drug induced activation of the rabbit aorta. *Pfluegers Arch.* **348**, 13–22.

Durbin, R. P., and Jenkinson, D. H. (1961). The effect of carbachol on the permeability of depolarized smooth muscle to inorganic ions. *J. Physiol. (London)* **157**, 74–89.

Edman, K. A. P., and Schild, H. O. (1962). The need for calcium in the contractile responses induced by acetylcholine and potassium in the rat uterus. *J. Physiol. (London)* **161**, 424–441.

Edman, K. A. P., and Schild, H. O. (1963). Calcium and the stimulant and inhibitory effects of adrenaline in depolarized smooth muscle. *J. Physiol. (London)* **169**, 404–411.

Evans, D. H. L., Schild, H. O., and Thesleff, S. (1958). Effects of drugs on depolarized plain muscle. *J. Physiol. (London)* **143**, 474–485.

Frandsen, E. K., Krishna, G. A., and Said, S. I. (1978). Vasoactive intestinal polypeptide promotes cyclic adenosine 3′5′-monophosphate accumulation in guinea-pig trachea. *Br. J. Pharmacol.* **62**, 367–369.

Gagnon, G., Regoli, D., and Rioux, F. (1980). Studies on the mechanism of action of various vasodilators. *Br. J. Pharmacol.* **70**, 219–227.

Golenhofen, K. (1981). Differentiation of calcium activation processes in smooth muscles using selective antagonists. *In* "Smooth Muscle: An Assessment of Current Knowledge" (E. Bulbring *et al.,* eds.), pp. 157–170. Arnold, London.

Haeusler, G., and Thorens, S. (1980). Effects of tetraethylammonium chloride on contractile, membrane and cable properties of rabbit artery muscle. *J. Physiol. (London)* **303**, 203–224.

Haeusler, G., Kuhn, H., and Thorens, S. (1980). The effect of tetraethylammonium chloride on calcium fluxes in smooth muscle from rabbit main pulmonary artery. *J. Physiol. (London)* **303**, 225–241.

Harbon, S., and Clauser, H. (1971). Cyclic adenosine 3′,5′-monophosphate levels in rat myometrium under the influence of epinephrine, prostaglandins, and oxytocin. Correlation with uterus motility. *Biochem. Biophys. Res. Commun.* **44**, 1496–1503.

Hardman, J. G. (1981). Cyclic nucleotides and smooth muscle contraction; some conceptual and experimental considerations. *In* "Smooth Muscle: An Assessment of Current Knowledge" (E. Bülbring *et al.,* eds.), pp. 249–262. Arnold, London.

Hinke, J. A. M. (1965). Calcium requirements for noradrenaline and high potassium ion contraction in arterial smooth muscle. *In* "Muscle" (W. M. Paul *et al.,* eds.), pp. 269–284, Pergamon, Oxford.

Ito, Y., Suzuki, H., and Kuriyama, H. (1977). On the roles of calcium ion during potassium induced contracture in the smooth muscle cells of the rabbit main pulmonary artery. *Jpn. J. Physiol.* **27**, 755–770.

Ito, Y., Kuriyama, H., and Suzuki, H. (1978). The effects of diltiazem (CRD-401) on the membrane and mechanical properties of vascular smooth muscles of the rabbit. *Br. J. Pharmacol.* **64**, 503–510.

Ito, Y., Kitamura, K., and Kuriyama, H. (1979). Effects of acetylcholine and catecholamines on the smooth muscle cell of the porcine coronary artery. *J. Physiol. (London)* **294**, 595–611.

Ito, Y., Kitamura, K., and Kuriyama, H. (1980). Actions of nitroglycerine on the membrane and mechanical properties of smooth muscles of the coronary artery of the pig. *Br. J. Pharmacol.* **70**, 197–204.

Keatinge, W. R. (1972). Mechanical response with reversed electrical response to noradrenaline by Ca-deprived arterial smooth muscle. *J. Physiol. (London)* **224**, 21–34.

Kitamura, K., and Kuriyama, H. (1979). Effects of acetylcholine on the smooth muscle cell of isolated main coronary artery of the guinea-pig. *J. Physiol.* (*London*) **293**, 119–133.

Kuriyama, H. (1981). Excitation-contraction coupling in various visceral smooth muscles. *In* "Smooth Muscle: An Assessment of Current Knowledge" (E. Bülbring *et al.*, eds.), pp. 171–197. Arnold, London.

Kuriyama, H., and Suzuki, H. (1978). The effects of acetylcholine on the membrane and contractile properties of smooth muscle cells of the rabbit superior mesenteric artery. *Br. J. Pharmacol.* **64**, 493–501.

Kukovetz, W. R., Holzmann, S., Wurm, A., and Pöch, G. (1979). Evidence for cyclic GMP-mediated relaxant effects of nitro-compounds in coronary smooth muscle. *Naunyn-Schmiedeberg's Arch. Pharmacol.* **310**, 129–138.

Mass, A. J. J., den Hertog, A., Ras, R., and van den Akker, J. (1980). The action of apamin on guinea-pig taenia caeci. *Eur. J. Pharmacol.* **67**, 265–274.

Mekata, F. (1980). Electrophysiological properties of the smooth muscle cell membrane of the dog coronary artery. *J. Physiol.* (*London*) **298**, 205–212.

Morgan, K. G., and Szurszewski, J. H. (1980). Mechanism of phasic and tonic actions of pentagastrin on canine gastric smooth msucle. *J. Physiol.* (*London*) **301**, 229–242.

Morgan, K. G., Muir, T. C., and Szurszewski, J. H. (1981). The electrical basis for contraction and relaxation in canine fundal smooth muscle. *J. Physiol.* (*London*) **311**, 475–488.

Mueller, E., and van Breemen, C. (1979). Role of intracellular Ca^{2+} sequestration in β-adrenergic relaxation of a smooth muscle. *Nature* (*London*) **281**, 682–683.

Ohashi, H., Takewaki, T., and Okada, T. (1974). Calcium and the contractile effect of carbachol in the depolarized guinea-pig taenia caecum. *J. Physiol.* (*London*) **24**, 601–611.

Ohashi, H., Takewaki, T., Shibata, N., and Okada, T. (1975). Effects of calcium antagonists on contractile response of guinea-pig taenia caecum to carbachol in a calcium deficient, potassium rich solution. *Jpn. J. Pharmacol.* **25**, 214–216.

Pöch, G., and Umfahrer, W. (1976). Differentiation of intestinal smooth muscle relaxation caused by drugs that inhibit phosphodiesterase. *Naunyn-Schmiedeberg's Arch. Pharmacol.* **293**, 257–268.

Shuba, M. F. (1977). The mechanism of the excitatory action of catecholamines and histamine on the smooth muscle of guinea pig ureter. *J. Physiol.* (*London*) **264**, 853–864.

Su, C., and Bevan, J. A. (1965). The electrical response of pulmonary artery muscle to acetylcholine, histamine, and serotonin. *Life Sci.* **4**, 1025–1029.

Tomita, T., and Watanabe, H. (1973). A comparison of the effects of adenosine triphosphate with noradrenaline and with the inhibitory potential of the guinea-pig taenia coli. *J. Physiol.* (*London*) **231**, 167–177.

van Breemen, C., Farinas, B. R., Gerba, P., and McNaughton, E. D. (1972). Excitation-contraction coupling in rabbit aorta studied by the Lanthanum method for measuring cellular calcium influx. *Circ. Res.* **30**, 44–54.

26

The Influence of Dietary Salt on Adrenergic Neuronal Function

THOMAS C. WESTFALL

There are a variety of control systems that regulate vascular function including humoral, neuronal, and local autoregulatory processes. One of the most important of the neuronal influences is carried out by adrenergic neurons of the sympathetic nervous system. Regulation of the adrenergically mediated effects on vascular smooth muscle can take place at several sites and by several processes including (1) nerve impulse frequency originating at several levels of the central nervous system (i.e., hypothalamus, nucleus tractus solitarii, etc.), (2) nerve impulse frequency via receptors located on the soma and dendrites of the sympathetic ganglion cell, (3) prejunctional events influencing synthesis, storage, or metabolism of norepinephrine (NE), (4) modulation of release by a variety of neuronal or hormonal substances acting prejunctionally at the level of the

371

THE ROLE OF SALT IN
CARDIOVASCULAR HYPERTENSION

neuroeffector junction, and (5) binding of NE or its metabolites to neuronal or extraneuronal sites, including postjuntional receptors.

The adrenergic neuroeffector junction is the final link which carries out the neuronally induced regulation of vascular smooth muscle function. The adrenergic varicosity is a complex biochemical and biophysical unit and for it to operate smoothly requires the interaction of several biophysical and biochemical systems involving transmitter synthesis, storage, release, metabolism, and interaction with appropriate receptors.

In the present chapter I will briefly review adrenergic neurotransmitter dynamics and then discuss the influence of dietary salt on adrenergic neuronal function in normal and hypertensive animals.

I. ADRENERGIC NEUROTRANSMITTER DYNAMICS

Figure 1 depicts a summary of the various dynamic events that take place at the adrenergic neuroeffector junction. Several comprehensive reviews are available which discuss this in greater detail (Smith, 1972; Smith and Winkler, 1972;

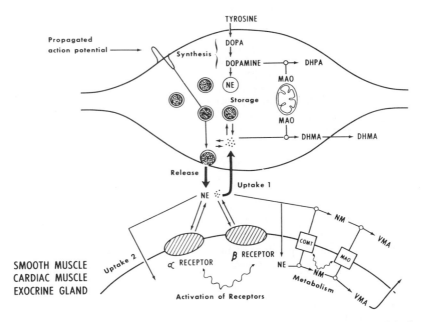

Fig. 1. The adrenergic nerve varicosity and the adrenergic neuroeffector junction. This figure also summarizes the various processes involved in adrenergic dynamics such as synthesis, storage, release, receptor activation (pre and post), and inactivation of NE.

Vanhoutte, 1978, 1980; Weiner *et al.*, 1972; Weinshilboum, 1979). A brief summary will be presented here.

The adrenergic neurotransmitter NE is synthesized by three enzymatically controlled steps starting with the uptake of tyrosine into the adrenergic varicosity and its conversion to dihydroxyphenylalanine (dopa), dopamine, and finally NE by the enzymes tyrosine-3-monooxygenase, aromatic L-amino acid decarboxylase, and dopamine-3-monooxygenase, respectively. The conversion of dopamine to NE takes place in the storage vesicles where the transmitter is stored in a complex with protein, ATP, and various ions. Upon the arrival of an action potential and depolarization of the terminal varicosity, NE is released, together with other soluble contents including dopamine β-hydroxylase, ATP, and chromogranins into the extracellular space. NE migrates to the vascular effector cell where it interacts with α_1 or β_2 adrenoceptors to cause vasoconstriction and in some cases vasodilation, respectively. NE is terminated by a specific carrier-mediated uptake system (uptake 1) across the neuronal membrane. This is an active transport process requiring Na^+ as well as energy. Following the recapture of NE inside the adrenergic varicosity, the amine is further transported into the storage vesicles for reuse or is metabolized by monoamine oxidase located on the outerlying membrane of the mitochondria. A second way of inactivation of NE is via the extraneuronal enzyme, catechol *O*-methyltransferase, following uptake into smooth muscle cells (uptake 2). The synthesis, storage, release, receptor activation, and inactivation of NE are obviously subject to various control mechanisms that must operate in concert for the smooth operation of the adrenergic neurons. Much information on the regulation of these processes is available.

Recently, it has been discovered that neural and hormonal substances can influence the quantitative release of NE per nerve impulse by an action on receptors located on the adrenergic varicosities and thereby influence the concentration of transmitter at the neuroeffector junction. Substances reported to decrease adrenergic neurotransmission include α-adrenoceptor agonists (α_2 agonists) including NE itself; purines such as ATP and adenosine; prostaglandins (PG) of the E series; acetylcholine (ACh), via muscarinic receptors; dopamine (DA); histamine; serotonin (5-HT); morphine and opioid peptides. Substances facilitating adrenergic neurotransmission include β-adrenergic agonists, ACh via nicotinic receptors, angiotensin (ANG), and possibly PG of the F series as well as thromboxanes. The site of origin of these various substances is depicted in Fig. 2. In addition to influencing adrenergic neurotransmission, they may also contribute to the regulation of vascular tone by acting directly on vascular smooth muscle and/or influencing the activity of other vasoactive substances. Several extensive reviews have appeared that discuss this aspect of control of adrenergic neuronal function in greater detail (Langer, 1977; Starke, 1977; Westfall, 1977, 1980; Rand *et al.*, 1980). Modulation by these substances are thought to have important physiological functions and may play important pathophysiological

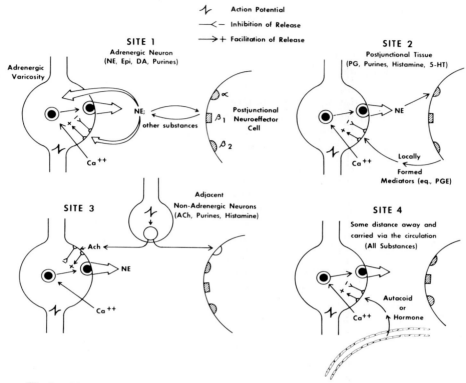

Fig. 2. The four sites of origin of neural and humoral substances which have been shown to increase or decrease the release of the adrenergic neurotransmitter during adrenergic neurotransmission. Site 1 represents the adrenergic nerve varicosity and "substances" may include NE, epinephrine, dopamine, and the purines ATP and adenosine. Site 2 represents the postjunctional tissue and may include prostaglandins, purines, histamine, and 5-hydroxytryptamine. Site 3 represents an adjacent noradrenergic neuron and "substances" may include acetylcholine, purines, or histamine. Site 4 represents "substances" that arrive at the adrenergic nerve varicosity via the circulation; these could include any of the substances already mentioned as well as angiotensin.

roles as well. Of particular importance is the negative feedback process mediated by the transmitter itself on prejunctional α_2 receptors. This is thought to be an important physiological control mechanism which regulates transmitter release. There is convincing evidence that during nerve stimulation, the level of NE in the neuroeffector junction continues to rise until a critical threshold is reached that shuts off further liberation of the transmitter by an action on α-adrenoceptors located on the adrenergic nerve varicosity. Also of great interest is the possibility that during stress the β-adrenoceptor and angiotensin facilitory systems may be functional.

Sodium is important in several of the various aspects of adrenergic dynamics including (1) the physiologically induced release of the transmitter due to membrane depolarization following the arrival of the action potential at the terminal varicosity, (2) neuronal uptake, and (3) retention and storage of NE. Dietary salt could potentially influence adrenergic neuronal function by acting on these three or at any other of the various processes involved in regulating adrenergic neuronal function.

II. INFLUENCE OF HIGH SALT ON ADRENERGIC NEURONAL FUNCTION

Little information is available on the influence of dietary salt alone on adrenergic neuronal function. An increase in dietary salt can apparently lead to an increase in urinary (Battarbee et al., 1979; Feuerstein et al., 1979) or plasma (Reid et al., 1975) catecholamines in rats and cats (Feuerstein et al., 1979). These changes could reflect an increase in adrenergic neuronal activity. In some cases the animals were hypertensive when the catecholamines were elevated, while in other cases they were normotensive. Similar studies in humans have led to conflicting results, however. For instance, Alexander et al. (1974) found a reduced urinary NE excretion and plasma dopamine β-hydroxylase activity in response to high sodium diets or saline infusion while Lake and Ziegler (1978) failed to demonstrate any change in plasma NE and dopamine β-hydroxylase.

Chronic sodium loading in dogs has been shown to enhance the faciltory effect that angiotensin has on catecholamine release due to sympathetic nerve stimulation (Carriere et al., 1980). This result could have important implications concerning the role of angiotensin and hypertension. Just the opposite appears to be the case in animals exposed to a low sodium diet. This will be discussed in detail below.

III. INFLUENCE OF LOW SALT ON ADRENERGIC NEURONAL FUNCTION

In dogs treated with a low, normal, or high sodium diet, it has been observed that the increase in mean arterial blood pressure following carotid artery occlusion was significantly less in the animals on the low sodium diet (Table I) (Rocchini et al., 1977). The small pressor response in the dogs on a low sodium diet was shown not to be related to changes in plasma renin activity, basal level of angiotensin II, to the degree of carotid hypotension, or to the vascular reaction to infused NE. On the other hand, the dose response to tyramine was shifted significantly to the right while that to NE was not different and suggests that the

TABLE I

Increase in Mean Arterial Blood Pressure following Carotid Artery Occlusion in Dogs Treated with Various Sodium Diets[a]

Treatment group	mEq/day	Increase in mean blood pressure (mm Hg ± SEM)
Low Sodium	10	14.1 ± 2.8[b]
Normal Sodium	70	28.6 ± 5.2
High Sodium	110	25.4 ± 7.5

[a] From Rocchini *et al.* (1977).
[b] $p < 0.007$.

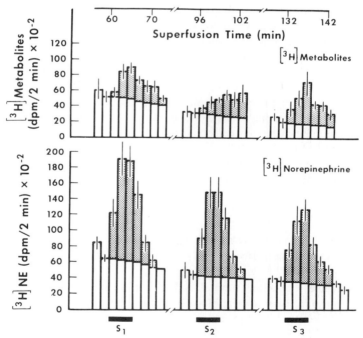

Fig. 3. The efflux of [³H]norepinephrine and [³H]metabolites from the superfused rat portal vein previously incubated with 10^{-7} M [³H]NE for 30 min. The tissue has been superfused for 60 min prior to three consecutive periods of field stimulation (5 Hz, 1 msec duration, supramaximal voltage) at 30-min intervals (S_1, S_2, and S_3). Desipramine (5×10^{-7} M) and metanephrine (4×10^{-5} M) are present in the superfusion fluid to block uptake 1 and uptake 2, respectively.

release of NE was decreased. These studies are consistent with the concept that a reduction in dietary sodium leads to a decreased responsiveness of the efferent sympathetic neurons. On the other hand, chronic restriction of sodium in humans has been reported to result in an increased urinary catecholamine excretion (Gordon *et al.*, 1964; Kelsch *et al.*, 1971).

Dietary salt restriction appears to blunt, while high salt diets appear to potentiate, the vascular effects of angiotensin. In addition, the neurogenic response to angiotensin (facilitation of transmitter release) also appears to be decreased in animals undergoing dietary salt restriction. The potentiation of the neurogenic responses to angiotensin II and III were depressed in portal veins of sodium restricted rabbits (Sybertz and Peach, 1980). In contrast, potentiation of neurogenic responses by angiotensin peptides in the vas deferens was not influence by changes in dietary sodium intake.

Direct *in vitro* evidence for this type of observation has been obtained in studies carried out by us on the superfused rat portal vein. Figure 3 shows the effect of three consecutive periods of field stimulation on the release of [^{3}H]NE from superfused rat portal vein previously incubated with the labeled transmitter. This procedure allows for the study of various drugs that can influence the stimulation-induced release of NE. In Fig. 4 various concentrations of angiotensin were added to the superfusion bath between the first and second stimulation and an S_2/S_1 ratio calculated. Figure 4 shows the concentration-dependent facilitation of NE release

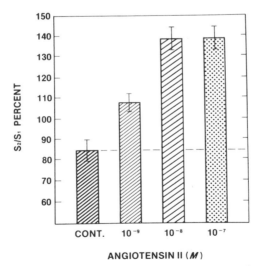

Fig. 4. The effect of three concentrations of angiotensin II (10^{-9}, 10^{-8}, and 10^{-7} M) on the electrically induced release of [^{3}H]norepinephrine from the superfused rat portal vein. The procedure was the same as depicted in Fig. 3. Angiotensin was added 20 min prior to the second stimulation (S_2) and the S_2 (in presence of angiotensin)/S_1 (in the absence of angiotensin) ratios plotted.

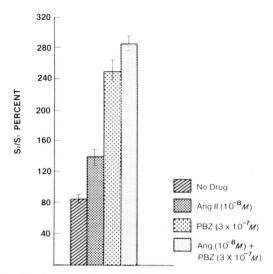

Fig. 5. The effect of angiotensin, phenoxybenzamine, and the combination of both agents on the electrically induced release of [³H]NE from the superfused rat portal vein. The experiment was carried out in a similar fashion as in Figs. 3 and 4 with drugs being added to the superfusion buffer 20 min prior to the second stimulation (S_2). Both angiotensin and phenoxybenzamine produced a significant enhancement of the field stimulation induced overflow of [³H]NE. The effect of the two drugs was nearly additive.

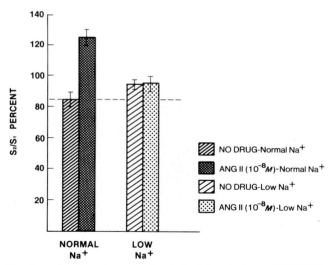

Fig. 6. The effect of angiotensin on the electrically induced release of [³H]NE from the superfused rat portal vein. Vessels were obtained from animals maintained on a normal (150 mEq/kg sodium) or low salt diet (22 mEq/kg sodium) for 10 days. The experiment was carried out in a similar fashion as Figs. 3–5. Angiotensin was added 20 min prior to the second stimulation (S_2). The normal facilitation on the field stimulation induced release of [³H]NE was significantly reduced in vessels obtained from animals maintained on the low sodium diet.

induced by angiotensin II. Figure 5 shows that such facilitation is additive with phenoxybenzamine which is well known to enhance NE release by blocking prejunctional α_2 receptors.

In Fig. 6 are depicted results of experiments carried out on vessels obtained from animals maintained on a low salt diet for 10 days. It can be seen that the normal facilitory effect of angiotensin on the electrically induced release of NE was not seen in vessels obtained from animals on a low sodium diet. These data directly confirm the observations of Sybertz and Peach (1980) and suggest that a decrease in dietary salt can have an important effect in blunting both the neurogenic as well as the direct vascular effect of angiotensin. The mechanism by which angiotensin produced this effect is yet to be established.

IV. DIETARY SALT AND EXPERIMENTAL HYPERTENSION

Increased ingestion of salt over prolonged periods of time has led to hypertension in normal rats in the absence of other kinds of interventions (Meneely and Ball, 1958; Battarbee and Meneely, 1978; Sapirstein *et al.*, 1950). Moreover, salt ingestion accelerates the development of hypertension in the spontaneously hypertensive rat as well as other models (Louis *et al.*, 1971; Ylitalo *et al.*, 1976; Vogel, 1966). In at least two models of hypertension ingestion of salt appears an absolute requirement for hypertension to develop. These are hypertension in the Dahl-sensitive rat (Dahl, 1961, 1972) and rats treated simultaneously with deoxycorticosterone acetate (DOCA)(Selye *et al.*, 1943). Of these various hypertensive models at least two have been shown to involve a neurogenic component which in turn appears dependent on increased intake of sodium chloride.

V. SODIUM-DEPENDENT HYPERTENSION INVOLVING A NEUROGENIC COMPONENT

The hypertension developed in both the Dahl-sensitive and DOCA/salt hypertensive rats appears to invoke an increase in adrenergic neuronal function.

Numerous investigators have presented evidence of increased peripheral sympathetic nerve activity in DOCA/salt hypertensive rats. There is an increase in NE turnover of adrenergically innervated tissues (de Champlain *et al.*, 1969; Kazda *et al.*, 1969; Nakamura *et al.*, 1970), an increase in plasma (Reid *et al.*, 1975) and urinary NE (de Champlain *et al.*, 1969), as well as an increase in monoamine oxidase activity (de Champlain *et al.*, 1968). These changes and other components of adrenergic neuronal function are summarized in Table II. Evidence has been presented suggesting that the increased turnover of NE is due to a reduced ability of the adrenergic storage vesicles to bind and store NE which

TABLE II

Adrenergic Neuronal Function in DOCA/Salt Hypertensive Rats

Activity	Change
Turnover of NE	Increased
Plasma NE	Increased
Urinary NE	Increased
MAO activity	Increased
Storage vesicle binding	Decreased
Tissue NE	Decreased
Extraneuronal NE uptake (uptake 2)	Decreased
NE uptake (uptake 1)	None
COMT activity	None
Electrically induced release from isolated hearts	None
Catecholamine synthesis (heart, etc.)	None

could lead to a continuous leakage onto vascular receptors (Krakoff *et al.,* 1967; de Champlain *et al.,* 1968). More recently, however, Giachetti *et al.* (1979) have challenged this view and have presented evidence suggesting that there was no difference in the storage capacity of adrenergic nerves in DOCA/salt hypertensive rats compared to normotensive animals. These investigators suggest that there is an increased rate of neuronal firing that is not compensated for by increased synthesis adequate to refill completely the storage vesicles.

Regardless of the precise mechanism, there is nevertheless strong evidence for increased adrenergic nerve activity that may participate in both the development and maintenance of hypertension. Further evidence is provided by the fact that both central and peripheral sympathectomy with 6-hydroxydopamine or neonatal guanethidine prevents the development of hypertension in DOCA/salt treated animals (Lewis *et al.,* 1975; Bell *et al.,* 1979).

Evidence also exists for an increase in adrenergic nerve activity in the salt-dependent Dahl-sensitive hypertensive rat. Takeshita and Mark (1978) have observed that neurogenic vasoconstriction was found to account for about 50% of the increase in vascular resistance produced by high salt in the salt-sensitive strain. Moreover, high salt intake potentiated responses to direct electrical sympathetic nerve stimulation, but not to exogenous NE in the salt-sensitive rats. These investigators and others have also observed that the administration of 6-hydroxydopamine peripherally in doses that reduced responses to direct sympathetic nerve stimulation and tyramine prevented the development of hypertension during high salt intake in the Dahl-sensitive strain (Takeshita *et al.,* 1979; Friedman *et al.,* 1979). These studies suggest that an intact sympathetic nervous system plays an essential role in the development of salt-induced hypertension in the Dahl-sensitive rat.

Although in both forms of hypertension it is apparent that salt is important and necessary in contributing to the increase in adrenergic nerve activity and development of hypertension, it is unclear if dietary salt is solely responsible for these developments. In the one case DOCA also appears necessary and in the other there is an unknown genetic component. However, it is of interest that dietary salt alone can cause hypertension although it appears unknown if it involves a neurogenic component. The mechanism by which sodium chloride produces these changes is also unclear.

VI. SUMMARY

Sodium is a necessary ingredient in several aspects of adrenergic neuronal function including release, uptake, and storage of the neurotransmitter norepinephrine. Dietary sodium could potentially influence adrenergic neuronal function by acting on these processes or any other of the various steps in adrenergic dynamics. Evidence exists that increasing dietary sodium may lead to an increased activity in adrenergic nerves and an enhancement of the normal facilitory action of angiotensin on adrenergic transmission. In addition, dietary sodium can cause the development of hypertension in Dahl-sensitive rats or rats simultaneously treated with DOCA. A neurogenic component consisting of increased activity of adrenergic nerves appears to be present in both forms of hypertension. It is unclear if sodium is causative or merely permissive in the neurogenic aspect of sodium-dependent hypertension. However, chronic dietary sodium intake can induce hypertension in the absence of other interventions. Low dietary salt may result in a decrease in efferent sympathetic nerve activity. Moreover, reduced dietary intake of salt appears to blunt the facilitory action of angiotensin on adrenergic neurotransmission.

ACKNOWLEDGMENT

Supported by grants from the National Institutes of Health, HL26317, DA02668, and N546215 from the Department of Health and Human Services.

REFERENCES

Alexander, R. W., Gill, J. R., Yamabe, H., Lovenberg, W., and Keiser, H. R. (1974). Effect of dietary sodium and acute saline infusion on the interrelationship between dopamine excretion and adrenergic activity in man. *J. Clin. Invest.* **54,** 194–200.

Battarbee, H. D., and Meneely, G. R. (1978). The toxicity of salt. *CRC Crit. Rev. Toxicol.* 355–376.

Battarbee, H. D., Funch, D. P., and Dailey, J. W. (1979). The effect of dietary sodium and potassium upon blood pressure and catecholamine excretion in the rat. *Proc. Soc. Exp. Biol. Med.* **161,** 32–37.

Bell, C., Elspeth, M., and McLachlan, M. (1979). Dependence of deoxycorticosterone/salt hypertension in the rat on the activity of adrenergic cardiac nerves. *Clin. Sci.* **57,** 203–210.

Carriere, S., Cardinal, J., and Le Grimellec, C. (1980). Influence of sodium intake on catecholamine release by angiotensin and renal nerve stimulation in dogs. *Can. J.Phsyiol. Pharmacol.* **58,** 1092–1101.

Dahl, L. K. (1961). Effects of chronic excess salt feeding: Induction of self-sustaining hypertension in rats. *J. Exp. Med.* **114,** 231–236.

Dahl, L. K. (1972). Salt and hypertension. *Am. J. Clin. Nutr.* **25,** 231–244.

de Champlain, J., Krakoff, L. R., and Axelrod, J. (1968). Relationship between sodium intake and norepinephrine storage during the development of experimental hypertension. *Circ. Res.* **23,** 479–491.

de Champlain, J., Meuller, R. A., and Axelrod, J. (1969). Turnover and synthesis of norepinephrine in experimental hypertension in rats. *Circ. Res.* **25,** 285–291.

Feuerstein, G., Boonyaviroj, P., and Gutman, Y. (1979). The effect of saline loading on blood pressure and catecholamine secretion in the rat and the cat. *Eur. J. Pharmacol.* **54,** 373–382.

Friedman, R., Tassinari, L. M., Heine, M., and Twai, J. (1979). Differential development of salt induced and renal hypertension in Dahl hypertensive sensitive rats after neonatal sympathectomy. *Clin. Exp. Hypertens.* **1,** 779–799.

Giachetti, A., Rubinstein, R., and Clark, T. L. (1979). Noradrenaline storage in deoxycorticosterone-saline hypertensive rats. *Eur. J. Pharmacol.* **57,** 99–106.

Gordon, R. D., Kuchel, O., Liddle, G. W., and Island, D. P. (1964). Role of the sympathetic nervous system in regulating renin and aldosterone production in man. *J. Clin. Invest.* **43,** 177–184.

Kazda, S. I., Pohlova, B., Bibr, B., and Cockova, S. (1969). Norepinephrine content of tissues in DOCA-hypertensive rats. *Am. J. Physiol.* **216,** 1472–1475.

Kelsch, R. C., Light, G. S., Luciano, J. R., and Oliver, W. J. (1971). The effect of prednisolone on plasma norepinephrine concentration and renin activity in salt-depleted man. *J. Lab. Clin. Med.* **77,** 268–277.

Krakoff, L. R., de Champlain, J., and Axelrod, J. (1967). Abnormal storage of norepinephrine in experimental hypertension in the rat. *Circ. Res.* **21,** 583–591.

Lake, C. R., and Ziegler, M. G. (1978). Effect of acute volume alterations on norepinephrine and dopamine β-hydroxylase in normotensive and hypertensive subject. *Circulation* **57,** 774–778.

Langer, S. Z. (1977). Presynaptic receptors and their role in the regulation of transmitter release. *Br. J. Pharmacol.* **60,** 481–497.

Lewis, P. J., Dargie, H., and Dollery, C. T. (1975). Role of saline consumption in the prevention of deoxycorticosterone hypertension in rats by 6-hydroxydopamine. *Clin. Sci. Mol. Med.* **48,** 327–330.

Louis, W. J., Taber, R., and Spector, S. (1971). Effects of sodium intake on inherited hypertension in the rat. *Lancet* **2,** 1283–1286.

Meneely, G. R., and Ball, C. O. T. (1958). Experimental epidemiology of chronic sodium chloride toxicity and the protective effect of potassium chloride. *Am. J. Med.* **25,** 713–720.

Nakamura, K., Gerold, M., and Thoenen, H. (1970). Experimental hypertension of the rat: Reciprocal changes of norepinephrine turnover in heart and brainstem. *Jpn. J. Pharmacol.* **20,** 605–607.

Rand, M. J., Majewski, H., Medgett, I. C., McCulloch, M. W., and Story, D. F. (1980). Prejunctional receptors modulating autonomic neuroeffector transmission. *Circ. Res.* **46,** Suppl. 1, 70–76.

Reid, J. L., Zivin, J. A., and Kopin, I. J. (1975). Central and peripheral adrenergic mechanisms in the development of deoxycorticosterone-saline hypertension in rats. *Circ. Res.* **37,** 569–579.

Rocchini, A. P., Cant, J. R., and Barger, A. C. (1977). Carotid sinus reflex in dogs with low to high sodium intake. *Am. J. Physiol.* **233,** 196–202.

Sapirstein, L. A., Brandt, W. L., and Drury, D. H. (1950). Production of hypertension in the rat by substituting hypertonic sodium chloride for drinking water. *Proc. Soc. Exp. Biol. Med.* **73,** 82–85.

Selye, H., Hall, C. E., and Rowley, E. M. (1943). Malignant hypertension produced by treatment with deoxycorticosterone acetate and sodium chloride. *Can. Med. Assoc. J.* **49,** 88–92.

Smith, A. D. (1972). Cellular control of the uptake, storage and release of noradrenaline in sympathetic nerves. *Biochem. Soc. Symp.* **36,** 103–131.

Smith, A. D., and Winkler, H. (1972). Fundamental mechanisms in the release of catecholamines. *Handb. Exp. Pharmacol.* [N.S.] **33,** 538–617.

Starke, K. (1977). Regulation of noradrenaline release by presynaptic receptor systems. *Rev. Physiol. Biochem. Pharmacol.* **77,** 1–124.

Sybertz, E. J., and Peach, M. J. (1980). In vitro neurogenic and musculotropic responses responses to angiotensin peptides in normal and sodium-restricted rabbits. *Circ. Res.* **46,** 836–842.

Takeshita, A., and Mark, A. L. (1978). Neurogenic contribution to hindquarters vasoconstriction during high sodium intake in Dahl strain of genetically hypertensive rat. *Circ. Res.* **43,** Suppl. 1, 86–91.

Takeshita, A., Mark, A. L., and Brody, M. J. (1979). Prevention of salt induced hypertension in the Dahl strain by 6-hydroxydopamine. *Am. J. Physiol.* **236,** 48–52.

Vanhoutte, P. M. (1978). Adrenergic neuroeffector interaction in the blood vessel wall. *Fed. Proc., Fed. Am. Soc. Exp. Biol.* **37,** 181–186.

Vanhoutte, P. M. (1980). The adrenergic neuroeffector interaction in the normotensive and hypertensive blood vessel wall. *J. Cardiovasc. Pharmacol.* **2,** Suppl. 3, 253–267.

Vogel, J. A. (1966). Salt-induced hypertension in the dog. *Am. J. Physiol.* **210,** 186–190.

Weiner, N., Cloutier, G., Bjur, R., and Pfeffer, I. (1972). Modification of norepinephrine synthesis in intact tissue by drugs and during short term adrenergic nerve stimulation. *Pharmacol. Rev.* **24,** 203–221.

Weinshilboum, R. M. (1979). Serum dopamine β-hydroxylase. *Pharmacol. Rev.* **30,** 133–166.

Westfall, T. C. (1977). Local regulation of adrenergic neurotransmission. *Physiol. Rev.* **57,** 659–728.

Westfall, T. C. (1980). Neuroeffector mechanisms. *Annu. Rev. Physiol.* **42,** 383–397.

Ylitalo, P., Hepp, R., Oster, P., Mohring, J., and Gross, F. (1976). Effects of varying sodium intake on blood pressure and renin angiotensin system in subtotally nephrectomized rats. *J. Lab. Clin. Med.* **88,** 807–816.

27

The Transmembrane Distribution of Sodium, Potassium, and Water in Vascular Smooth Muscle and the Hormonal Regulation of Vascular Tone and Reactivity

SYDNEY M. FRIEDMAN

THE ROLE OF SALT IN
CARDIOVASCULAR HYPERTENSION

I. INTRODUCTION

Five years ago, we advanced the view that "net Na pumping activity, that is, the resultant of passive Na^+ influx and active efflux, stands at the center of both the acute vasoconstrictive response and the sustained hypertensive state" (Friedman and Friedman, 1976). This was based on the recognition that in salt-dependent hypertension, at least in the SHR and DOCA-induced forms, both permeability and Na^+ transport activity are increased. Since then, we have studied the interplay of these factors in regulating the transmembrane distribution of Na in vascular smooth muscle and have obtained added precision and support for this thesis (Friedman and Nakashima, 1978; Friedman, 1979).

II. THE TRANSMEMBRANE SODIUM GRADIENT

The transmembrane distribution of Na may be defined as the ratio $[Na]_o/[Na]_i$, or operationally as the sodium gradient across a membrane of finite thickness. At this time, some of the basic principles underlying the maintenance of the Na gradient in steady state can be defined.

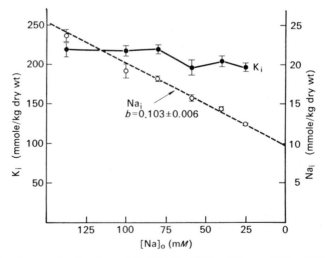

Fig. 1   Arteries were incubated overnight (18 hr) at 10°C and for an additional 3 hr at 37°C in media with sucrose as replacement for NaCl. They were then transferred to Na-free, Li-substituted medium (LiPSS) at 3°C for 45 min for the measurement of cell Na and K. Each point is the average for six arteries and verticals indicate SE. (Reprinted with permission from the *J. Physiol.*, Friedman, 1977.)

A. Constancy

The Na gradient remains constant over a wide range of change of $[Na]_o$. This operational principle can be seen in its simplest form in the incubated artery when $[Na]_o$ is reduced by replacement with sucrose (Friedman, 1977). In the example shown in Fig. 1, arteries were incubated overnight at 10°C in K-free PSS (physiological salt solution) in order to dissipate transmembrane ion gradients. They were then allowed to recover for 3 hr at 37°C in media of varying Na concentration. Each point represents the average of six arteries. One component of Na_i is evidently free in solution, since it falls linearly in direct proportion to $[Na]_o$, while another is evidently constrained or bound, since it remains constant. As expected, cell K falls only as much as is necessary to satisfy Donnan forces.

It is important to recognize that the same constancy of the Na gradient obtains whatever the replacement, even, for example, when Na is replaced with K. In the experiment shown in Fig. 2, KCl is used to replace NaCl, and not surprisingly

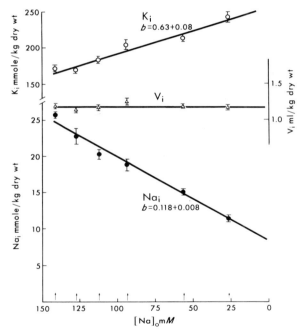

Fig. 2. Arteries were incubated overnight (18 hr) at 10°C in K-free PSS and for an additional 3 hr at 37°C in media with KCl as replacement for NaCl. They were then transferred to matching Li-substituted media at 3°C for 45 min for the measurement of cell Na and K. Cell water was calculated from Li uptake (Friedman and Nakashima, 1978). Each point is the average for six arteries and verticals indicate SE.

cell K rises rather than falls as in the previous example. Even so, cell Na falls in linear relation to [Na]$_o$ and the zero intercept is much as it was in the previous illustration. Evidently then, the Na gradient is maintained by an efficient pumping system at some preset optimal level characteristic for a given tissue. This is associated with a constant value for cell water.

B. Equilibration

The Na gradient adjusts rapidly to an imposed change. This can be readily demonstrated by continuously measuring [K]$_i$ and hence indirectly [Na]$_i$ while imposing changes in [K]$_0$. For this we have used double-barreled glass microelectrodes sufficiently small (<0.3 μm) to impale smooth muscle cells in the tail artery. One barrel is filled with a K$^+$-selective exchanger (valinomycin, Corning #477317) and the other with 1.0 M NaCl for recording the membrane potential. In the experiment shown in Fig. 3, a normal vascular smooth muscle cell in the rat tail artery, bathed in PSS at 37°C, was impaled. KCl was then used as before to replace equimolar amounts of NaCl. The increase in [K]$_i$ which follows an increase in [K]$_0$ can be seen to occur within a few minutes. As expected, of course, this is associated with an abrupt fall in E_m.

C. Determinants

These and other similar experiments show that not only do monovalent cations redistribute themselves to establish a new equilibrium in response to a change in the ionic environment, but do so rapidly. It follows then that if the sodium gradient is to be changed, the characteristics of one or more of its determinants must be altered. There are four basic functional determinants of the Na gradient apart from the geometric or structural features of the cell membrane: the metabolic activity of the cell, the mode of operation of the Na$^+$,K$^+$-ATPase which is the Na transport enzyme, the amount and/or efficiency of the transport enzyme, and the permeability of the membrane to Na$^+$ and K$^+$. We shall consider these in order.

1. Dependence on Metabolism

It has long been known that the transmembrane Na gradient falls when temperature is reduced, or when appropriate metabolic substrate is denied to the transport enzyme. The rate of fall is slow, and probably limited by the rate for passive Na$^+$ influx. As shown in Fig. 4, which typifies the effect of depriving the cell of utilizable substrate, the cell accumulates Na in exchange for K (Palatý *et al.*, 1971). In this experiment, lactose was used as replacement for glucose during anaerobic incubation of the rat tail artery. Whether the Na gradient can be sustained at step levels by set levels of substrate deprivation is not yet known, nor

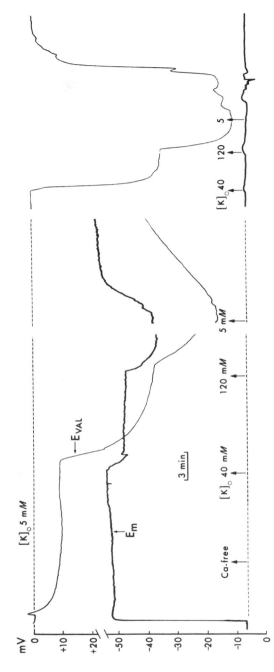

Fig. 3. A typical record of responses of the K⁺-selective side (E_{VAL}) and indifferent side (E_m) of a double-barreled microelectrode during sustained impalement of a smooth muscle cell in the rat tail artery at room temperature. On impalement, a sharp negative E_m is recorded coincident with a positive E_{VAL} response. The apparent delay indicates the pen override. First arrow indicates change of solution from PSS to Ca-free PSS with EGTA. Subsequent arrows indicate changes of $[K]_o$ to 40 and 120 mM and then return to 5 mM. This continuous run is here compressed for presentation (gap = 5 min). The responses of the same electrode to the same sequence of solution changes in the bathing medium is shown in the final panel.

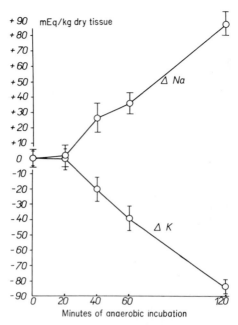

Fig. 4. The effect of anaerobic incubation in the absence of utilizable exogenous substrate (lactose PSS) on the Na and K content of the rat tail artery. Each point is the average for six arteries and verticals indicate SE. (Reprinted with permission from the *Can. J. Physiol. Pharmacol.*, Palatý *et al.*, 1971).

is it known whether, conversely, the Na gradient can be enhanced by supranormal metabolic activity, although, as will appear later, this calls to mind Fregly's observations concerning the relation of thyroid activity to the hypertensive process (Fregly, 1975).

2. Dependence on Transport Mode

It is apparent that if $[K]_o$ is reduced, even if replaced by $[Na]_o$, the transport enzyme is denied one of its primary components, and must progressively shift its mode of operation as $[K]_o$ falls below some critical level necessary to sustain a normal Na^+-K^+ exchange (Brading, 1979). This principle has long been recognized, but the quantitative changes that result from applying it to vascular tissue have not previously been described in detail (Jones and Karreman, 1969).

In the experiment shown in Fig. 5, tissues were incubated for 3 hr at 37°C in physiological media in which step amounts of KCl were replaced with NaCl. They were then washed as usual in cold LiPSS containing the same limited amounts of KCl as had been used for incubation. To begin with, as $[K]_o$ is reduced from the usual 5 mM level, both K_i and Na_i remain unchanged until a

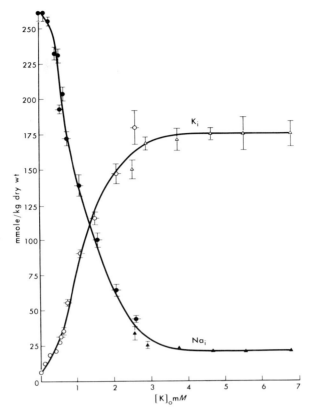

Fig. 5. Arteries were incubated overnight at 10°C in K-free medium and then returned to media containing 0–7 mM [K]$_o$ for a further 3 hr at 37°C. Na$_i$ and K$_i$ were measured after removal of extracellular components by a final 45-min wash at 2°C in K-free Li-substituted medium (LiPSS). The three experiments required for this range are indicated by the symbols: exp. 1, ●○; exp. 2, ◐○; exp. 3, ▲ △. Each point is the average of six arteries. SE of the mean is indicated by verticals where it exceeds symbol size.

critical level is reached at about 3 mM [K]$_o$. Below this, K$_i$ falls steeply in exchange for Na$_i$. Each step level in [K]$_o$ evidently results in a sustained steady-state step change in both Na$_i$ and K$_i$. (Time does not permit discussion here of the apparent disequilibrium in this exchange at levels below 0.7 mM [K]$_o$.) As shown in Figs. 6 and 7, no change in cell water was observed except at very low levels of [K]$_o$, and consequently E_K actually increases during most of this range, that is, the cells hyperpolarize. This change has, in fact, been observed in experiments with intracellular microelectrodes (Casteels *et al.*, 1977). Thus, in this case, although the Na gradient is reduced, Na transport activity is well maintained throughout.

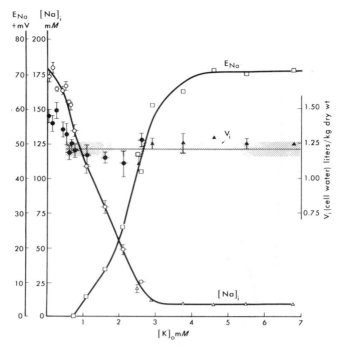

Fig. 6. Recalculation of Na$_i$ values shown in Fig. 1. Cell water, V_i, is calculated from the measured values for Li taken up extracellularly during the final 45 min cold LiPSS wash. The three experiments of the series are indicated by the symbols: exp. 1, ● ○; exp. 2, ◖○; exp. 3, ▲ △. Each point is the average of six arteries with SE of the mean indicated by verticals, except for E_{Na} which is derived from calculated averages. The shaded bar indicates ± 1 SD for the series of V_i values.

3. Dependence on Membrane Permeability

It has long been recognized that vasoconstrictors and stretch increase membrane permeability and allow both the Na$^+$ and K$^+$ gradients to run downhill. We have recently attempted to quantify this exchange using p-chloromercuribenzene sulfonate (PCMBS), an agent now used conventionally in red cell studies to increase membrane permeability and so reversibly discharge transmembrane gradients of monovalent cations (Garrahan and Rega, 1967; Garay and Meyer, 1979). We have found that the degree of increase in permeability induced by PCMBS in vascular tissue is dose dependent and can be limited to produce step levels of change. Typical results are shown in Fig. 8. In this experiment, tissues were incubated for 3 hr at 37°C in PSS containing very small amounts of PCMBS ranging from 1 to 5 μM. They were washed as usual in cold LiPSS to remove extracellular Na. Such low doses of this agent increase the permeability of the

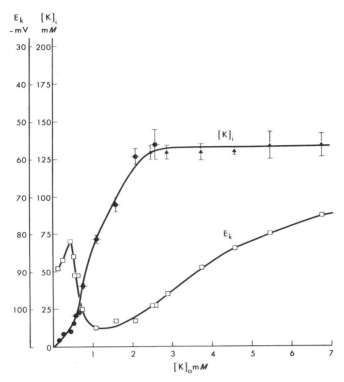

Fig. 7. Recalculation of K_i values shown in Fig. 1 in terms of V_i shown in Fig. 2. The three experiments of the series are indicated by the symbols: exp. 1, ●; exp. 2, ●; exp. 3 ▲. Each point is the average of six arteries with SEM indicated by verticals, except for E_K which is derived from calculated averages.

membrane sufficiently to increase Na_i without much change in cell water so that, in effect, the Na^+ gradient is reduced. They cause no serious damage since the process is reversible. In separate experiments, we have found that a new steady state can be reasonably well maintained for at least 3 hr. Since hydrated K^+ is so much smaller than hydrated Na^+, the loss of K^+ under the same circumstances is considerably more dramatic than the gain of Na^+. There is clearly no reduction in transport activity here. Indeed, since no change in cell water, V_i, is observed, the pump may actually be working overtime to maintain relatively low levels of Na_i despite the excessive inward leak. As expected, membrane permeability is a determinant of the Na gradient. An important corollary of this is that K^+ uptake may be disproportionately reduced and could erroneously be attributed to pump failure. It follows then that when a reduction in K^+ uptake is measured directly, or inferred from the Rb^+ uptake, this cannot in itself provide evidence of di-

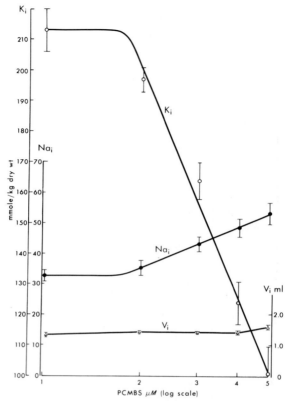

Fig. 8. Arteries were incubated overnight at 10°C in K-free PSS and for an additional 3 hr at 37°C in PSS containing p-chloromercuribenzene sulfonate (PCMBS). They were then transferred to LiPSS at 3°C for 45 min for the measurement of cell Na, K, and water. Each point is the average for six arteries and verticals indicate SE.

minished transport activity. This may underlie some of the recent observations of Haddy and associates (Haddy *et al.*, 1978) in experimental hypertension, and we will return to this later. Conversely, we may also note that cell Na_i may increase, and a fall in the Na gradient thereby be indicated, while at the same time the cell may be hyperpolarized, depolarized, or unaffected.

4. Dependence on Na^+,K^+-ATPase Activity

It is well recognized that the Na gradient is produced and maintained by the activity of the Na^+,K^+-ATPase, familiarly called the Na^+ pump. Thus, the gradient falls if the enzyme is specifically blocked with ouabain, or if the energy requirements for enzyme activity are not met. It is probable also that the normal physiological activity of the pump requires a normal background of adrenal steroid production, since in the nephrectomized rat plasma $[Na]_o$ falls and $[K]_o$ rises within 90 min of adrenalectomy, indicating that the adrenal controls the transmembrane distribution of Na and K at the cellular level and apart from the kidney (Friedman *et al.*, 1958). Conversely, *in vitro*, in the incubated artery the Na gradient appears to be enhanced by very low doses of aldosterone (Friedman, 1980). This is shown in Fig. 9. In this experiment, tissues were incubated in our standard procedure in the presence of aldosterone. They were then washed in cold LiPSS for 45 or 90 min. Cell Na is obviously diminished in arteries exposed to aldosterone and this change is not an artifact produced by excessive leaching out in exchange for Li during the cold wash. Since cell water remains unchanged or, at most, slightly diminished, it is probable that the Na gradient is enhanced. Similar results can be produced by as little as 10^{-9} M aldosterone, as low a dose as has been found effective with other methods used to examine its effects on the Na^+,K^+-ATPase. Many such studies have already established that aldosterone stimulates Na^+ transport, measured chemically in terms of Na^+,K^+-ATPase activity directly (Edelman and Marver, 1980), or measured electrically in terms of the short circuit current in frog skin or toad bladder (Sharp and Leaf, 1966). What was previously unknown is that this effect can also be measured directly in terms of a steady-state decrease in cell Na.

These observations with aldosterone now explain our findings in DOCA-saline treated rats. In this latter case we observed that cell Na in arteries maintained *in vitro* in steady state becomes subnormal within 2 weeks of treatment. As illus-

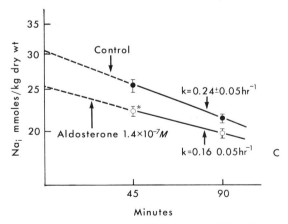

Fig. 9. Arteries were incubated overnight at 10°C in K-free PSS and for an additional 3 hr at 37°C in PSS in the presence or absence of aldosterone. Cell Na was measured after 45- or 90-min wash in LiPSS at 3°C. Loss of Na by exchange with Li is described by a single exponential rate constant. Symbols as above for groups of nine arteries.

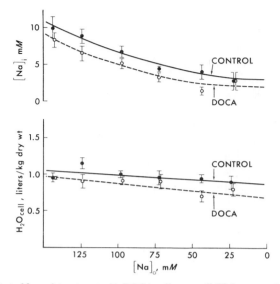

Fig. 10.   Effect of 3-week treatment with DOCA-saline on cell [Na] measured at varying [Na]$_o$ in incubated rat tail arteries. Calculation of [Na]$_i$ was based on measured values for free Na$_i$ and cell water. (Reprinted with permission from the *Can. J. Physiol. Pharmacol.*, Friedman and Nakashima, 1978.)

trated in Fig. 10, it was later shown that this change primarily involves the free Na$_i$ component and is associated with a modest reduction of cell water.

We conclude this discussion of basic principles underlying Na distribution with some general statements concerning cell water. No method at present in use provides an absolute measure of cell water, or partitions it into free and structured phases. At best, the methods available permit an estimate of change, and even here can miss small and perhaps critical effects. Within these constraints, we have noticed that cell water tends to rise when Na transport activity diminishes, and to decrease when pump activity increases.

III. TRANSMEMBRANE SODIUM GRADIENT IN HYPERTENSION

It is in the context of the general principles I have outlined that I now propose to consider the present situation with regard to Na distribution in experimental hypertension. It is essential here to distinguish between tissues taken from hypertensive animals and allowed to reach a new steady state *in vitro* by prolonged incubation in physiological salt solution, and those taken more or less directly from *in vivo* conditions, although at times this distinction may blur.

In the first case, in incubated tissues, there is considerable agreement that Na transport activity is enhanced in both the SHR and in DOCA-induced hypertension. At first, radioisotope flux data indicated only diminished ability of vascular tissue to accumulate K and extrude Na, and an increased turnover of K (Jones, 1973). Chemical analytic as well as electrometric data from our laboratory (Friedman *et al.*, 1975; Friedman and Friedman, 1976) then showed that both increased permeability and increased Na transport were involved. Studies of K-induced relaxation in Bohr's laboratory (Webb and Bohr, 1978), microelectrode data from Hermsmeyer (1976), and enzyme studies in Daniel's laboratory (Wei *et al.*, 1976) have also indicated that Na transport is enhanced.

In a typical electrometric study, the transmembrane Na^+ and K^+ gradients in the rat tail artery are first dissipated by prolonged overnight exposure to K-free

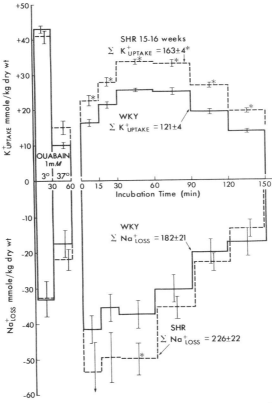

Fig. 11. Changes of K^+ and Na^+ recorded during a continuous sequence of incubations of nine matched pairs of SHR and WKY arteries. Active exchanges were preceded by passive exchanges in the presence of 1 mM ouabain and then initiated by washout of ouabain at 3°C followed by rapid transfer of the tissue from 3° to 37°C. (Reprinted with permission from *Hypertension*, Friedman, 1979.)

PSS at 10°C. The artery is then connected for perfusion and chilled to 3°C so that the artery can be ouabainized and K^+ readmitted while the tissue is not metabolically active. In a typical experiment such as shown in Fig. 11, temperature is then raised to 37°C in the continuing presence of ouabain, so that passive exchanges of Na^+ and K^+ can be monitored and measured. Ouabain is then washed out and the ensuing active exchange of Na^+ and K^+ monitored continuously, or in a sequence of 60-μl aliquots as in the experiments shown here. Enhanced active exchange of Na^+ and K^+ is directly observed and consistently characterizes the tail artery of the SHR and DOCA-induced hypertensive rat (Friedman and Friedman, 1976; Friedman and Nakashima, 1978; Friedman, 1979). This change is not a simple consequence of the existence of the hypertensive state, since as seen in Fig. 12 it is not observed in arteries obtained from rats with a similar degree of blood pressure elevation induced by renal artery constriction.

A wholly different type of ion distribution is observed, however, in arteries taken for examination from the *in vivo* state. This shows up clearly when fresh arteries are taken from either the SHR (Friedman and Friedman, 1976) or

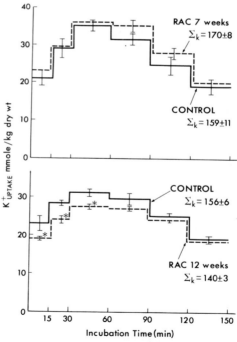

Fig. 12. Changes in K^+ recorded as in Fig. 11 during a continuous sequence of incubations of 12 arteries from rats with one clipped renal artery and six normal controls at 7 and 12 weeks of hypertension. (Reprinted with permission from *Hypertension*, Friedman, 1979.)

DOCA-hypertensive rat (Friedman, 1974), immersed at once in cold LiPSS to allow for the washout of extracellular Na, and subsequently taken for analysis at a sequence of intervals covering the period 30–90 min. As shown in Fig. 13, this procedure reveals two facts: first, that cell Na is higher than normal in the hypertensive artery *in vivo,* and second, that cell Na exchanges with Li more rapidly than normal even at low temperature. This change is the same in the DOCA-treated animal (Fig. 14) as in the SHR.

The conclusion is obvious: in these forms of hypertension, these vascular smooth muscle cells are abnormally permeable to Na^+ to a degree sufficient to allow an increase of cell Na^+ despite the enhanced activity of the Na transport system. This change is not observed in renovascular hypertension. Jones (1973) has come to the same conclusion with entirely different methods.

When we consider these findings, it is apparent that we can account for certain of our observations on the basis of enhanced mineralocorticoid activity. This explains the subnormal sodium in the incubated or *in vitro* preparation as well as the indications of enhanced transport activity observed with many methods in many different laboratories. Some additional factor or factors, however, must be invoked to account for the increased permeability which is just as solidly based a finding in these salt-dependent forms of hypertension. If we are correct in proposing that "net Na pumping activity" is the central theme of the hypertensive state, then the SHR and DOCA-hypertensive rat represent to varying degrees the

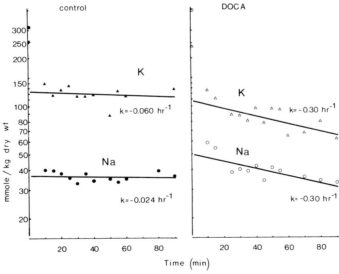

Fig. 13.   Cell Na and K in freshly excised tail arteries from control and DOCA-saline treated rats at various intervals after incubation in LiPSS at 2°C. (Reprinted with permission from *Circ. Res.*, Friedman, 1974.)

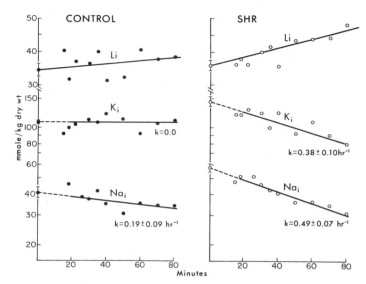

Fig. 14. Cell Na and K in freshly excised tail arteries from control and spontaneously hypertensive rats (SHR) at various intervals after incubation in LiPSS at 2°C. (Reprinted with permission from *Circulation Research,* Friedman and Friedman, 1976.)

situation where permeability and Na transport are both increased. It is not difficult to envisage other combinations, many of which will produce evidence of diminished uptake of K^+ or Rb^+ not necessarily indicative of pump suppression so much as of an imbalance between the leak and the pump. It seems to us, then, that now more than ever before we can still say, in words we used 25 years ago, "that peripheral vascular resistance depends on the 'sodium transfer systems' broadly defined, which govern the dynamic equilibrium between the entrance and extrusion of sodium, potassium, and water in vascular smooth muscle" (Friedman *et al.,* 1957). The apparent disagreement between those of us actively engaged in this field may stem more from the way we interpret our methods and stress either the pump or the leak, rather than from any real difference in our observations.

ACKNOWLEDGMENTS

This work was carried out with the aid of grants from the British Columbia Heart Foundation and the Medical Research Council of Canada.

REFERENCES

Brading, A. F. (1979). Maintenance of ionic composition. *Br. Med. Bull.* **35**, 227–234.

Casteels, R., Kitamura, K., Kuriyama, H., and Suzuki, H. (1977). The membrane properties of the smooth muscle cells of the rabbit main pulmonary artery. *J. Physiol. (London)* **271**, 41–61.

Edelman, I. S., and Marver, D. (1980). Mediating events in the action of aldosterone. *J. Steroid Biochem.* **12**, 219–224.

Fregly, M. J. (1975). Thyroid activity of spontaneous hypertensive rats. *Proc. Soc. Exp. Biol. Med.* **149**, 124–132.

Friedman, S. M. (1974). An ion exchange approach to the problem of intracellular sodium in the hypertensive process. *Circ. Res.* **34, 35**, Suppl. 1, I-123–I-128.

Friedman, S. M. (1977). The effects of external sodium substitution on cell sodium and potassium in vascular smooth muscle. *J. Physiol. (London)* **270**, 195–208.

Friedman, S. M. (1979). Evidence for enhanced sodium transport in the tail artery of the spontaneously hypertensive rat. *Hypertension* **1**, 572–582.

Friedman, S. M. (1980). Direct effects of aldosterone on cell Na in the rat tail artery in vitro. *In* "Intracellular Electrolytes and Arterial Hypertension" (H. Zumkley and H. Losse, eds.), pp. 122–127. Thieme, Stuttgart.

Friedman, S. M., and Friedman, C. L. (1976). Cell permeability, sodium transport, and the hypertensive process in the rat. *Circ. Res.* **39**, 433–441.

Friedman, S. M., and Nakashima, M. (1978). Evidence for enhanced Na transport in hypertension induced by DOCA in the rat. *Can. J. Physiol. Pharmacol.* **56**, 1029–1035.

Friedman, S. M., Friedman, C. L., and Nakashima, M. (1957). Cationic shifts and blood pressure regulation. *Circ. Res.* **5**, 261–267.

Friedman, S. M., Nakashima, M., and Friedman, C. L. (1958). The extrarenal effect of adrenalectomy on sodium and potassium distribution in the rat. *Endocrinology* **62**, 259–267.

Friedman, S. M., Nakashima, M., and Friedman, C. L. (1975). Cell Na and K in the rat tail artery during the development of hypertension induced by desoxycorticosterone acetate. *Proc. Soc. Exp. Biol. Med.* **150**, 171–176.

Garay, R. P., and Meyer, P. (1979). A new test showing abnormal net Na^+ and K^+ fluxes in erythrocytes of essential hypertensive patients. *Lancet* **1**, 349–353.

Garrahan, P. J., and Rega, A. F. (1967). Cation loading of red blood cells. *J. Physiol. (London)* **193**, 459–466.

Haddy, F., Pamnani, M., and Clough, D. (1978). The sodium-potassium pump in volume expanded hypertension. *Clin. Exp. Hypertens.* **1**, 295–336.

Hermsmeyer, K. (1976). Electrogenesis of increased norepinephrine sensitivity of arterial vascular muscle in hypertension. *Circ. Res.* **38**, 362–367.

Jones, A. W. (1973). Altered ion transport in vascular smooth muscle from spontaneously hypertensive rats. Influences of aldosterone, norepinephrine, angiotensin. *Circ. Res.* **33**, 563–572.

Jones, A. W., and Karreman, G. (1969). Potassium accumulation and permeation in the canine carotid artery. *Biophys. J.* **9**, 910–924.

Palatý, V., Gustafson, B., and Friedman, S. M. (1971). Maintenance of the ionic composition of the incubated artery. *Can. J. Physiol. Pharmacol.* **49**, 106–112.

Sharp, G. W. G., and Leaf, A. (1966). Studies on the mode of action of aldosterone. *Recent Prog. Horm. Res.* **22**, 431–465.

Webb, R. C., and Bohr, D. F. (1978). Potassium-induced relaxation as an indicator of Na^+-K^+ ATPase activity in vascular smooth muscle. *Blood Vessels* **15**, 198–207.

Wei, J. W., Janis, R. A., and Daniel, E. E. (1976). Studies on subcellular fractions from mesenteric arteries of spontaneously hypertensive rats: Alterations in both calcium uptake and enzyme activities. *Blood Vessels* **13**, 293–308.

28

The Role of an Ouabain-Like Humoral Factor in the Genesis of Low Renin Hypertension

FRANCIS HADDY, STEPHEN HUOT, DAVID CLOUGH, AND MOTILAL PAMNANI

I. INTRODUCTION

The mechanism of volume-expanded, salt-dependent hypertension is particularly difficult to understand. The increased pressure cannot be explained by the

403

THE ROLE OF SALT IN
CARDIOVASCULAR HYPERTENSION

volume expansion per se. Renin levels are low and the blood pressure responses to converting enzyme inhibitors and angiotensin antagonists are minimal. Catecholamine levels are not helpful; in fact catecholamine levels, like angiotensin levels, decrease as a function of salt intake in normal subjects. Long-term autoregulation, subsequent to increased cardiac output and overperfusion of tissues, has been considered but this cannot be the complete explanation because increases in total peripheral resistance and blood pressure have been observed in the absence of an increase in cardiac output.

Recent studies in our laboratory suggest that Na^+,K^+-ATPase and sodium potassium pump activities are reduced in the cardiovascular muscle of animals with experimental low renin hypertension and that these abnormalities result from a circulating ouabain-like agent. These findings are of interest because induced suppression of Na^+, K^+-ATPase and sodium–potassium pump activities in the cardiovascular muscle of normal animals and man with the cardiac glycosides reproduces some of the changes seen in experimental low renin hypertension. These changes include vasoconstriction, increased vascular sensitivity to vasoactive agents, increased cardiac contractility, and raised blood pressure (particularly if diuresis cannot occur).

In this review, we summarize the evidence that suggests that experimental low renin hypertension is related to the release of a ouabain-like humoral agent which acts by suppressing Na^+,K^+-ATPase and hence sodium–potassium pump activity in vascular and cardiac muscle. Relevant studies in the human are also summarized.

II. EVIDENCE FOR SODIUM–POTASSIUM PUMP SUPPRESSION

We have used two indices of sodium–potassium pump activity in animals with low renin hypertension, ouabain-sensitive rubidium-86 uptake by blood vessels and Na^+,K^+-ATPase activity of cardiac microsomes.

Rubidium can substitute for potassium in active transport by the sodium–potassium pump across cell membranes. It is used in the study of pump activity because its radioactive form has a longer half-life and a lower energy emission than the radioactive form of potassium. The ouabain-sensitive rubidium-86 uptake is that fraction of the uptake related to active transport because ouabain inhibits the sodium–potassium pump which is responsible for active transport. Pamnani in our laboratory adapted the rubidium uptake technique to blood vessels and we first applied the technique to mesenteric arteries and veins of dogs with one-kidney, one wrapped hypertension (Overbeck *et al.*, 1976). After at least four weeks of sustained significant hypertension in the experimental animal and at the same time interval in the sham operated control animal, blood vessels were obtained simultaneously from the pair for measurements of ouabain-sensitive and ouabain-insensitive rubidium-86 uptakes. First, the vessels were incubated at 0°C in potassium free Krebs–Henseleit solution to depress the sodium–potassium pump and load the cells with sodium. Next, to stimulate the pump, the vessels were incubated at 37°C in potassium free Krebs–Henseleit solution containing 2 mM nonradioactive rubidium. The solution also contained radioactive rubidium-86 and its uptake was measured 18 min later. Each vessel was divided in half, one half placed in media without ouabain and the other in media with ouabain.

Ouabain-sensitive rubidium-86 uptake, which reflects membrane sodium-potassium pump activity, was calculated as the difference between rubidium-86 uptake without and with ouabain. The rubidium-86 uptake in the presence of ouabain (ouabain-insensitive uptake) reflects distribution in extracellular space and passive penetration into cells (determined by cell wall permeability and surface area).

We found that ouabain-sensitive uptake by both arteries and veins from the hypertensive animals was less than that by arteries and veins from the sham operated normotensive animals. The ouabain-insensitive uptake was not different in the two groups of animals. Thus, the defect was only in the ouabain-sensitive sodium–potassium pump. Since the defect was also present in veins, it did not appear to be secondary to increased pressure.

We next examined cardiac microsomal Na^+,K^+-ATPase activity in a similar model of low renin hypertension. Like sodium-potassium pump activity in intact cells, the ability of isolated cell membranes to split adenosine triphosphate, i.e., the total ATPase activity, is partially inhibited by addition of ouabain to and removal of potassium from the incubating medium. The residual activity is due to Mg^{2+}-ATPase. Na^+,K^+-ATPase activity is then the difference between the total ATPase and the Mg^{2+}-ATPase activities. Practical problems preclude the routine measurement of Na^+,K^+-ATPase activity in microsomes from vascular smooth muscle. Clough in our laboratory therefore measured Na^+,K^+-ATPase activity in microsomes isolated from the left and right ventricles of rats with one-kidney, one clip hypertension and found it suppressed in both chambers (Clough *et al.*, 1977a,b). Since the defect was also present in the right ventricle, it did not appear to be secondary to increased pressure.

We have subsequently examined ouabain-sensitive rubidium-86 uptake by blood vessels and the Na^+,K^+-ATPase activity of cardiac microsomes in a variety of models of experimental hypertension, some investigator induced and others genetic in origin. We found that ouabain-sensitive rubidium-86 uptake and Na^+,K-ATPase activity are reduced in the investigator induced, low renin, presumably volume-expanded forms of hypertension. These include one-kidney, one wrapped hypertension in the dog (Overbeck *et al.*, 1976) and one-kidney, one clip (Clough *et al.*, 1977a,b; M. B. Pamnani, D. L. Clough, and F. J. Haddy, unpublished observation), one-kidney, DOCA, saline (Pamnani *et al.*, 1978a;

Clough *et al.*, 1978), and reduced renal mass (Huot *et al.*, 1980a,b; Clough *et al.*, 1980) hypertensions in the rat. On the other hand, ouabain-sensitive rubidium-86 uptake is increased in two genetic forms of hypertension, SHR relative to WKY (Pamnani *et al.*, 1979) and Dahl S on high salt relative to Dahl S on normal salt (Pamnani *et al.*, 1980a). Na^+,K^+-ATPase activity is normal in SHR relative to WKY (Clough *et al.*, 1980) and decreased in Dahl S on high salt relative to Dahl S on normal salt (D. L. Clough, M. B. Pamnani, and F. J. Haddy, unpublished observation). Ouabain-insensitive rubidium-86 uptake by blood vessels is normal in all forms of low renin hypertension studied except one-kidney, DOCA, saline hypertension, where it is increased. It is also increased in both forms of genetic hypertension.

These findings suggest that sodium–potassium pump activity is suppressed in the low renin models and that the one-kidney, DOCA, saline model may have the additional defect of increased permeability. The latter suggestion is compatible with the observations of other investigators (Jones and Hart, 1975; Friedman 1974) and studies in toad urinary bladder which indicate that aldosterone increases the permeability of the apical plasma membrane to sodium (Leaf, 1980). The findings also suggest that sodium–potassium pump activity is increased in the genetic models but that this results secondarily from increased permeability of the cell membrane to sodium. This suggestion for SHR is compatible with the findings of other investigators (Jones, 1973; Friedman, 1979).

III. EVIDENCE FOR AN OUABAIN-LIKE HUMORAL AGENT

Since decreased pump activity was seen only in the investigator induced low renin forms of hypertension and because the defect was also observed on the low pressure side of the circulation, we questioned the roles of volume expansion and a ouabain-like humoral agent. We reasoned that if the decreased pump activity is in fact a consequence of expansion of the extracellular fluid volume, acute volume expansion of animals should reproduce the changes in rubidium-86 uptake. Furthermore, if the changes result from a humoral agent, they should be reproduced in the arteries of another animal on application of plasma from the volume expanded animal. We therefore acutely volume expanded normal anesthetized rats with normal saline and maintained the expansion for 2 hr. Paired control rats were sham-expanded for an equal period of time. Tail arteries were removed for measurement of rubidium-86 uptake. Blood was also collected and plasma supernates prepared by boiling the plasma. Ouabain-sensitive rubidium-86 uptake was significantly suppressed in the tail arteries from the volume-expanded rats and the degree of suppression was similar to that seen in the low renin models of hypertension (Pamnani *et al.*, 1978b, 1980b). Ouabain-insensitive uptake was unaffected, as is the case in most models of low renin hypertension. Furthermore, total rubidium-86 uptake was suppressed in tail arteries from normal rats on application of plasma supernates from the volume expanded rats (relative to the uptake seen on application of plasma supernates from the sham-expanded rats). The sodium and potassium concentrations and the osmolalities of the two supernates were not significantly different. Plasma supernates from acutely expanded dogs had the same effect on the rat tail arteries (Pamnani *et al.*, 1978b, 1980b).

In another study in rats, extracellular fluid volume was expanded with an isoosmotic solution of mannitol rather than saline and the changes in rubidium uptake by tail arteries of the expanded rats were the same as those seen in the saline-expanded rats, i.e., decreased ouabain-sensitive rubidium-86 uptake without change in ouabain-insensitive rubidium-86 uptake (Pamnani *et al.*, 1980b).

These findings encouraged us to examine the plasma in animals with low renin hypertension (Pamnani *et al.*, 1980b,c). We therefore prepared a new series of dogs with one-kidney, one wrapped hypertension. Supernates of boiled plasma from these animals and their sham operated control animals were then applied to tail arteries from normal rats. Ouabain-sensitive rubidium-86 uptake by the rat tail arteries was suppressed by the supernates from the hypertensive dogs and ouabain-insensitive rubidium-86 uptake was unaffected, just as is the case in the hypertensive animal's own vessels. Plasma supernate from rats with one-kidney, one clip hypertension was also active (M. B. Pamnani, D. L. Clough, and F. J. Haddy, unpublished observation); so was plasma supernate from rats with reduced renal mass hypertension (S. Huot, M. B. Pamnani, and F. J. Haddy, unpublished observation). In both cases it reduced total rubidium-86 uptake when applied to the tail artery taken from another rat (the amount of supernate was not sufficient to segregate total uptake into its ouabain-sensitive and insensitive components). Plasma supernate from the hypertensive dogs also reduced short circuit current across the toad bladder, as did plasma supernate from acutely saline expanded dogs (W. T. Chen, M. B. Pamnani, S. Huot, D. L. Clough, and F. J. Haddy, unpublished observation).

These findings indicate that sodium–potassium pump activity in animals with low renin hypertension is suppressed by a heat stable humoral agent released by the volume expansion per se.

IV. SOURCE OF THE OUABAIN-LIKE HUMORAL AGENT

Brody *et al.* (1978) have recently shown that lesions of the anteroventral third ventricle (AV3V) both prevent and ameliorate one-kidney, DOCA, saline, and one-kidney, renal hypertension in rats, models in which we observed decreased ouabain-sensitive rubidium-86 uptake. Bealer *et al.* (1979) observed that antinatriferic activity is absent in the acutely volume-expanded rat with the AV3V lesion. We therefore wondered whether the lesion would influence rubidium-86 uptake by blood vessels. James Buggy prepared rats with AV3V lesions and sham lesions and we acutely volume-expanded them with saline. Ouabain-sensitive rubidium-86 uptake by the tail artery was higher in the lesioned than in the sham-lesioned animal (M. B. Pamnani, J. Buggy, S. Huot, and F. J. Haddy, unpublished observation). Furthermore, total rubidium-86 uptake by arteries from normal rats was greater when incubated in plasma supernates prepared from lesioned rats than when incubated in supernates from sham-lesioned rats. Apparently the AV3V area influences the plasma level of the heat stable factor which is active on vascular rubidium-86 uptake.

V. NATURE OF THE HUMORAL AGENT

In our previous reviews (Haddy and Overbeck, 1976; Haddy *et al.*, 1978, 1979), we suggested that the pump suppression in blood vessels and heart of animals with low renin hypertension results from natriuretic factor because its plasma level rises with volume, it inhibits Na^+,K^+-ATPase, and it suppresses sodium pump activity in the renal tubule. The natriuretic factor in plasma appears to be a low molecular weight acidic peptide, formed from a larger precursor molecule (Gruber and Buckalew, 1978). Like the humoral pump suppressor observed in our studies, it is heat stable. It may be released in response to distention of the pulmonary vascular bed (Epstein, 1978) and it appears to come from brain (Bealer *et al.*, 1979). Our studies in the AV3V lesioned animal and in the toad bladder (see above) strengthen the possibility that the vascular pump suppressor observed in our studies is in fact natriuretic factor. However, much more work is required before this can be stated with certainty. Recent attempts at purification of natriuretic factor have met with some success (see Raghaven and Gonick, 1980, for example). It would be of interest to apply such a partially purified preparation to the rat tail artery to see whether it reduces ouabain-sensitive rubidium-86 uptake without influencing ouabain-insensitive rubidium-86 uptake, as is the case for plasma supernates from animals with experimental low renin hypertension (see above). It would also be of interest to see whether it constricts blood vessels and raises blood pressure when administered to the normal animal. One preparation of natriuretic factor does appear to sensitize arterioles to norepinephrine (Plunkett *et al.*, 1980).

The old and recent literature in fact suggests that presence of an unknown, slowly acting pressor and sensitizing agent in the blood of animals with low renin hypertension (see references in Haddy *et al.*, 1979). The agent, which was first observed in 1940 (Solandt *et al.*, 1940), appears to have a molecular weight of about 1000 and, like natriuretic factor and the humoral pump suppressor observed in our studies, is heat stable. Dahl *et al.* (1969) published one of the papers in support of an unknown pressor agent. In it, almost as an afterthought, they speculated that a common pathogenic mechanism exists in both salt and renal hypertension and suggested that many of the apparent anomalies of the angiotensin–aldosterone system in hypertension could be explained if a sodium-excreting hormone were postulated which had the capacity of also inducing hypertension when produced by a hypertension-prone subject. They apparently never pursued this possibility.

VI. HOW PUMP SUPPRESSION MIGHT RAISE BLOOD PRESSURE

Suppression of the sodium–potassium pump in cardiovascular muscle, with the cardiac glycosides for example, has long been known to increase cardiac contractility and constrict blood vessels (Haddy et al., 1978, 1979, 1980). It has more recently been shown that it also increases the responses of blood vessels to vasoactive agents (Leonard, 1957; Brender et al., 1969, 1970; O'Neill et al., 1980) and raises blood pressure. With respect to the latter, Vatner et al. (1971) showed that ouabain raises blood pressure in the normal conscious dog due entirely to a rise in total peripheral resistance and De Mots et al. (1978) showed that the same is the case for normal man. We have observed that ouabain produces a large rise in arterial blood pressure in the anesthetized dog given fluid intravenously at the rate of the urine flow so that extracellular fluid volume cannot change (Haddy and Scott, 1973). This simulates the abnormal arterial pressure–urine flow relationship seen in hypertensive states, as emphasized by Guyton et al. (1974). Thus, subjects with normal hearts respond to the cardiac glycosides with elevated pressure, particularly if diuresis cannot occur.

These changes are not unlike those seen in experimental low renin hypertension (Haddy et al., 1978, 1979). Increased cardiac contractility, vasoconstriction, and increased vascular responses to vasoactive agent all occur in low renin hypertension. Increased cardiac contractility has been observed by Hawthorne et al. (1974) during the development of one-kidney, one clip hypertension in dogs.

While it is clear that pump suppression stimulates the muscle cells in heart and blood vessels, the cellular mechanism is not so clear. A direct effect on muscle cell sarcolemma, independent of effects on the adrenergic nerve terminals, seems to account for part of the stimulation because some smooth muscle preparations still contract in response to ouabain or potassium-free media following sympathectomy, adrenergic blockade, or reserpinization (van Breeman et al., 1978; Fleming, 1980; Lang and Blaustein, 1980; Toda, 1980). This contraction apparently results from inhibition of sarcolemmal Na^+,K^+-ATPase and sodium-potassium pump activities (Chen et al., 1972), resulting in an increase in the intracellular calcium concentration. The mechanism of the increased intracellular calcium concentration in vascular smooth muscle is not clear. Both increased calcium influx due to electrogenic depolarization (Thomas, 1972; Chen *et al.*, 1972; Hendrickx and Casteels, 1974; Anderson, 1976; Siegel *et al.*, 1976; Fleming, 1980) and decreased calcium efflux via the sodium–calcium exchange mechanism (Reuter *et al.*, 1973; Blaustein, 1977; van Breeman *et al.*, 1978; Lang and Blaustein, 1980) have been postulated. In the first case the extra calcium enters the muscle cell through voltage-dependent calcium channels and in the second case the decreased sodium gradient (due to the increase in internal sodium concentration) provides less energy for sodium efflux.

Indirect actions via the sympathetic nervous system may also be involved in the stimulation because in some preparations of smooth muscle the responses to ouabain and potassium-free media are modified or inhibited by mechanical or chemical sympathectomy, adrenergic blockade, and reserpine (van Breeman *et al.*, 1978; Lorenz *et al.*, 1980; Toda, 1980). These findings should come as no surprise because norepinephrine uptake into adrenergic nerve terminals is linked to Na^+,K^+-ATPase and the sodium-potassium pump; uptake is sodium and potassium dependent and inhibited by ouabain and release is increased by ouabain (Sharma and Banerjee, 1977; Nakazato *et al.*, 1978; Gillis and Quest, 1979). Inhibition of uptake and increase of release should increase the concentration of norepinephrine in the neuroeffector cleft and therefore enhance the contractile response. The long-term effects could be different, however. Some investigators report that chronic administration of digitalis results in decreased tissue content of catecholamines (Gillis and Quest, 1979), as if the nerve terminal has been depleted of norepinephrine.

Animals with low renin hypertension in fact have decreased tissue norepinephrine content and catecholamine fluorescence and the vascular response to sympathetic nerve stimulation is decreased while the response to injected norepinephrine is increased (de Champlain *et al.*, 1969; LeLorier *et al.*, 1976; Constantopoulos, 1977; Fink and Brody, 1978, 1980). There is also a decreased capacity of the sympathetic nervous system to take up and retain norepinephrine (de Champlain *et al.*, 1969; LeLorier *et al.*, 1976). Of particular interest is the observation that the retention and store of cardiac norepinephrine correlate negatively with the sodium intake in the rat, i.e., the higher the sodium intake, the lower the retention and store of norepinephrine and the higher the blood pressure (de Champlain *et al.*, 1969). We have therefore suggested that consideration should be given the possibility that the sodium–potassium pump defect extends to the adrenergic nerve terminals and baroreceptors (Haddy *et al.*, 1978, 1979). Were this the case, impaired reflex compensation would result in higher pressures (there would be less reflex opposition to the directly mediated vasoconstriction). Catecholamine depletion also introduces the question of denervation supersensitivity (Fleming, 1976; Fleming and Westfall, 1975; Haddy *et al.*, 1978, 1979; Abel *et al.*, 1980).

VII. SODIUM–POTASSIUM PUMP ACTIVITY IN HYPERTENSIVE HUMANS

There have been no studies of the sodium–potassium pump activity in the cardiovascular tissues of hypertensive humans but increased sodium content in arterial wall (Tobian, 1960) and studies of white and red cells (see references in Haddy *et al.*, 1978) suggest that a pump defect may exist in some hypertensive subjects. Of particular interest is the observation that the ouabain-sensitive rate constant for sodium-22 efflux from leukocytes isolated from patients with essential hypertension is suppressed (Edmondson *et al.*, 1975). This defect is accompanied by increased intracellular sodium and water contents. It appears to be more severe in patients with low renin hypertension (Edmondson and McGregor, 1980). The hypertension of pre-eclampsia is also associated with a reduced ouabain-sensitive rate constant for sodium-22 efflux and elevated sodium content in leukocytes (Forrester and Alleyne, 1980).

Certain observations suggest that this defect results from a plasma factor. Fitzgibbon *et al.* (1980) recently reported that the sodium-22 efflux from red cells incubated in plasma decreases as a function of sodium excretion in hypertensive but not normotensive subjects. The ouabain sensitivity of the abnormality was not indicated. Wessels and Zunkley (1980) reported that the increased sodium influx characteristic of the red blood cells of hypertensive subjects is transmissable by the plasma of some patients with essential hypertension to the red blood cells of normotensive subjects. While Clarkson *et al.* (1980) failed to find that plasma from hypertensive subjects is active on the red blood cells of normotensive subjects, Poston *et al.* (1980) found that white blood cells from normal subjects exhibit reduced ouabain-sensitive sodium-22 efflux when incubated in plasma from hypertensive subjects.

The important question, however, is not whether there is a plasma factor that affects the sodium–potassium pump of blood cells but rather whether there is a plasma factor that affects the sodium–potassium pump in vascular and cardiac cells, as our studies suggest is the case in animals with low renin hypertension. The practical problems associated with studying blood vessels and heart muscle in the hypertensive human, along with the renin status, are formidable but not insurmountable.

From many population surveys, it appears that the prevalence of hypertension in the diabetic population is greater than in the nondiabetic population. Certain observations suggest that this may be related to suppressed function of the sodium–potassium pump. Insulin has been shown to increase sodium and potassium flux in a series of tissues; the lack of insulin does the reverse (Weismann *et al.*, 1976). Furthermore, there is evidence that the hypertensive diabetic with nephropathy is hypervolemic due to decreased free water clearance and to the osmotic effect of hyperglycemia (Christlieb, 1980). Clearly, most of these patients have low renin hypertension. Low or normal plasma renin activity is also found in most hypertensive diabetics without clinically evident renal disease, possibly related to hyperglycemia (Christlieb, 1980). The hypervolemia diabetic may have two reasons for suppressed sodium–potassium pump activity: subnormal insulin levels and increased natriuretic factor level. Diabetes of long standing is associated with only 10% of normal norepinephrine in cardiovascular tissues (Neubauer and Christensen, 1976), similar to animals with low renin hypertension (see above). Diabetic children appear to be more sensitive to dietary salt, responding promptly to increased intake with increased blood pressure (McQuarrie *et al.*, 1936). Studies should be conducted to determine whether these observations are related to suppressed sodium–potassium pump activity in cardiovascular muscle and adrenergic nerve terminals.

Population surveys also indicate that the prevalence of hypertension in the obese population is greater than in the nonobese population. Recent studies suggest reduced activity of the red cell sodium–potassium pump in the obese human (De Luise *et al.*, 1980). Studies should be conducted to see if this is also the case for cardiovascular muscle.

VIII. SUMMARY

Ouabain-sensitive ^{86}Rb uptake, a measure of sodium–potassium pump activity, is suppressed in the blood vessels of animals with low renin, presumably volume-expanded hypertension. These include dogs with one-kidney, one wrapped hypertension and rats with (1) one-kidney, one clip, (2) one-kidney, DOCA, salt, and (3) reduced renal mass hypertension. The same is the case for rats and dogs following acute volume expansion with saline or mannitol and supernates of boiled plasma from these rats and dogs reduce ^{86}Rb uptake when applied to tail arteries from normal rats. This latter observation invited the search for similar activity in the plasma of the hypertensive animals. A new series of paired dogs with one-kidney, one wrapped hypertension and a sham operation was therefore prepared. After at least 4 weeks of sustained significant hypertension in the experimental animal and a similar time period in its paired sham-operated normotensive control animals, supernates of boiled plasma were prepared and applied to tail arteries from normal rats. Ouabain-sensitive ^{86}Rb uptake by the tail artery was significantly suppressed by the hypertensive plasma supernate relative to the normotensive plasma supernate whereas ouabain-insensitive ^{86}Rb uptake was unaffected, just as is the case for the hypertensive animal's own blood vessels. Supernates of boiled plasma were also prepared from rats with one-kidney, one clip and reduced renal mass hypertension and appropriate normotensive control animals and applied to tail arteries from normal rats. In both cases, total ^{86}Rb uptake by the tail artery was suppressed by the hypertensive plasma supernate relative to the normotensive plasma supernate. When normotensive rats with an AV3V lesion and a sham lesion were acutely volume-expanded with saline, ouabain-sensitive ^{86}Rb uptake by the tail artery was higher in the lesioned than in the sham lesioned animals and total ^{86}Rb uptake by arteries from normal rats was greater when incubated in supernates prepared from volume-expanded lesioned rats than when incubated in supernates from the expanded sham-lesioned rats.

We conclude that plasma from dogs with one-kidney, one wrapped and rats with one-kidney, one clip, and reduced renal mass hypertension contains a heat stable factor that suppresses vascular sodium–potassium pump activity. It appears in response to volume expansion per se and apparently the AV3V area of the brain influences the plasma concentration. It is known that suppression of the vascular sodium–potassium pump, with ouabain for example, increases contractile activity and the contractile responses to vasoconstrictor agents. Thus, the humoral pump inhibitor may be involved in the genesis and maintenance of the hypertension.

REFERENCES

Abel, P. W., Trapani, A., Aprigliano, O., and Hermsmeyer, K. (1980). Trophic effect of norepinephrine on the rat portal vein in organ culture. *Circ. Res.* **47,** 770–775.

Anderson, D. K. (1976). Cell potential and sodium-potassium pump in vascular smooth muscle. *Fed. Proc., Fed. Am. Soc. Exp. Biol.* **35,** 1294–1297.

Bealer, S., Haywood, J. R., Johnson, A. K., Gruber, K. A., Buckalew, V. M., and Brody, M. J. (1979). Impaired natriuresis and secretion of natriuretic hormone in rats with lesions of the anteroventral 3rd ventricle. *Fed. Proc., Fed. Am. Soc. Exp. Biol.* **38,** 1232.

Blaustein, M. (1977). Sodium ions, calcium ions, blood pressure regulation and hypertension: A reassessment and a hypothesis. *Am. J. Physiol.* **232,** C165–C173.

Brender, D., Vanhoutte, P. M., and Shepherd, J. T. (1969). Potentiation of adrenergic venomotor responses in dogs by cardiac glycosides. *Circ. Res.* **25,** 597–606.

Brender, D., Strong, C. G., and Shepherd, J. T. (1970). Effects of acetylstrophanthidin on isolated veins of the dog. *Circ. Res.* **26,** 647–655.

Brody, M. J., Fink, G. D., Buggy, J., Haywood, J. R., Gordon, F. J., and Johnson, A. K. (1978). The role of the anteroventral third ventricle (AV3V) region in experimental hypertension. *Circ. Res.* **43,** Suppl. I, 2–13.

Chen, W. T., Brace, R. A., Scott, J. B., Anderson, D. K., and Haddy, F. J. (1972). The mechanism of the vasodilator action of potassium. *Proc. Soc. Exp. Biol. Med.* **140,** 820–824.

Christlieb, A. R. (1980). Diabetes and hypertension. *Cardiovasc. Rev. Rep.* **1,** 606–616.

Clarkson, E. M., MacGregor, G. A., and de Wardener, H. E. (1980). Observations using red cells on the natriferic properties of plasma from normotensive and hypertensive individuals, and of the low molecular weight natriuretic substance obtained from human urine. *In* "Intracellular Electrolytes and Arterial Hypertension" (H. Zunkley and H. Losse, eds.), pp. 95–97. Thieme, Stuttgart.

Clough, D. L., Pamnani, M. B., and Haddy, F. J. (1978). Decreased Na,K-ATPase activity in left ventricular myocardium of rats with one-kidney DOCA-saline hypertension. *Clin. Res.* **26,** 361.

Clough, D. L., Pamnani, M. B., Overbeck, H. W., and Haddy, F. J. (1977a). Decreased myocardial Na,K-ATPase in rats with one-kidney Goldblatt hypertension. *Fed. Proc., Fed. Am. Soc. Exp. Biol.* **36**, 491.

Clough, D. L., Pamnani, M. B., Overbeck, H. W., and Haddy, F. J. (1977b). Decreased Na,K-ATPase in right ventricular myocardium of rats with one-kidney Goldblatt hypertension. *Physiologist* **20**, 18.

Clough, D. L., Pamnani, M. B., Huot, S., and Haddy, F. J. (1980). Left ventricular Na,K-ATPase activity in rats with reduced renal mass hypertension and spontaneous hypertension. *Physiologist* **23**, 91.

Constantopoulos, G. (1977). *In* "Hypertension" (J. Genest, E. Koiw, and O. Kuchel, eds.), pp. 452–470. McGraw-Hill, New York.

Dahl, L. K., Knudsen, K. D., and Iwai, J. (1969). Humoral transmission of hypertension: Evidence from parabiosis. *Circ. Res.* **24, 25**, Suppl. 1, 21–33.

de Champlain, J., Krakoff, J., and Axelrod, J. (1969). Interrelationship of sodium intake, hypertension, and norepinephrine storage in the rat. *Circ. Res.* **24, 25**, Suppl. 1, 75–92.

De Luise, M., Blackburn, G. L., and Flier, J. S. (1980). Reduced activity of the red cell sodium-potassium pump in human obesity. *N. Engl. J. Med.* **303**, 1017–1022.

De Mots, H., Rohimtoola, S. H., McAnulty, J. H., and Porter, G. A. (1978). Effects of ouabain on coronary and systemic vascular resistance and myocardial oxygen consumption in patients without heart failure. *Am. J. Cardiol.* **41**, 88–93.

Edmondson, R. P. S., and MacGregor, G. A. (1980). Leucocyte cation transport in essential hypertension. Its relationship to the renin angiotensin system. *In* "Intracellular Electrolytes and Arterial Hypertension" (H. Zunkley and H. Losse, eds.), pp. 187–193. Thieme, Stuttgart.

Edmondson, R. P. S., Thomas, R. D., Hilton, P. J., Patrick, J., and Jones, N. F. (1975). Abnormal leucocyte composition and sodium transport in essential hypertension. *Lancet* **1**, 1003–1009.

Epstein, M. (1978). Renal effects of head-out water immersion in man. *Physiol. Rev.* **58**, 529–581.

Fink, G. D., and Brody, M. J. (1978). Neurogenic control of renal circulation in hypertension. *Fed. Proc., Fed. Am. Soc. Exp. Biol.* **37**, 1202–1206.

Fink, G. D., and Brody, M. J. (1980). Impaired neurogenic control of renal vasculature in renal hypertensive rats. *Am. J. Physiol.* **238**, H770–H775.

Fitzgibbon, W., Myers, J., and Morgan, T. (1980). Red cell ^{22}Na efflux and urine sodium excretion in essential hypertension. *Proc. Meet. Int. Soc. Hypertens., 7th,1980*, p. 33.

Fleming, W. W. (1976). Variable sensitivity of excitable cells:possible mechanisms and biological significance. *Rev. Neurosci.* **2**, 43–90.

Fleming, W. W. (1980). The electrogenic Na^+,K^+ pump in smooth muscle:physiologic and pharmacologic significance. *Annu. Rev. Pharm. Toxicol.* **20**, 129–149.

Fleming, W. W., and Westfall, D. P. (1975). Altered resting membrane potential in the supersensitive vas deferens of the guinea-pig. *J. Pharmacol. Exp. Ther.* **192**, 381–389.

Forrester, T. E., and Alleyne, G. A. O. (1980). Leukocyte electrolytes and sodium efflux rate constants in the hypertension of pre-eclampsia. *Proc. Meet. Int. Soc. Hypertens., 7th, 1980* p. 35.

Friedman, S. M. (1974). An ion exchange approach to the problem of intracellular sodium in the hypertensive process. *Circ. Res.* **34, 35**, Suppl. 1, 123–128.

Friedman, S. M. (1979). Evidence for enhanced sodium transport in the tail artery of the spontaneously hypertensive rat. *Hypertension* **1**, 572–582.

Gillis, R. A., and Quest, J. A. (1979). The role of the nervous system in the cardiovascular effects of digitalis. *Pharmacol. Rev.* **31**, 19–97.

Gruber, K. A., and Buckalew, V. M., Jr. (1978). Further characterization and evidence for a precursor in the formation of plasma antinatriferic factor. *Proc. Soc. Exp. Biol. Med.* **159**, 463–467.

Guyton, A. C., Coleman, T. G., Cowley, A. W., Jr., Manning, R. D., Jr., Norman, R. A., Jr., and Ferguson, J. D. (1974). A systems analysis approach to understanding long-range arterial blood pressure control and hypertension. *Circ. Res.* **35,** 159–176.

Haddy, F. J., and Overbeck, H. W. (1976). The role of humoral agents in volume expanded hypertension. *Life Sci.* **19,** 935–948.

Haddy, F. J., and Scott, J. B. (1973). Mechanism of the acute pressor action of hypokalemia, hypomagnesemia, and hypo-osmolality. *Am. Heart J.* **85,** 655–661.

Haddy, F. J., Pamnani, M. B., and Clough, D. L. (1978). The sodium-potassium pump in volume expanded hypertension. *Clin. Exp. Hypertens.* **1,** 295–336.

Haddy, F. J., Pamnani, M. B., and Clough, D. L. (1979). Humoral factors and the sodium-potassium pump in volume expanded hypertension. *Life Sci.* **24,** 2105–2118.

Haddy, F. J., Pamnani, M. B., and Clough, D. L. (1980). Volume overload hypertension: A defect in the Na-K pump? *Cardiovasc. Rev. Rep.* **1,** 376–385.

Hawthorne, E. W., Hinds, J. E., Crawford, W. J., and Tearney, R. J. (1974). Left ventricular myocardial contractility during the first week of renal hypertension. *Circ. Res.* **34, 35,** Suppl. I, 223–234.

Hendrickx, H., and Casteels, R. (1974). Electrogenic sodium pump in arterial smooth muscle cells. *Pfluegers Arch.* **346,** 299–306.

Huot, S., Pamnani, M., Clough, D., and Haddy, F. (1980a). Depressed Na^+-K^+ pump activity in tail arteries of reduced renal mass hypertensive rats. *Fed. Proc., Fed. Am. Soc. Exp. Biol.* **39,** 1188.

Huot, S. J., Pamnani, M. B., Clough, D. L., and Haddy, F. J. (1980b). Vascular Na^+-K^+ pump activity and development of reduced renal mass hypertension. *Physiologist* **23,** 91.

Jones, A. W. (1973). Altered ion transport in vascular smooth muscle from spontaneously hypertensive rats. *Circ. Res.* **33,** 563–572.

Jones, A. W., and Hart, H. G. (1975). Altered ions transport in aortic smooth muscle during deoxycorticosterone acetate hypertension in the rat. *Circ. Res.* **37,** 333–341.

Lang, S., and Blaustein, M. P. (1980). The role of the sodium pump in the control of vascular tone in the rat. *Circ. Res.* **46,** 463–470.

Leaf, A. (1980). Sodium transport by isolated toad urinary bladder. *Proc. Int. Union Physiol. Sci.* **14,** 176.

LeLorier, J., Hedtke, J. L., and Shideman, F. E. (1976). Uptake of and response to norepinephrine by certain tissues of hypertensive rats. *Am. J. Physiol.* **230,** 1545–1549.

Leonard, E. (1957). Alteration of contractile response of artery strips by a potassium-free solution, cardiac glycosides and changes in stimulation frequency. *Am. J. Physiol.* **189,** 185–190.

Lorenz, R. R., Powis, D. A., Vanhoutte, P. M., and Shepherd, J. T. (1980). The effects of acetylstrophantidin and ouabain on the sympathetic adrenergic neuroeffector junction in canine vascular smooth muscle. *Circ. Res.* **47,** 847–854.

McQuarrie, I., Thompson, W. H., and Anderson, J. A. (1936). Effects of excessive ingestion of sodium and potassium salts on carbohydrate metabolism and blood pressure in diabetic children. *J. Nutr.* **11,** 77–101.

Nakazato, Y., Okga, A., and Onoda, Y. (1978). The effect of ouabain on noradrenaline output from peripheral adrenergic neurones of isolated guinea pig vas deferens. *J. Physiol. (London)* **278,** 45–54.

Neubauer, B., and Christensen, N. J. (1976). Norepinephrine, epinephrine and dopamine contents of the cardiovascular system in long-term diabetics. *Diabetes* **25,** 6–10.

O'Neill, J., Inciarte, D., Swindall, B., and Haddy, F. (1980). Effect of ouabain on norepinephrine vasoconstriction in the dog forelimb. *Fed. Proc., Fed. Am. Soc. Exp. Biol.* **39,** 582.

Overbeck, H. W., Pamnani, M. B., Akera, T., Brody, T. M., and Haddy, F. J. (1976). Depressed function of a ouabain-sensitive sodium-potassium pump in blood vessels from renal hypertensive dogs. *Circ. Res.* **38** Suppl. 2, 48–52.

Pamnani, M. B., Clough, D. L., and Haddy, F. J. (1978a). Altered activity of the sodium-potassium pump in arteries of rats with steriod hypertension. *Clin. Sci. Mol. Med.* **55**, 41s–43s.

Pamnani, M. B., Clough, D. L., Steffen, R. P., and Haddy, F. J. (1978b). Depressed Na^+-K^+ pump activity in tail arteries from acutely volume expanded rats. *Physiologist* **21**, 88.

Pamnani, M. B., Clough, D. L., and Haddy, F. J. (1979). Na^+-K^+ pump activity in tail arteries of spontaneously hypertensive rats. *Jpn. Heart J. (Suppl. 1)* **20**, 228–230.

Pamnani, M. B., Clough, D. L., Huot, S. J., and Haddy, F. J. (1980a). Vascular Na^+-K^+ pump activity in Dahl S and R rats. *Proc. Soc. Exp. Biol. Med.* **165**, 440–444.

Pamnani, M. B., Clough, D. L., Huot, S. J. and Haddy, F. J. (1980b). Sodium-potassium pump activity in experimental hypertension. *In* "Mechanisms of Vasodilation" (P. Vanhoutte, ed.), pp. 391–403. Raven, New York.

Pamnani, M., Huot, S., Steffen, R., and Haddy, F. (1980c). Evidence for a humoral Na^+ transport inhibiting factor in one-kidney, one wrapped hypertensive dogs. *Physiologist* **23**, 91.

Plunkett, W. C., Gruber, K. A., Hutchins, P. M., and Buckalew, V. M., Jr. (1980). Vascular reactivity is increased by factors in plasma of volume expanded dogs. *Clin. Res.* **28**, 827A.

Poston, L., Sewell, R. B., Williams, R., Richardson, P., and de Wardener, H. E. (1980). The effect of (1) a low molecular weight natriuretic substance and (2) serum from hypertensive patients on the sodium transport of leucocytes from normal subjects. *In* "Intracellular Electrolytes and Arterial Hypertension" (H. Zunkley and H. Losse, eds.), pp. 93–95. Thieme, Stuttgart.

Raghaven, S. R. V., and Gonick, H. C. (1980). Partial purification and characterization of natriuretic factor from rat kidney. *Proc. Soc. Exp. Biol. Med.* **164**, 101–104.

Reuter, H., Blaustein, M. P., and Haeusler, G. (1973). Na-Ca exchange and tension development in arterial smooth muscle. *Philos. Trans. R. Soc. London, Ser. B* **265**, 87–94.

Sharma, V. K., and Banerjee, S. P. (1977). Inhibition of [^{3}H] norepinephrine uptake in peripheral organs of some mammalian species by ouabain. *Eur. J. Pharmacol.* **41**, 417–429.

Siegel, G., Roedel, H., Nolte, J., Hofer, H. W., and Bertsche, O. (1976). *In* "Physiology of Smooth Muscle" (E. Bülbring and M. F. Shuba, eds.), pp. 19–39. Raven, New York.

Solandt, D. Y., Nassim, R., and Cowan, C. R. (1940). Hypertensive effect of blood from hypertensive dogs. *Lancet* **1**, 873–874.

Thomas, R. C. (1972). Electrogenic sodium pump in nerve and muscle cells. *Physiol. Rev.* **52**, 563–594.

Tobian, L. (1960). Interrelationship of electrolytes, juxtaglomeruler cells and hypertension. *Physiol. Rev.* **40**, 280–312.

Toda, N. (1980). Mechanisms of ouabain-induced arterial muscle contraction. *Am. J. Physiol.* **239**, H199–H205.

van Breeman, C., Aaronson, P., and Loutzenhiser, R. (1978). Sodium-calcium interactions in mammalian smooth muscle. *Pharmacol. Rev.* **30**, 167–208.

Vatner, S. F., Higgins, C. B., Franklin, D., and Braunwald, E. (1971). Effects of a digitalis glycoside on coronary and systemic dynamics in conscious dogs. *Circ. Res.* **28**, 470–479.

Weismann, W. R., Sinha, S., and Klahr, S. (1976). Insulin stimulates active sodium transport in toad bladder by two mechanisms. *Nature (London)* **260**, 546–547.

Wessels, F., and Zunkley, H. (1980). Sodium metabolism in red cells in hypertensive patients. *In* "Intracellular Electrolytes and Arterial Hypertension" (H. Zunkley and H. Losse, eds.), pp. 59–68. Thieme, Stuttgart.

29

Sodium–Calcium Exchange in Vascular Smooth Muscle: Key to the Genesis of Essential Hypertension

MORDECAI P. BLAUSTEIN

I. INTRODUCTION

The central role of sodium in the genesis of essential hypertension, so well documented in the literature, has provided the natural and obvious focus for this symposium. Needless to say, it is important for us to understand the role of sodium as a causative agent in this disease which is so prevalent in the United

417

THE ROLE OF SALT IN
CARDIOVASCULAR HYPERTENSION

States and other accultured societies. Recently, a comprehensive hypothesis was enunciated (Blaustein, 1977, 1980; deWardener and MacGregor, 1980) that provides a rational explanation for the role of sodium in the manifestation of this disease. In this article, I review the hypothesis, focusing on possible peripheral vascular mechanisms that lead to the increased vascular resistance in hypertension.

II. THREE KEY FACTORS IN ESSENTIAL HYPERTENSION

As reviewed by MacGregor in this symposium, there appear to be three key factors in the genesis of essential hypertension: a genetic factor, a humoral factor, and an environmental factor (namely, sodium). The inherited factor may be a defect in the body's ability to excrete a sodium load. Although such a defect remains to be identified in humans with the disease, the Dahl sodium-sensitive strain of rats may be an excellent model system in which to explore this possibility (deWardener and MacGregor, 1980). Chronic renal transplantation experiments have demonstrated that, in the Dahl rats, the primary defect appears to reside in the kidneys (Tobian et al., 1966; Dahl et al., 1974).

With an inherited (renal) defect in sodium excretion, excessive sodium ingestion will tend to increase extracellular fluid volume. The normal homeostatic response may then be increased secretion of a hormone that promotes sodium excretion, namely, natriuretic hormone (cf. deWardener, 1978). This may be the humoral factor first recognized by Dahl in his rat model of essential hypertension (Dahl et al., 1967). This hormone may inhibit sodium reabsorption by blocking sodium pumps at the peritubular (basolateral) borders of renal tubular cells (e.g., Fine, 1976). Moreover, this could be the agent that greatly enhances excretion of a sodium load in patients with essential hypertension (e.g., Viskoper et al., 1971). There is accumulating evidence (e.g., Edmundson and MacGregor, 1981; Poston et al., 1981) to support the hypothesis (Haddy and Overbeck, 1976; Blaustein, 1977) that a circulating sodium transport inhibitor plays a central role in essential hypertension in humans.

Clearly, with a restricted sodium intake, there will be no need for secretion of the natriuretic agent. A large sodium intake may be necessary to raise the level of natriuretic hormone above normal.

III. NATRIURETIC HORMONE AS INHIBITOR OF SODIUM TRANSPORT IN NONRENAL CELLS

Nearly 30 years ago, Tobian and Binion (1952) showed that the sodium content of arterial smooth muscle was elevated in hypertension. In the past 20 years, numerous investigators have documented the fact that the sodium concentration in erythrocytes and leukocytes is elevated in patients with essential hypertension (e.g., Losse *et al.*, 1960; Gessler, 1962; Edmondson *et al.*, 1975). Recently, Poston *et al.* (1981) demonstrated that blood plasma from hypertensive patients contains a substance that inhibits sodium transport in leukocytes from normal individuals; this could of course provide the explanation for the elevated sodium content in the various cells from hypertensive patients.

All these studies imply that natriuretic hormone levels may be elevated in the plasma of hypertensive patients. This may be the agent responsible for the high intracellular sodium concentrations in various types of cells, including vascular smooth muscle cells, in these individuals. Furthermore, it is important to stress the fact that the sodium concentration gradient will be reduced in the cells that are affected because plasma sodium concentrations remain normal in these patients.

IV. NATRIURETIC HORMONE AND ITS RELATIONSHIP TO THE INCREASED PERIPHERAL RESISTANCE

If there is, indeed, a genetic renal defect and, as a consequence of excessive sodium intake, an elevated level of natriuretic hormone in the plasma of hypertensive patients a fundamental question remains: How is this translated into the increased peripheral resistance that is the hallmark of this disease? Two hypotheses have been put forth to explain this interrelationship between elevated natriuretic hormone levels and increased peripheral vascular resistance. According to the hypothesis of Haddy and Overbeck (cf. Haddy and Overbeck, 1976; Haddy *et al.*, 1978; Overbeck, 1979), the main manifestation of the circulating sodium pump inhibitor may be a steady depolarization of the vascular smooth muscle cells that should enhance their permeability to calcium. As a result, calcium influx would increase because the large electrochemical gradient for calcium, across the plasma membrane, favors calcium entry; this causes the cytoplasmic calcium concentration to rise, thereby promoting muscle contraction. Haddy and Overbeck attribute the depolarization to inhibition of the electrogenic sodium pumps in the smooth muscle cells (Hendrickx and Casteels, 1974). However, as pointed out elsewhere (Blaustein, 1981), the Haddy–Overbeck hypothesis is implausible on theoretical grounds. There can be no significant reduction in the electrogenic sodium pump's contribution to the resting membrane potential in the steady state, when the pumps are *partially* inhibited. This is due to the fact that, when the pumps are *partially* inhibited, the pumped sodium efflux (including the electrogenic component) must rise until the efflux again equals the leak influx. This will occur when the cell sodium concentration rises appropriately.

The alternative hypothesis is that it is this rise in cytoplasmic sodium concentration, per se, that contributes to the increased peripheral vascular resistance (Blaustein, 1977, 1980). There are several possible ways in which this may occur, and each must be evaluated in turn.

One possibility is that the natriuretic hormone also inhibits sodium pumps in sympathetic neurons. In this case, the reduced sodium gradient across the plasma membrane of sympathetic nerve terminals may then contribute to the increased sympathetic tone that apparently plays a role in hypertension. This will result from the fact that, in nerve terminals, sodium and calcium transport are coupled by a counterflow transport mechanism (e.g., sodium ions enter in exchange for exiting calcium) (Blaustein and Ector, 1976). Under these circumstances, the calcium concentration gradient across the plasma membrane will be tightly linked to the sodium concentration gradient. Therefore, a reduction in the sodium gradient, for example as a result of a rise in cell sodium, will cause the cytoplasmic calcium concentration to rise as well (see Blaustein, 1974). Then, because neurotransmitter release is triggered by a rise in the cytoplasmic calcium concentration, we might expect both tonic (spontaneous) as well as depolarization-evoked catecholamine release to be enhanced. This increased transmitter release could be expected to activate the smooth muscle contraction to a greater extent than normal. Obviously, increased contraction of the smooth muscle in the walls of the small resistance vessels will directly increase peripheral vascular resistance.

This cannot be the only mechanism, however, because there is evidence that vascular smooth muscle contractility (the contractile response to a given stimulus) is enhanced in patients with hypertension. Thus, the smooth muscle itself must be altered.

V. SODIUM–CALCIUM EXCHANGE AND VASCULAR SMOOTH MUSCLE TONE

As we have shown previously (Reuter et al., 1973; Blaustein et al., 1980; Lang and Blaustein, 1980; also see Blaustein, 1977), vascular smooth muscle also possesses a sodium–calcium exchange transport system. Therefore, in this tissue, too, a rise in the cytoplasmic steady-state sodium concentration will produce a concomitant rise in the cytoplasmic calcium concentration. As a result, there will also be increased storage of calcium in the sarcoplasmic reticulum (i.e., both free and stored calcium levels will rise).

In smooth muscle, as in other types of muscle, the immediate trigger for contraction is appropriate elevation of the cytoplasmic free (ionised) calcium concentration (cf. Filo et al., 1965). However, vascular smooth muscle is known to maintain constant tension or "tone" (e.g., Uchida and Bohr, 1969). Two possible mechanisms could account for this tone: (1) the steady-state free calcium concentration may be maintained above contraction threshold, so that the muscle fibers are always partially contracted, or (2) there may be spontaneous, asynchronus activation of the smooth muscle fibers so that, at any given moment, at least some of the fibers are partially or completely contracted. With either mechanism, the increased cytoplasmic calcium that would result from sodium pump inhibition and the rise in cell sodium would be expected to increase vascular smooth muscle tone and contractility. As mentioned above, the increased tone is manifested as an increase in peripheral resistance and observed as an elevation of blood pressure. Vascular smooth muscle tension is a graded function of the calcium concentration (cf. Filo *et al.*, 1965). Therefore, if the calcium concentration is constantly maintained above the contraction threshold, any increase in the calcium level will be immediately translated into an increase in tension. However, if the second explanation for tone (i.e., spontaneous, asynchronous activity) is correct, then the calcium that enters the cytoplasm from the extracellular fluid and/or the intracellular stores (sarcoplasmic reticulum) during depolarization will be superimposed on an elevated baseline. Moreover, if the stores are more fully saturated than normal, more calcium will be released from the intracellular stores in response to a given stimulus. The net result will be a higher free calcium level and, therefore, greater tension when the smooth muscle fibers are activated.

VI. SUMMARY

The hypothesis described above shows how, in the presence of an inherited defect in renal sodium handling, excessive sodium intake may be translated into an increase in peripheral vascular resistance. To compensate for the sodium overload and tendency to blood volume expansion, large amounts of natriuretic hormone will be secreted into the plasma. This will have the salutary effect of promoting natriuresis and keeping plasma volume normal, as a result of the inhibition of sodium pumps in renal tubular cells. However, the hormone will, as a side effect, inhibit sodium pumps in other cells as well. Unfortunately, as a consequence of the inhibition of sodium pumps in vascular smooth muscle cells (and, perhaps, sympathetic nerve terminals), the sodium concentration in these cells will rise. Then, as a result of sodium–calcium exchange, the calcium concentration in these cells will also increase. This rise in cell calcium will be translated, either directly or indirectly, into an increase in smooth muscle tone. Thus, peripheral vascular resistance and, therefore, blood pressure, will increase.

Perhaps the most interesting feature of this hypothesis is that it lends itself directly to experimental testing and verification. Clearly, we should look for (1) a specific inherited defect in renal tubular handling of sodium; (2) identification and isolation of the natriuretic hormone, and proof of its elevation in the plasma of patients with essential hypertension; (3) proof that the natriuretic hormone inhibits sodium pumps, including those in vascular smooth muscle cells; and finally (4) more direct evidence that the sodium–calcium exchange mechanism functions in vascular smooth muscle cells.

ACKNOWLEDGMENTS

I thank Mrs. D. Ayers for preparing the typescript. Supported by NSF grant PCM-7911704 and a grant from the Muscular Dystrophy Association.

REFERENCES

Blaustein, M. P. (1974). The interrelationship between sodium and calcium fluxes across cell membranes. *Rev. Physiol. Biochem. Pharmacol.* **70**, 33–82.

Blaustein, M. P. (1977). Sodium ions, calcium ions, blood pressure regulation and hypertension: A reassessment and a hypothesis. *Am. J. Physiol.* **232**, C165–C173.

Blaustein, M. P. (1980). How does sodium cause hypertension? An hypothesis. *In* "Intracellular Electrolytes and Arterial Hypertension" (H. Zumkley and H. Losse, eds.), pp. 151–157. Thieme, Stuttgart.

Blaustein, M. P. (1981). What is the link between vascular smooth muscle sodium pumps and hypertension? *Clin. Exp. Hypertens.* **3**, 173–178.

Blaustein, M. P., and Ector, A. C. (1976). Carrier-mediated sodium-dependent and calcium-dependent calcium efflux from pinched-off presynaptic nerve terminals (synaptosomes) in vitro. *Biochim. Biophys. Acta* **419**, 295–308.

Blaustein, M. P., Lang, S., and James-Kracke, M. (1980). Sodium ions, calcium transport, and the control of vascular tone. *In* "Intracellular Electrolytes and Arterial Hypertension" (H. Zumkley and H. Losse, eds.), pp. 24–30. Thieme, Stuttgart.

Dahl, L. K., Knudsen, D. K. D., Hein, M., and Leitl, G. (1967). Effects of chronic excess salt ingestion. Genetic influence on the development of salt hypertension in parabiotic rats: Evidence of a humoral factor. *J. Exp. Med.* **126**, 687–699.

Dahl, L. K., Heine, M., and Thompson, K. (1974). Genetic influences of the kidneys on blood pressure. Evidence from chronic renal homografts in rats with opposite predispositions to hypertension. *Circ. Res.* **34**, 94–101.

deWardener, H. E. (1978). The control of sodium excretion. *Am. J. Physiol.* **235**, F163–F173.

deWardener, H. E., and MacGregor, G. A. (1980). Dahl's hypothesis that a saluretic substance may be responsible for a sustained rise in arterial pressure: Its possible role in essential hypertension. *Kidney Int.* **18**, 1–9.

Edmondson, R. P., and MacGregor, G. A. (1981). Leucocyte cation transport in essential hypertension: It relation to the renin-angiotensin system. *Br. Med. J.* **282**, 1267–1269.

Edmondson, R. P. S., Thomas, R. D., Hilton, P. J., Patrick, J., and Jones, N. F. (1975). Abnormal leucocyte composition and sodium transport in essential hypertension. *Lancet* **i**, 1003–1005.

Filo, R. S., Bohr, D. F., and Reugg, J. C. (1965). Glycerinated skeletal and smooth muscle. Calcium and magnesium dependence. *Science* **147**, 1581–1583.

Fine, L. G., Bourgoignie, J. J., Hwang, K. H., and Bricker, N. S. (1976). On the influence of natriuretic factor from patients with chronic uremia on the bioelectrical properties and sodium transport of the isolated mammalian collecting tubule. *J. Clin. Invest.* **58**, 590–597.

Gessler, V. (1962). Intra- und extracellulare Elektrolytveranderungen bei essentieller Hypertonie vor und nach Behandlung. *Z. Kreislaufforsch.* **51,** 177–183.

Haddy, F. J., and Overbeck, H. W. (1976). The role of humoral agents in volume expanded hypertension. *Life Sci.* **19,** 935–948.

Haddy, F. J., Pammnani, M., and Clough, D. (1978). The sodium-potassium pump in volume expanded hypertension. *Clin. Exp. Hypertens.* **1,** 295–336.

Hendrickx, H., and Casteels, R. (1974). Electrogenic sodium pump in arterial smooth muscle cells. *Pfluegers Arch.* **346,** 299–306.

Hilton, J. P., and Jones, N. F. (1975). Abnormal leucocyte composition and sodium transport in essential hypertension. *Lancet* **1,** 1003–1005.

Lang, S., and Blaustein, M. P. (1980). The role of the sodium pump in the control of vascular tone. *Circ. Res.* **46,** 463–470.

Losse, H., Wehmeyer, H., and Wessels, F. (1960). Der Wasser- und Elektrolytgehalt von Erythrozyten bei arterieller Hypertonie. *Klin. Wochenschr.* **38,** 393–395.

Overbeck, H. T. (1979). The sodium pump in cardiovascular muscle in hypertension: Whose hypothesis? *Clin. Exp. Hypertens.* **1,** 551–556.

Poston, L., Sewell, R. B., Wilkinson, S. P., Richardson, P. J., Williams, R., Clarkson, E. M., MacGregor, G. A., and deWardener, H. E. (1981). Evidence for a circulating sodium transport inhibitor in essential hypertension. *Br. Med. J.* **282,** 847–849.

Reuter, H., Blaustein, M. P., and Haeusler, G. (1973). Na-Ca exchange and tension development in arterial smooth muscle. *Philos. Trans. R. Soc. London, Ser. B* **265,** 87–94.

Tobian, L., and Binion, J. T. (1952). Tissue cations and water in arterial hypertension. *Circulation* **5,** 754–758.

Tobian, L., Coffee, K., McCrea, P., and Dahl, L. (1966). Comparison of the antihypertensive potency of kidneys from one strain of rats susceptible to salt hypertension and kidneys from another strain resistant to it. *J. Clin. Invest.* **45,** 1080 (abstr.).

Uchida, E., and Bohr, D. F. (1969). Myogenic tone in isolated perfused resistance vessels. Occurrence among vascular beds and along vascular trees. *Circ. Res.* **25,** 549–555.

Viskoper, J. R., Czaczkes, J. W., Schwartz, N., and Ullmann, T. D. (1971). Natriuretic activity of a substance isolated from human urine during excretion of a salt load. Comparison of hypertensive and normotensive subjects. *Nephron* **8,** 540–548.

30

Effects of Changing the Sodium Gradient on Calcium Fluxes in Smooth Muscle

CORNELIS VAN BREEMEN, MICHAEL KOLBER, AND PHILIP AARONSON

I. INTRODUCTION

The preceding chapters have amply stressed the importance of the involvement of Na ions in the genesis of arterial hypertension. Knowledge of the mechanisms linking Na to altered vascular smooth muscle contractility could thus conceivably be utilized in the therapeutic control of blood pressure. Since Ca is the main regulator of smooth muscle force development, we have studied in some detail the Na,Ca interactions in two standard smooth muscle preparations: the guinea pig taenia coli (GPTC) and the rabbit aorta (RA). This study begins to describe

425

THE ROLE OF SALT IN
CARDIOVASCULAR HYPERTENSION

how Na affects the Ca transport and binding sites which regulate cytoplasmic Ca activity and consequently smooth muscle contraction and relaxation.

Several theories have been proposed to explain the cellular interplay between Na and Ca. The simplest of these involves a Na,Ca exchange carrier of the type postulated by Reuter and Seitz (1968) as the sole Ca transport system linking the extracellular space (ECS) to the cytoplasm. Blaustein (1977) has applied this model to vascular smooth muscle in order to obtain a quantitative relationship between intracellular Na concentration ($[Na]_i$) and peripheral resistance. Alternatively Na,Ca interactions may be more complex involving a number of cellular sites (van Breemen et al., 1979). Na may compete with Ca for negative groups in membrane pores and cytoplasmic membrane surfaces (Kolber and van Breemen, 1981) and in addition may affect the turnover rate of the Ca-ATPase. The complexity of smooth muscle Ca regulation is further increased by the presence of sarcoplasmic reticulum (Devine et al., 1972) which uses ATP to pump Ca out of the myoplasm (Hurwitz et al., 1973).

Owing to its simplicity, the former theory is amenable to testing in smooth muscle. Even without assigning a turnover number or specific affinities to the carrier, the assumption of an obligatory exchange of n Na per Ca across the membrane gives the following equilibrium relationship (Baker, 1972):

$$\frac{[Ca]_o}{[Ca]_i} = \left(\frac{[Na]_o}{[Na]_i} \right)^n e^{(2-n)} \frac{EF}{RT} \tag{1}$$

where E = membrane potential, F = Faraday, R = gas constant, and T = absolute temperature. If it is further assumed that Na and Ca compete at both inner and outer membrane surfaces for access to the carrier, then the theory predicts a fall in Ca efflux and rise in Ca influx when $[Na]_i$ is increased (Na,K pump inhibition) or when $[Na]_o$ is decreased (substitution).

Our data, as well as a number of other studies, show that Eq. (1) is not obeyed in smooth muscle (van Breemen et al., 1979). In addition, we find that the simple kinetic predictions are not observed. Instead, we report transient phenomena which are not explained by the Na,Ca exchange carrier.

We will now describe our experiments in detail and suggest alternative explanations based on the postulates provided by the second theory above.

II. METHODS

The objective of this chapter is to provide an overview of our work performed during the last 4 years. The experimental procedures essentially consist of rapid isolation of the smooth muscle preparations (rabbit aorta and guinea pig taenia coli), incubation in PSS (in mM: NaCl, 140; KCl, 5; $CaCl_2$, 1.5; $MgCl_2$, 1; glucose, 10; HEPES buffer, 5; bubbled with 100% O_2 at 37°C), modifying the

PSS by isotonic substitutions or addition of drugs and measuring contractile activity, cellular cation contents, and transplasmalemmal ^{45}Ca fluxes (after removal of extracellular cations in ice cold "quenching solutions" containing La^{3+} or EGTA). The analytical methods have been described in detail elsewhere (Aaronson et al., 1979; Aaronson and van Breemen, 1981; Meisheri et al., 1981) while the experimental protocols will be given with results below.

III. RESULTS AND DISCUSSION

In order to test if the transmembrane Na^+ gradient (∇Na) provides the energy for Ca extrusion we examined the possibility of dissociating the ∇Na^+ from the ∇Ca^{2+}. Two main procedures exist for altering ∇Na^+: inhibition of the Na,K

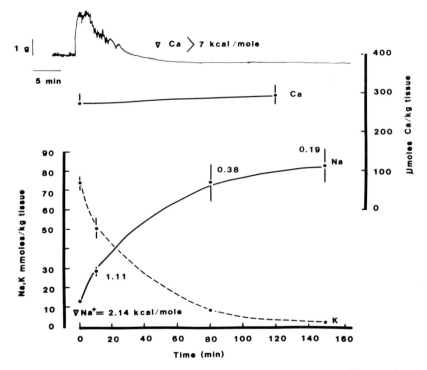

Fig. 1. The effect of ouabain treatment on total cellular Na, K (lower), Ca (middle), and tension development (upper). Values at time zero represent control values measured immediately prior to the addition of 10^{-5} M ouabain to PSS bathing guinea pig taenia coli. The values shown next to the Na tracing indicate the calculated magnitude of the electrochemical Na gradient at each time point, assuming that all cellular Na was free in solution. The value for ∇Ca was calculated assuming that $[Ca]_i \leq 10^{-7}$ M, and $E_m \leq 15$ mV.

pump and substitution of [NaCl]$_e$ (extracellular NaCl concentration) with other
electrolytes or sucrose. Both approaches were used. Figure 1 illustrates the
results obtained when GPTC was incubated in PSS containing 10^{-5} M ouabain:
(1) the intracellular Na and K concentrations approach their extracellular values,
(2) the cellular Ca content does not change, and (3) the muscle undergoes a
transient contraction which is followed by complete relaxation. The numbers
associated with the Na curve give approximate values for the ∇Na^+ in kcal/mole
Na during the ouabain exposure. They were calculated from the cellular Na
concentrations using values for the membrane potential obtained during ouabain
exposure of GPTC by Casteels (1966) and Matthews and Sutter (1967). We have
also found that the GPTC contains very little intracellular bound Na (Aaronson
and van Breemen, 1981). The activation curve for smooth muscle myofilaments
dictates that the [Ca]$_i$ must remain below 10^{-7} M for complete relaxation (Filo et
$al.$, 1965). Thus the $\nabla Ca \geq 9$ kcal/mole Ca^{2+} at rest under physiological conditions and decreases to approximately 7 kcal/mole Ca^{2+} after 2 hr in ouabain due
to membrane depolarization. Since the ∇Na decreases to < 200 cal/mole Na, a
Ca extrusion process driven by Na influx would need a stoichiometry of 35 Na^+
exchanged for each Ca^{2+} in order to explain the maintenance of the ∇Ca during
Na,K pump inhibition. Such a stoichiometry, which in addition would have to be

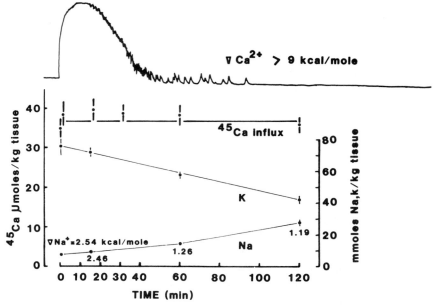

Fig. 2.   The effect of K-free PSS upon total cellular Na,K (lower), ^{45}Ca influx (middle), and
tension development (upper) of guinea pig taenia coli. "Ca influx" is equivalent to ^{45}Ca uptake into
cells during a 3-min labeling period. Values for the electrochemical Na gradient at each time point are
shown below the Na measurements; the Ca gradient is indicated above the tension tracing.

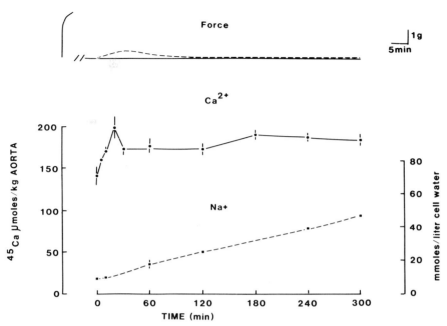

Fig. 3. The effect of incubation of rabbit aorta in K-free PSS on total cellular Na (bottom line, right ordinate), Ca (middle line, left ordinate), and tension development. A maximal (10^{-5} M norepinephrine) contracture is shown to the left of the zero K tension experiment.

variable, seems unreasonable. Furthermore we have previously shown that a reduction of cellular ATP by metabolic inhibition with iodoacetic acid and dinitrophenol will induce a large Ca gain approaching equilibrium (van Breemen *et al.*, 1981). The conclusion therefore is that the Ca extrusion mechanism which maintains Ca homeostasis inside the smooth muscle cells is energized by ATP and not by the ∇Na^+. The Na,K pump may also be inhibited by removal of extracellular K^+ which is illustrated in Fig. 2. The inhibition is not complete such that the intracellular monovalent cation concentrations change more slowly than in ouabain. We again see a transient activation of the myofilaments concomitant with an initial depolarization. This is followed by a hyperpolarization (Casteels *et al.*, 1973) and relaxation while the Ca influx rate remains equal to control values. In experiments not shown here it was found that ^{45}Ca efflux was slightly elevated resulting in a 33% reduction in the Ca content at 2 hours. Comparison of the ∇Ca with the ∇Na during zero K treatment again leads to the conclusion that Na influx does not drive the Ca extrusion pump in GPTC. In addition the net Ca loss during an increase in $[Na]_i$ runs counter to the concept of ∇Na mediating Ca extrusion.

The results of Na pump inhibition in rabbit aortic smooth muscle are essentially the same. Figure 3 illustrates the effects of K removal in RA. The Na gain does not induce a parallel Ca accumulation. The transient contraction appears to be due to norepinephrine release from the nerve terminals since it is prevented by 10^{-6} M phentolamine. As seen before in the GPTC ouabain induces a rapid accumulation of $[Na]_i$ in the RA but in addition caused a nonspecific leak (measured by $[^{14}C]$sorbitol penetration) after 2 hr. The transient ouabain induced contraction was inhibited by phentolamine.

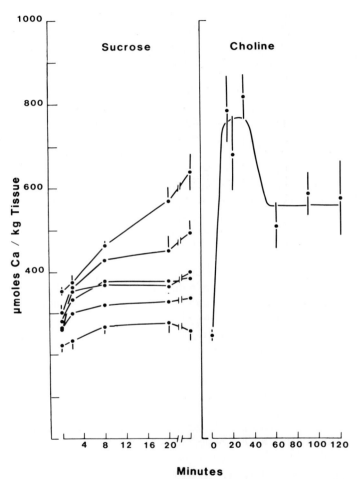

Fig. 4. The effect of medium Na depletion on total exchangeable cellular Ca in guinea pig taenia coli. The values at time zero represent control values for each experiment. In the experiments in which sucrose was used as a Na substitute, cellular Ca was measured following a reduction of [Na] to 80, 40, 20, 10, 1, or 0 mM. The right side of the figure shows combined data from three separate experiments in which [Na] was reduced to zero, with choline as an isotonic substitute.

In the light of the above dissociation of the ∇Ca^{2+} from the ∇Na^+ it becomes impossible to explain active Ca extrusion solely by means of a Na,Ca exchange carrier in smooth muscle plasmalemma. This conclusion motivated us to search for alternate mechanisms to account for the important interactions between Na^+ and Ca^{2+} in smooth muscle.

The ∇Na was also changed by substituting sucrose or choline Cl for NaCl. Graded reductions in $[Na]_o$ led to increasing values of cellular Ca (Fig. 4). The cellular Ca content reached a new steady state between 20 and 60 min, during which time the muscle was relaxed. The changes were due to alterations in $[Na]_e$, and not to lowered ionic strength since similar results were obtained with choline Cl substitution. In experiments not shown here the time course of $[Na]_i$ loss (corrected for bound cellular Na) in the above media were followed (Aaronson and van Breemen, 1981). The ratios of the new steady rate values, $[Na]_e/[Na]_i$, were then plotted as a function of $[Na]_e$. It is evident from Fig. 5 that extracellular Na depletion results in diminished Na^+ gradients. The results again did not support the Na,Ca exchange carrier hypothesis in that the $[Ca]_i$ values were below that predicted from Eq. (1). An alternative theory is explored in Fig. 6 which shows the dependency of total cellular Ca on $[Na]_i$. If we postulate that intracellular membranes possess negatively charged sites and that Ca^{2+}, Na^+, and K^+ compete for adsorption to these sites, then we could fit the experimental

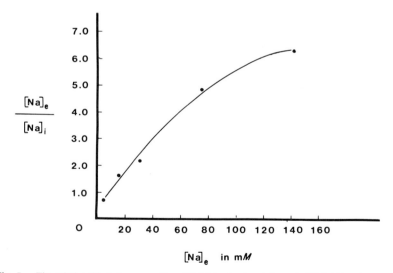

Fig. 5. The relationship between medium [Na] (abscissa) and the ratio $[Na]_e/[Na]_i$ in guinea pig taenia coli. Tissues were exposed to various low-Na media for 30 min, a time sufficient to allow cellular Na to drop to a stable value. Total cellular Na, tissue dry/wet weight ratio, and the extracellular space were then measured and used to calculate $[Na]_i$; the assumption was made that all cellular Na was free in solution.

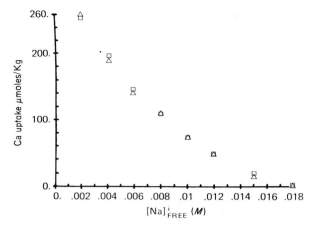

Fig. 6. The relationship between free intracellular Na and cellular Ca uptake observed in guinea pig taenia coli ($\triangle$), and predicted by the model ($\square$) of Kolber and van Breemen (1981) for Na–Ca competition at intracellular anionic binding sites.

data ($\triangle$) with calculated values ($\square$). The method of solution consisted of solving the Boltzman, Langmuir and Gouy–Chapman equations self-consistently using K_D values for Ca, Na, and K binding of 4×10^{-8} M, 9×10^{-3} M, and 1 M, respectively, and a charge density of 0.005 $e/Å^2$ (Kolber and van Breemen, 1981). Thus, as the $[Na]_i$ is lowered, Na desorption from the negative sites is thought to make new binding sites available for Ca. This will lead to an increase in total cellular Ca while the free intracellular Ca concentration is maintained constant by an ATP-fueled Ca pump.

When Na^+ is reintroduced into the sucrose medium bathing GPTC, Ca^{2+} is displaced from the cells as shown in Fig. 7. Ca extrusion was also effected by adding LiCl instead of NaCl. Under appropriate conditions even K^+ may be used to reverse the sucrose-induced Ca again (Fig. 8). Figure 8 shows that when GPTC is exposed to sucrose PSS, it gains Ca. A subsequent exposure to K^+ substituted PSS (145 mM K^+) induces an additional net Ca gain which is accompanied by a large contraction. The high K^+-induced Ca gain results from the opening of D600 sensitive membrane potential operated Ca channels (Aaronson and van Breemen, 1981; Ozaki and Urakawa, 1979). The lower curve was obtained by exposing GPTC to the same sequence of solutions in the presence of 10^{-5} M D600. Blockade of the potential-dependent Ca channels reversed the high K^+-induced Ca gain but did not affect the Ca gain induced by sucrose. This experiment provides two arguments against the hypothesis that the Ca loss is energized by a Na,Ca exchange carrier: (1) K^+ can substitute for Na and (2) $[K^+]_0$ displaces cellular Ca in the virtual absence of any monovalent cation gradient since only a small portion of cellular K^+ was lost in the sucrose solution.

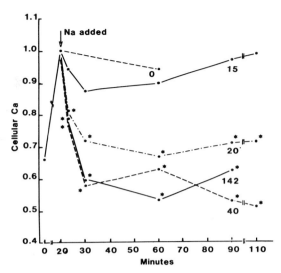

Fig. 7. The effect of Na repletion on total exchangeable cellular Ca in guinea pig taenia coli. Tissues were placed in a zero Na (sucrose) PSS at time zero and allowed to gain cellular Ca for 20 min. Subsequently, tissues were placed in media containing the Na concentrations shown. Since these data are collected from four separate experiments, all values within each experiment were normalized to that measured after 20 min in the zero Na medium in order to facilitate comparison. Asterisks denote measurements of cellular Ca during Na repletion that were significantly lower than the zero Na value.

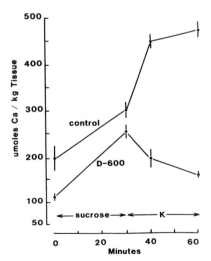

Fig. 8. The effect of successive exposure of tissues to sucrose PSS and K PSS on total cellular Ca. The upper line represents cellular Ca in tissues that were incubated in zero Na (sucrose) PSS for 30 min and then placed into zero Na(K) PSS. The lower line represents an identical protocol, except that 10^{-5} M D600 was added during the last hour of ^{45}Ca labeling, and was present in both zero Na media.

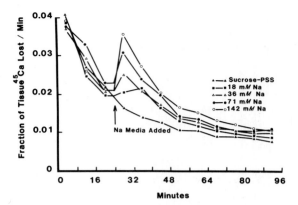

Fig. 9. The effect of Na repletion on ^{45}Ca efflux. Tissues were labeled with ^{45}Ca in PSS for 150 min, and then in zero Na (sucrose) PSS for 30 min. Tissues were then washed for 45–50 min in an ice cold PSS containing 5.0 mM EGTA and 6.5 mM Ca in order to selectively remove extracellular label. Efflux at 37°C was subsequently initiated in zero Na (sucrose) PSS. After 24 min, this solution was replaced with one of several Na-containing media.

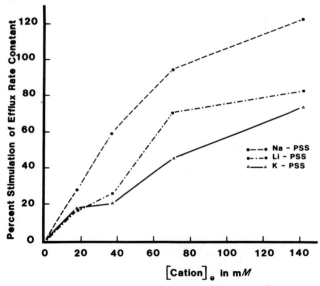

Fig. 10. The percentage stimulation of the apparent rate constant of ^{45}Ca efflux on replacement of Na, Li, or K into the efflux medium. Tissues were treated as described for Fig. 8, except that in some cases, media containing Li or K instead of Na were substituted for sucrose PSS at 24 min. The difference between the rate constant observed during the first 8 min of cation repletion and that observed during the same time in tissues which were left in sucrose PSS (control value) is expressed as percentage of the control value, and is shown on the ordinate.

The displacement of cellular Ca by monovalent cations was also demonstrated as a transient stimulation of ^{45}Ca efflux. Figure 9 shows this effect upon restitution of graded Na$^+$ concentrations after sucrose. If the stimulated ^{45}Ca efflux had resulted from activation of an extrusion mechanism a more sustained elevation of the ^{45}Ca efflux rate would have been anticipated (Baker and McNaughton, 1976). Both Li$^+$ and K$^+$ induced similar transient stimulations of ^{45}Ca efflux although peak ^{45}Ca efflux rates were somewhat lower (Fig. 10). Further evidence against a specific Na,Ca exchange carrier being responsible for the above stimulation of ^{45}Ca efflux was obtained by substituting a number of cations including choline and Tris ions for sucrose after pretreatment in zero Ca, 2 mM EGTA (Fig. 11). In this case all monovalent cations caused similar increases in ^{45}Ca efflux. The reason for this may be that EGTA induced some membrane leakiness which would facilitate entry of the larger monovalent cations.

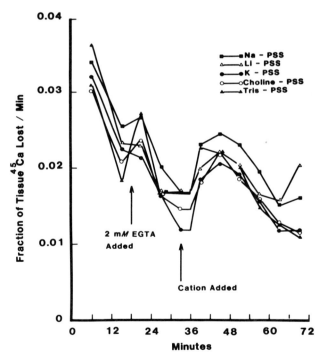

Fig. 11.   Stimulation of ^{45}Ca efflux by monovalent cations in the presence of 2 mM EGTA. Tissues were labeled with ^{45}Ca and extracellular label was washed out as described for Fig. 8. Efflux was initiated into sucrose PSS. After 18 min, all tissues were switched to a zero Ca sucrose PSS containing 2 mM EGTA. After an additional 12 min, this medium was replaced by one of several monovalent cation containing zero Ca media containing 2 mM EGTA.

Summing up our work on the GPTC we have achieved complete dissociation of the ∇Ca^{2+} from the ∇Na^+ and provided strong evidence for Na^+,Ca^{2+} competition for intracellular sites. It was of interest to note that in the Na^+ substitution experiments discussed above relatively large quantities of Ca (200–300 μmoles/ kg wet wt) could be introduced with only a submaximal transient contracture while subsequent displacement of the same amount of Ca did not induce any tension development. A possible explanation for this observation is that Na^+ and Ca^{2+} compete for binding sites which are separated from the myoplasm. Such sites could be located within superficially located SR (Aaronson and van Breemen, 1981).

In the context of this symposium the possibility still remains that a Na,Ca exchange carrier determines $[Ca]_i$ in smooth muscle of the resistance arterioles even though evidence from the GPTC excludes this possibility for intestinal smooth muscle. The difficulty of obtaining adequate amounts of pure arteriolar smooth muscle precludes the application of our analytical techniques to this tissue. For this reason we decided to examine Na,Ca interactions in the rabbit aorta under the assumption that the basic cellular mechanism of Ca extrusion would not change as one proceeds down the arterial circulation. We have already

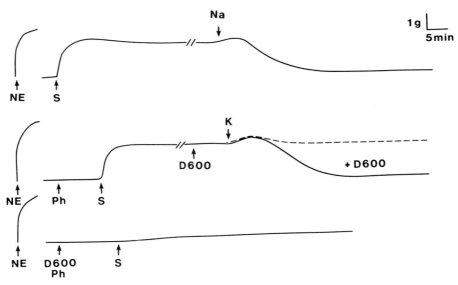

Fig. 12.   Effects of Na, K, and 10^{-5} M D600 on the zero Na (sucrose) contracture. Tissues were first exposed to 10^{-5} M norepinephrine to determine maximal tension development, and then washed with PSS until tension returned to the resting level. Ph represents the addition of 10^{-6} M phentolamine to the medium; S indicates the isotonic replacement of medium Na by sucrose. The middle tracing shows that replacement of sucrose with isotonic K-PSS caused a transient increase in tension which was followed by a relaxation to resting level in the presence of 10^{-5} M D600.

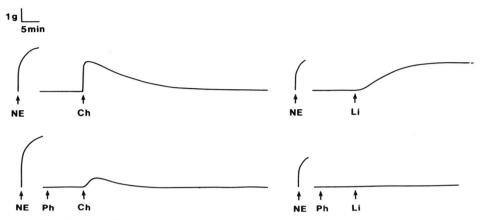

Fig. 13. The effect of isotonic replacement of medium Na with Li or choline on tension development in the presence or absence of 10^{-6} M phentolamine. Maximal contractures induced by 10^{-5} M NE are shown to the left.

shown a dissociation of ∇Ca^{2+} from ∇Na^+ during Na,K pump inhibition in RA (Fig. 3). In Figure 12 the contractile effects of monovalent cation depletion and restitution are shown. The aorta responded with a Ca gain accompanied by a maintained submaximal contracture when Na was replaced by sucrose, and subsequently relaxed if Na was replaced, or if the sucrose was replaced by K in the presence of 10^{-5} M D600. The relaxation by the monovalent cations was associated with the loss of cellular Ca. Phentolamine, which was introduced to block effects due to the release of endogenous norepinephrine, only partially inhibited the sucrose contracture. Since the remainder of the contracture was blocked by D600, it is likely that sucrose caused some depolarization in the RA.

In contrast to the results obtained in sucrose, phentolamine (10^{-6} M) blocked contractions induced by replacement of Na by Li or choline (Fig. 13). This indicates that in the rabbit aorta, the rise in Ca_i during Na substitution [which in any case is vastly smaller than the steady-state values predicted by Eq. (1)] is not directly related to reversal of the ∇Na but is due to neurotransmitter release and depolarization. Figures 14 and 15 show the Ca gains in various Na-free media in the absence and presence of 10^{-6} M phentolamine. Li and K induced smaller Ca gains than did sucrose or choline. Note also that an initial transient Ca uptake seen when Na was replaced by K in the presence of 10^{-5} M D600 (Fig. 14) was abolished if phentolamine was added to the medium. These data indicate that this initial Ca gain was due to a release of norepinephrine from nerve endings induced by the Na substitution.

We also measured the relative magnitudes of ^{45}Ca efflux stimulation which could be induced when Na, Li, or K were substituted in a Na-free (sucrose)

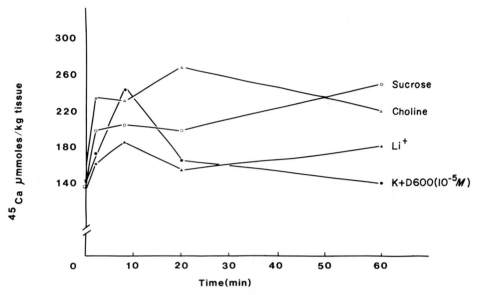

Fig. 14. The cellular uptake of Ca induced by the isotonic replacement of Na with sucrose, choline, Li, or K. 10^{-5} M D600 was included in K-PSS.

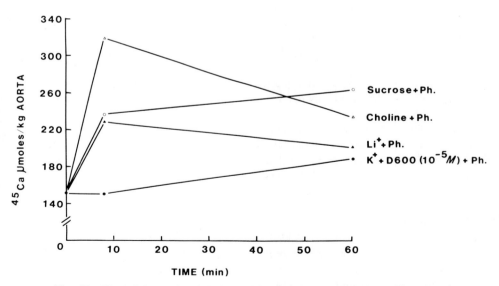

Fig. 15. The cellular uptake of Ca induced by the isotonic replacement of Na with sucrose, choline, Li, or K in the presence of phentolamine (Ph). Ph was added 10 min before Na substitution and was present during the remainder of the experiment. K-PSS also contained 10^{-5} M D600.

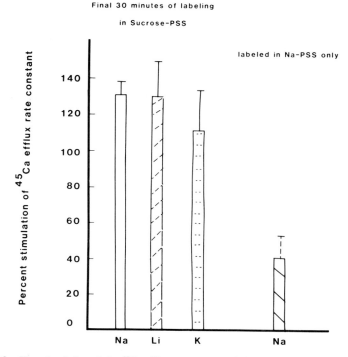

Fig. 16. The stimulation of the ^{45}Ca efflux rate constant induced by replacement of zero Na (sucrose) PSS by isotonic media containing Na, Li, or K. Efflux stimulation was calculated by subtracting the rate constant measured during the last 5-min efflux period in sucrose PSS (control efflux) from that observed in the next efflux period, where either Na, Li, or K was present. This difference was then expressed as a percentage of the control efflux. Monovalent cation mediated stimulation was increased by pretreatment of tissues in a zero Na medium during the last 30 min of labeling (left).

medium, as was described for GPTC (Figs. 9 and 10). Figure 16 shows that in RA all three monovalent cations were equipotent in transiently stimulating ^{45}Ca efflux, thus eliminating the possibility that this effect was due to a specific Na,Ca exchange carrier.

IV. SUMMARY

We have tested the hypothesis that the ∇Na and ∇Ca are obligatorily linked through a Na,Ca exchange carrier in both visceral and arterial smooth muscle. The abolition or reversal of the ∇Na in both types of smooth muscle by either Na,K pump inhibition or Na substitution did not result in a corresponding decrease in the ∇Ca. Since the plasmalemma is permeable to Ca and a large electrochemical Ca gradient persists as long as the ATP phosphate potential is maintained, we postulate that Ca is extruded from the cells by a Ca-ATPase mechanism.

Cellular Ca (not cytoplasmic free Ca) increased upon removal of $[Na]_e$ and was lost upon Na restitution. This effect was not specific for Na (both Li and K could replace Na) and could be explained by competitive adsorption of Na and Ca to negatively charged membrane surfaces within the cells. The contractile effects of Na,K pump inhibition or Na substitution in the rabbit were related to norepinephrine release from the nerve terminals (Bonaccorsi *et al.*, 1977; Karaki and Urakawa, 1977) and in one case to membrane depolarization.

The deleterious effects of excessive Na intake and/or retention on blood pressure regulation can therefore not be explained by a simple Na,Ca exchange carrier hypothesis. Na,Ca interactions in smooth muscle are clearly much more complex involving altered rates of neurohormone secretion and competitive adsorption to a number of intracellular sites.

The transmembrane electrochemical Na gradient (∇Na) was altered in the smooth muscle of guinea pig taenia coli (GPTC) and rabbit aorta (RA) by Na,K pump inhibition and $[Na]_e$ substitution. In GPTC, 10^{-5} M ouabain caused an increase in $[Na]_i$, a decrease in $[K]_i$, but no change in cell Ca. Zero K caused similar Na and K changes but induced a 33% loss of cell Ca. Transient contractions could be explained by depolarization. In the RA treated with 10^{-6} M phentolamine, ouabain, or zero K did not induce a significant Ca uptake nor a contraction.

Na substitution with sucrose or choline induced a transient contraction and maintained cell Ca gain in the GPTC. The Ca gain could be reversed by Na, Li, or K in the presence of the Ca antagonist, D600. The reversal of the sucrose-induced Ca gain by monovalent cations was mainly due to a transient stimulation of Ca efflux. Na substitution experiments in the RA bore essentially similar results. Contractions caused by Li and choline substitution could be blocked by phentolamine and the sucrose contraction was abolished by D600 plus phentolamine. The results rule out the possibility that Ca homeostasis in smooth muscle is effected by a Na,Ca exchange carrier. The data were, however, consistent with an ATP fuelled Ca extrusion pump, and a new theory of Na,Ca competition for intracellular negatively charged membrane sites.

REFERENCES

Aaronson, P., and van Breemen, C. (1981). Effects of Na gradient manipulation upon cellular Ca, ^{45}Ca fluxes, and cellular Na in the guinea pig taenia coli. *J. Physiol.* (*London*) (in press).

Aaronson, P., van Breemen, C., Loutzenhiser, R., and Kolber, M. (1979). A new method for measuring the kinetics of transmembrane ^{45} Ca efflux in the smooth muscle of the guinea pig taenia coli. *Life Sci.* **25**, 1781–1790.

Baker, P. F. (1972). Transport and metabolism of calcium ions in nerve. *Prog. Biophys. Mol. Biol.* **24,** 177–223.

Baker, P. F., and McNaughton, P. A. (1976). Kinetics and energetics of calcium efflux from intact squid giant axons. *J. Physiol. (London)* **259,** 103–144.

Blaustein, M. P. (1977). Sodium ions, calcium ions, blood pressure regulation, and hypertension: A reassessment and a hypothesis. *Am. J. Physiol.* **232,** c165–c173.

Bonaccorsi, A., Hermsmeyer, K., Smith, C. B., and Bohr, D. F. (1977). Norepinephrine release in isolated arteries induced by K-free solution. *Am. J. Physiol.* **232,** H140–H145.

Casteels, R. (1966). The action of ouabain on the smooth muscle cells of the guinea pig's taenia coli. *J. Physiol. (London)* **184,** 131–142.

Casteels, R., Droogmans, G., and Hendrickx, H. (1973). Membrane potential of smooth muscle cells in K-free solution. *J. Physiol. (London)* **228,** 733–748.

Devine, C., Somlyo, A. P., and Somlyo, A. V. (1972). Sarcoplasmic reticulum and excitation-contraction coupling in mammalian smooth muscles. *J. Cell Biol.* **52,** 690–718.

Filo, R., Bohr, D., and Ruegg, J. C. (1965). Glycerinated skeletal and smooth muscle; calcium and magnesium dependence. *Science* **147,** 1581–1583.

Hurwitz, I., Fitzpatrick, D. F., Debbas, G., and Landon, E. J. (1973). Localization of calcium pump activity in smooth muscle. *Science* **179,** 384–386.

Karaki, H., and Urakawa, N. (1977). Possible role of endogenous catecholamines in the contractions induced in rabbit aorta by ouabain, sodium-depletion and potassium-depletion. *Eur. J. Pharmacol.* **43,** 65–72.

Kolber, M. A., and van Breemen, C. (1981). Competitive membrane adsorption of Na^+, K^+, and Ca^{2+} in smooth muscle cells. *J. Membr. Biol.* **58,** 115–121.

Matthews, E. K., and Sutter, M. C. (1967). Ouabain induced changes in contractile and electrical activity, potassium content and response to drugs, of smooth muscle cells. *Can. J. Physiol. Pharmacol.* **45,** 509–520.

Meisheri, K. D., Hwang, O., and van Breemen, C. (1981). Evidence for two separate Ca^{2+} pathways in smooth muscle plasmalemma. *J. Membr. Biol.* **59,** 19–25.

Ozaki, H., and Urakawa, N. (1979). Na-Ca exchange and tension development in guinea pig aorta. *Naunyn-Schmiedegerg's Arch. Pharmacol.* **309,** 171–178.

Reuter, H., and Seitz, N. (1968). The dependence of calcium efflux from cardiac muscle on temperature and external ion composition. *J. Physiol. (London)* **195,** 450–470.

van Breemen, C., Aaronson, P., and Loutzenhiser, R. (1979). Sodium-calcium interactions in mammalian smooth muscle. *Pharmacol. Rev.* **30**(2); 167–208.

van Breemen, C., Aaronson, P., and Loutzenhiser, R. (1981). The influence of Na on Ca fluxes in the guinea pig taenia coli. *In* "Vascular Neuroeffector mechanisms" (J. A. Bevan, T. Godfraind, R. A. Maxwell, and P. M. Vanhoutte, eds.), pp. 227–236. Raven, New York.

31

The Implementation of Public Health Policy: Science and Reality

SANFORD A. MILLER

It is fortunate that the organizers of this conference decided to discuss the issue of what to do about sodium and hypertension after the technical conference had taken place. Whether they knew it or not, what they really did was separate science from reality. The last few days have dealt with the issues of science. In this arena investigators can discuss these subjects, with very strong disagreement, and still be willing to discuss further, in a nonadversarial way, how these differences can be resolved. In the arena of implementation of public health policy, this is rarely true. Earlier Dr. Hunt referred to the widespread public concern regarding the sodium content of processed foods and also to the fact that some 5000 health professionals and others signed a petition which was forwarded to the FDA urging it to take action to restrict the sodium content of processed foods. The problem is that the petition fundamentally ignored what government agencies can or cannot do. More importantly, it ignored the realities of the process by which such health related regulatory activities evolve.

First, there is a vast difference between making recommendations to, or demands of, government and the ways government can implement these proposals. I have had the experience of being on both sides of this issue. Prior to joining the FDA, I served on the Select Committee on GRAS Substances convened by the Federation of American Societies for Experimental Biology. One of its functions was the assessment of sodium chloride as a generally regarded as safe (GRAS)

443

THE ROLE OF SALT IN
CARDIOVASCULAR HYPERTENSION

However, the greatest area of our ignorance is the interaction among the various substances added to, or present in, our food supply as well as in the recognition of degrees of susceptibility among people exposed to these substances. There are a large number of toxic substances in the food we eat. We are exposed to as much as 10 g of solanine, a potent alkaloid, in sprouted potatoes each year. We are exposed each year to about 40 mg of hydrogen cyanide in lima beans and about 14 mg of arsenic in seafood, etc. One of the most potent carcinogens known (aflatoxin) is produced naturally by mold growth on cereals and nuts. Clearly, we could carry this to the ridiculous. The fact is that most of us can deal with these substances in food, particularly at the low levels at which they are found. However, there are individuals in our population who cannot handle the small amount of the toxic substances which they ingest. For unknown reasons, they are sensitive to one or more substances in their food supply. The government has problems dealing with issues of this kind. First of all, as I suggested earlier, we find difficulty in regulating food (containing such toxic substances) as compared to food additives largely because the legal requirement to prove harm is much more rigorous in the case of food. To regulate food, the government must prove that the food causes harm to a substantial portion of the population under ordinary conditions of use. This might be called the "bodies in the street" hypothesis! There is little that can be done about a particular food if one cannot prove that people are going to be harmed under ordinary conditions of use. On the other hand, for substances classified as food additives, only a presumption of harm under any possible condition of use is usually sufficient to take regulatory action. All one needs is a strong suspicion, supported by reasonable data. The reason for this is simple. In 1958, Congress amended the Food, Drug, and Cosmetic Act to place the burden of proof for proving safety on the person or company promoting the use of an additive who then must show that it does not harm anybody. This is an easier standard to challenge than the one for foods.

Another point of some importance is that the law also states that, in addition to the safety standard, to remove a food, one must also show that removing it from the market is not going to endanger the food supply. The definition of "endangering the food supply" is one that has been argued in many courts, but, on occasion, substances such as aflatoxin are permitted in foods even though the risk of aflatoxin may be one in ten to the minus fourth or fifth power. This is a substantial risk when one considers that the government is being asked to ban things when the risk is less than one in ten to the minus sixth power. On the other hand, if we tried to ban all foods containing aflatoxin from the market, we would end up with no corn, no peanuts, etc. That is a problem of some significance since without peanut butter, the entire American food system may very well come to a screeching halt!

A second reason for difficulty in dealing with these problems concerns the traditional philosophy on which food safety policy has been based. In general,

FDA regulatory actions have been concerned primarily with the safety of the entire population. Because of the magnitude of the problems, we have often been forced to treat people as statistical entities, not as individuals. In the last couple of decades a fundamental shift has taken place in that philosophy which is basically related to a change in social philosophy in the United States. Individuals have become a major concern of government. This revolution against the dictatorship of the majority is the end result of a very successful growth in affluence in the United States. Nevertheless, while this may be a very useful and very important social philosophy, there has not yet been provided any help to regulatory agencies in developing regulatory options incorporating these concepts to deal with their problems.

Thus, there are substantial problems in dealing with issues such as sodium and hypertension. Not only does regulation of the sodium content of food go directly against a fundamental hedonic desire of people who want foods that have a salty taste, it is also the center of the philosophic debate of the rights of the majority versus the needs of a minority in the sense that the number of salt-sensitive individuals is relatively few compared to the totality of the population. It also deals with important economic issues because it costs money to resolve these problems, i.e., to change a formulation, to label a product, etc. Hence, the resolution of this issue is not really as simple as signing a petition that says, "We must do something about the salt in our diet."

It is important to understand all dimensions of this complex problem. The FDA believes now (and has for some time) that the sodium content of the American diet represents a potential hazard to a significant part of the population. Seven years ago, we were developing a labeling approach to this problem but it became a part of the larger labeling activities of the Agency. Because of its specific importance, for three years we tried to separate the issue of sodium in foods from the other issues of food labeling. We have been able to convince at least two commissioners, including the current one, that this is a useful thing to do. Indeed, he is totally in support of this effort which has resulted in an FDA program to reduce sodium intake in the United States.

In the development of this program, two problems have had to be resolved. First, what can we do to help the salt-sensitive people in the population? Second, what, if anything, shall we do to modify the sodium intake of the "general population"? Clearly, one option might be to forget the population as a whole and allow salt intake to continue until it reaches that "salt price" at which hypertension increases in a sufficient number of individuals to require action. We believe this is not a viable solution. For a public health problem of this magnitude, the only justifiable strategy is prevention. Clearly then two strategies are needed.

The strategy for salt-sensitive individuals involves three different components. First, there is need for identification of the salt-sensitive population. This is a responsibility of those who are in both the clinical and research areas of this field. Second, such individuals must be provided with appropriate education to motivate them to make proper food choices. This may be where FDA can play a role, i.e., in providing information. People need information at the time of purchase in order to make the right choices. When combined with the extensive education programs of the NHLBI, this may prove to be of significant impact. Third, we need to increase the availability of organoleptically acceptable low-sodium foods to aid in compliance with prescribed low-sodium diets. Again FDA may play a role in permitting greater latitude in formulating such products and labeling them.

For the bulk of the population, there are also several areas to be considered. First, provision of information is as important to the population as a whole as it is to the salt-sensitive group. Second, we also need to make an effort to reduce the content of salt in all current food products to the lowest level necessary to perform the functional task for which the sodium salts are intended. With these two approaches, reduction of the current intake of sodium from 6–9 g/day to 3–4 g/day is a reasonable goal.

To address these issues, the FDA will develop a strategy that will include the following points. First, it is very clear that any formal government action to restrict the intake of salt directly in foods will be a very formidable task. It might be accomplished, but under the legal options open to the Agency, we would have to take each processed food product, one at a time, and show that each product in particular was a significant contributor to the salt load of the population. We would also be required to state the level to which sodium could be reduced. We might accomplish this using the GMP (Good Manufacturing Practice) regulations which state that any food additive can be used only at the minimal level at which it is effective. However, we would have to do this food by food (a very difficult, time-consuming task). Moreover, it would only apply to those uses of sodium classified as food additive uses. This option would also be a tremendous drain on the resources of an agency that has been shrinking in size for at least the past three years. This then does not appear to be a useful approach at this time. Second, the Agency will propose, in the very near future, the nutritional labeling of the sodium content of food as an addition to the nutritional labeling of the product. This will cover about half of the processed food supply. In addition, we will propose to the industry that they make a voluntary effort to label the sodium content of all foods without necessarily triggering full nutritional labeling. One of the questions that is raised in our proposal is whether the label should report both sodium and potassium content or just sodium alone, leaving potassium as a separate issue.

The second part of the strategy directly challenges industry not only to promote voluntary labeling but also to begin the process of reducing the sodium content of the food supply. This does not mean that every food requires reduction of sodium content but rather that, overall, the entire food supply should show a reduction in sodium.

The third part of the strategy will involve monitoring of sodium exposure and intake. The Agency has begun to monitor both the concentration of sodium in food products and the intake of sodium by the population as a whole. If there is no change after some reasonable period of time, e.g., 1–3 years, then we will move to further, more restrictive regulatory action. If there are reductions in the sodium content of food and in sodium intake, then there will be little need for regulation. The ball is now in the court of industry. It is their opportunity to do what they have always claimed that they would do if they were not bothered by Federal regulations.

In addition to the specific question of sodium, the Agency has also been considering a change in the whole philosophy of labeling which would give a great deal more flexibility to industry in how this information is to be presented.

If none of this works, we would next move into a phase of mandatory labeling in which all foods would be required to be labeled with their sodium content. If the industry fails in its voluntary labeling and in the reduction in sodium content of processed food, it would give further impetus and support to the need for mandatory labeling. A bill to accomplish this has been introduced into the Congress. A still more rigorous regulatory step might include the concept of a warning label. In this option, those foods that contribute significantly to sodium intake would have to contain some kind of warning for salt-sensitive individuals. If this still did not work, we would then consider restriction of that segment of the food supply that contains high sodium levels and provides a substantial portion of the sodium intake.

To accomplish the goal of reducing sodium intake and hypertension, there are really two significant things that must be done over the next several years. First, the kind of research now going on, with respect to the role of sodium in hypertension, must continue. It is essential to reduce the areas of controversy which confuse and obfuscate the regulatory and political issues. Second, those of us in the profession who are concerned with these issues must let these concerns continue to be heard. When there are hearings and the opportunity to testify is offered, we must voluntarily ask the committees to testify and not wait to be invited. Ultimately an effective program to reduce the incidence of hypertension must involve the professions, industry, consumers, and government acting together in the interests of public health and not as adversaries promoting narrow self-interest.

32

Labeling the Sodium Content of Processed Foods: The View of a Food Processor

ROBERT A. STEWART*

The current Federal regulations specify that any label bearing the statement "no salt added" or "prepared without added salt" must be considered a special dietary purpose food for persons who wish to reduce their sodium intake or are persons on a restricted sodium diet. Such foods must carry a statement on the label indicating the amount of sodium in the food. The amount must be expressed in multiples of 5 mg of sodium per 100 g of food and per serving of the food. The amount of sodium must be determined by laboratory analyses, the results of which must be included when the label is submitted for approval. Further, the control procedures must meet the approval of a government agency.

Compliance to the current regulations requires an overstatement of sodium rather than understatement. In other words, a given jar of baby food must not contain more sodium than indicated on the label. This poses a real problem when one considers the natural variation in the sodium content of the many ingredients of baby foods. For example, we have found that the sodium content of beets ranges from 87.6 mg to 139 mg per 100 g with an average of 118.5 mg/100 g with a standard deviation of 17.31 mg/100 g. Taking into account the possible

*Consultant, Gerber Products Company.

THE ROLE OF SALT IN
CARDIOVASCULAR HYPERTENSION

levels of sodium that might be encountered, the declaration on the label must reflect the high end of the range resulting in a declaration of 140 mg/100 g for strained beets. Thus, the label indicates that a baby would get 21 mg Na per jar more than he would get from the average jar and 52 mg of Na more from the jar of beets containing the minimal level of sodium.

The agreement reached with the Federal inspector regarding baby foods containing meat is that the declaration on the label may be equal to the mean plus 3 or 4 standard deviations depending on the number of samples analyzed in determining the mean.

Examples	Samples analyzed	Label	Mean	Difference
Jr. turkey and broth	15	80	51.7	29.3
Jr. beef and broth	28	85	56.0	29.0
Jr. chicken and broth	32	55	38.6	16.4

I will not attempt to cover the details of all the 133 baby foods carrying a mandatory declaration of sodium content, but all of them carry an overstatement that is likely to be present in 95% or more of the baby foods on the grocers' shelves.

In addition to the problems of inaccurate statements on labels, the process of preparing the label is costly. The laboratories and special analytical instruments are expensive. When we add to this the technician's time for collecting representative samples from each of the plants, carrying out the chemical tests and then statistically analyzing the results, the cost really begins to mount. Throw in the time of the label coordinator, the nutritionists, the legal department, and management, and a consideration of alternatives becomes mandatory.

What are the alternatives?

1. Eliminate the need for sodium analyses on the label by removing any reference to "no salt added" on the label.

2. Change the regulation so that average values, determined from representative composited samples, could be used for declarations on labels.

The first alternative has a serious marketing disadvantage in that mothers have been conditioned to look for the "no salt" declaration to assure themselves that they are following the so-called best practices for feeding their babies. Sales personnel are confident it would be more costly to remove the declaration than keep the present system in operation.

The second alternative has the advantage of furnishing more accurate information for controlling the average sodium intake, and in reality, does not pose any demonstrable risk when the label understates the sodium level of a given jar. In addition, the final cost to the consumer would be reduced.

Our dietary surveys indicate that at 7 to 8 months, the age when infants are consuming their maximal caloric intakes from baby foods, their total sodium intake is 26.6 mEq per day.

If we were to use average analytical values instead of upper limit sodium content on strained carrots, which incidentally is the baby food showing the widest natural variation in sodium and has a relatively high sodium content, a jar containing the maximal level of sodium could supply 84 mg or 3.7 mEq of sodium more than would be listed on the label. This amounts to 14% of the total sodium intake of an infant 7–8 months of age.

Our long-term feeding studies have demonstrated that feeding 81.1 mEq Na per day for 5 months did not increase blood pressure over a low sodium intake of 15.2 mEq Na per day. In other words, there was no demonstrable effect of a 434% increase in sodium intake fed continuously for 5 months. It would appear, therefore, that an occasional increase of 14% would not present a risk insofar as inducing hypertension is concerned.

We in the baby food industry recommend the second alternative in that it will provide more accurate information to the consumer at less cost and will not introduce a risk factor.

33

The Role of Salt in Cardiovascular Hypertension: A Summation

JAMES C. HUNT

An International Conference on Biological and Behavioral Aspects of Sodium Chloride Intake was held at the Monell Chemical Senses Center, January 24–26, 1979, and the proceedings have been published by Academic Press. The previous symposium has provided an excellent foundation for our current discussions, and I wish to recommend this publication to all of the participants in the current conference.

This symposium has been divided into three major sections: (1) the intake of sodium and the factors influencing sodium intake; (2) the excretion of sodium and the factors influencing sodium excretion, and (3) the interaction of sodium with peripheral adrenergic neuroeffector mechanisms and the regulation of vascular smooth muscle tone.

Recently, there has been a major surge of interest in the role of dietary sodium in the hypertensive process. The public has become aware that sodium is an aggravating, if not a causative, factor in the development of high blood pressure. Efforts are being made to decrease the sodium content of processed foods. Literally thousands of biomedical scientists in this country recently signed a petition concerning the labeling of the sodium content of processed food. This petition was forwarded to the Food and Drug Administration for consideration. I believe that we are going to hear more of such things from the public in the near future. It is for this and many other reasons that this symposium is timely.

Early in the symposium, we heard comments concerning primitive man and the fact that his diet had a low sodium to potassium ratio. Meneely emphasized that salt was a rare and prized commodity in ancient times. Up to the time of the Roman Empire, it was still considered to be a highly valuable and prized commodity. Indeed, the salary of the Roman Legion was paid in salt at one time. Only in the past 50 years has salt been readily available at low cost to most peoples of the world. It is over this span of time that we must look at salt with respect to its potential role in the etiology and development of hypertension.

The populations with low blood pressure in the world are now relatively few. They are unacculturated peoples such as the Eskimos, the Aborigines, the Indians, and certain South Sea Islanders. Dietary intake of sodium by these peoples is uniformly less than 75 mEq/day with the exception of a tribe of recently discovered Indians in Mexico who consume about 85 mEq/day. It is thought that this group is normotensive because of their extreme physical activity. When unacculturated man is subjected to high sodium intake, blood pressure rises to the levels of that of western man. The prevalence of high blood pressure in these people during exposure to the diet of an acculturated society is about the same as it is in a western society; i.e., somewhere between 15 and 20% of the population becomes susceptible to high blood pressure.

The use of sodium in acculturated societies is excessive to the extreme. It is most difficult to find either prepared food or food products without added sodium in some form at the present time. This, when associated with a major change in the eating habits of individuals in this country, including the use of prepackaged foods and dining out, adds 100 to 200 mEq of sodium to our daily intake. This is totally inconsistent with a susceptible person remaining normotensive. The diet of the average American at the present time, at least in the midwest, exceeds 225 mEq of sodium per day. There is no reason to suspect that other parts of the country differ in this respect. An accurate estimate of the daily sodium intake by an individual is difficult to make. Unfortunately, in most determinations, only sodium chloride is considered although sodium enters the body associated with other anions as well. Since free-living subjects have great variability from day to day in their sodium intake, the most accurate measurements that one can obtain is by a 24-hr urine collection, and even then, one needs to collect urine on several successive days because of the wide variation in the daily intake of sodium. However, such a measurement still does not define for us where the sodium intake comes from, and it is important in medicine and in health care delivery to determine the sources of dietary sodium. This is important if one wishes to change the dietary sodium intake of a patient as part of a treatment program or in preventive health maintenance. Thus, a detailed dietary history is essential, and this requires interaction among the dietician or clinical nutritionist and the other health care providers. Computer programs or computer assisted programs for determination of the amounts and source of the dietary sodium intake are also often required to handle a large volume of patients. Most institutions at which this service is available use a 7-day dietary history, completed by the patient and analyzed by the dietitian with computer assistance.

To look at this question, Marilyn Fregly reported on the estimated sodium intake of the average American from the amount of sodium used by the food processing industry, the HANES I study and the FDA Market Basket Survey. Estimates of daily sodium chloride intake by these studies ranged from 10 to 14 g. Fregly noted that most of these studies emphasized that breads, meats, and milk products were the principal sources of dietary sodium and accounted for approximately 70% of daily intake. This will vary greatly from part to part of the country. In the Midwest, for example, meats will account for more than 50% of the dietary sodium intake because Midwesterners eat a great deal of bacon, ham, and sausage and other prepared meats that are very high in sodium. Our studies indicate that approximately 225 mEq is an average intake of dietary sodium by Midwesterners, and this would be quite consistent with the 10–14 g of sodium chloride that Fregly estimated to be ingested by Americans. Interestingly, females ingest less sodium than men at any age, and peak intakes of salt apparently occur in girls 6 to 11 years of age. In men, the peak salt intake will range from 18 to 44 years of age.

Berenson carried this further, and reported on the sodium intake by school children in Bogalusa, Louisiana, a town of 22,000 people with approximately 5000 school children, of which approximately one-third were black. He found much the same sort of dietary sodium intake, except that in his study, the intake of sodium from soups contributed significantly. He noted that in Louisiana the dietary intake of potassium by blacks is considerably less than for whites and commented on the potential importance of this observation. In a neighboring town of approximately 7000 individuals, his group undertook to treat hypertensive school children. A public and patient education program was used to control sodium intake and this was combined with the use of a diuretic agent and a β-adrenergic blocking drug. He noted that there was a 7 mm Hg decrease in diastolic blood pressure in those children who were initially above the 90th percentile of blood pressures for their age. The decrease in blood pressure occurred very promptly. He did not have data to determine whether urinary sodium output had changed but was of the judgment that the reduction in blood pressure was entirely a drug-related effect. Berenson believes that the children had not decreased their dietary sodium intake and that effecting a behavioral change in this population would be very difficult.

Calabrese reported on the effect of the sodium concentrations of the water supply to two nearby communities in Massachusetts on the blood pressures of public school students. The sodium content in the drinking water of one community was strikingly low; that is, it contained about 10 mg/liter. The drinking water of the second community contained approximately 200 mg/liter. Although this difference in the sodium concentrations of the drinking water really is a difference of only about 7 mEq/liter of water, he noted an elevation in the blood pressures of the students from the community with the higher sodium concentration in their drinking water. We will look forward to a continuation of this study.

Allen reported on a five year intervention study that she and members of Stamler's group are undertaking in Chicago with aspirations to reduce dietary sodium intake to 75 mEq per day. Preliminary observations from this group indicate that it is possible to restrict calories, reduce weight, and effect some reduction in dietary sodium intake. Indeed, Allen noted a 3- to 5-g decrease in NaCl intake, i.e., a reduction from about 225 mEq to 150 mEq of sodium in the diet. This group is also looking for markers to identify hypertension-susceptible individuals and is studying red blood cell sodium transport. The Chicago study is imaginative, is being conducted by an experienced team including clinical nutritionists, and certainly should bring forth important new information. The potential for long-term lowering of blood pressure without antihypertensive drug therapy needs to be more fully explored.

Stewart reported on balance studies in infants less than 1 year of age. The levels of sodium intake in the two groups of infants were 15 and approximately 80 mEq/day. There were really few differences between the two groups in blood pressure and in weight in the short-term follow-up. There were some differences in salt and water balances in these infants but they were not impressive. There were the expected differences in urinary aldosterone and sodium excretion. I am uncertain whether it would be possible to predict long-term influences of an increased sodium intake over the relatively short period of exposure (5 months) used by these investigators. However, it is clear that their follow-up of these children 8 years later showed no really noteworthy differences between the two groups.

Schachter emphasized the limited ability of the infant kidney to excrete sodium during the first year of life. This is exactly opposite to what I had always thought and been told. The infant kidney had been portrayed to me as a sodium-wasting kidney rather than a kidney which has a maximum in terms of sodium excretion. Schachter also pointed out the role of potassium in preventing the elevation of blood pressure and the potential importance of the sodium to potassium ratio in this regard. This is not a new concept, but it is being pursued in this group of infants which he and his colleagues are following on a long-term basis.

Mickelsen studied various combinations of sodium and potassium chloride and demonstrated that 90% of his test population could not distinguish between a one-to-one ratio of these two substances. He strongly advocated the use of this mixture in those instances where sodium intake should be diminished. Interestingly, the one-to-one mixture is by weight, which means that there is more sodium than potassium because of their difference in molecular weight. In those instances where sodium control cannot be effected by reduction of dietary sodium, there may be a justification for the substitution of "light salt" which is the one-to-one mixture recommended by Mickelsen.

Bertino was of the impression that the taste of sodium chloride is learned from childhood and that this taste dictates sodium intake. She also suggested that sodium balance influences the taste for salt.

Fregly noted that hypertensive rats have an aversion to sodium. They differentiate between water and NaCl solutions at lower concentrations of NaCl solution than do normotensive rats. The aversion does not develop until blood pressure has reached maximal levels. The mechanism of this differentiation by hypertensive rats is unknown. It is also interesting that the rat apparently does not have a discriminatory taste with respect to the sodium content of its diet. This was new to me, and I found it most interesting.

Phillips noted that there is an important central action of angiotensin II in all models of hypertension, including secondary hypertension. He feels that high blood pressure affects the brain in some way. When the brain is injected with angiotensin II, a characteristic vasoconstriction, water retention, thirst, and an appetite for sodium are induced. He noted that the receptors for angiotensin II are in the anterior portion of the third ventricle of the brain and that the binding sites for angiotensin II are influences by a low sodium diet.

Battarbee demonstrated the importance of potassium and the sodium to potassium ratio in food on vascular resistance. He noted that the potassium content of the diet modulated the effects of the sympathetic nervous system on vascular resistance in rats.

Now with respect to the excretion of sodium and the factors influencing sodium excretion, Knox did not commit himself as to whether there is a natriuretic hormone. He discussed several possible mechanisms that could be involved in the escape from the sodium-retaining effects of mineralocorticoid hormones. He feels that the available evidence does not allow one to distinguish among a variety of factors, including a possible natriuretic factor, the influence of the renin–angiotensin system, certain physical factors (such as wall thickness), the renal adrenergic system, and the vasodepressor systems. We must look to future research for clarification of this issue.

Grekin studied the role of dietary sodium in the establishment and maintenance of high blood pressure in deoxycorticosterone acetate (DOCA)-treated pigs. There was a prompt sodium retention with an increased cardiac output in some of his pigs; others had only an increased peripheral vascular resistance while still others had an increase in both. He felt that the hypokalemia observed in the treated animals resulted from a shift of potassium into cells since there was no evidence of increased kaliuresis. He noted that with a diet limited to 20 mEq of sodium, there occurred a decrease in blood pressure and decrease in the peripheral vascular resistance in approximately half of his pigs. Sodium restriction from the outset of the experiment prevented the development of hypertension in all of the pigs studied. Grekin and associates have established an interesting model for future study.

Hall studied the effects of captopril, the angiotensin I converting enzyme inhibitor, in blocking both adrenal regeneration and sodium-induced hypertension in rats. Captopril was not effective in blocking hypertension induced following adrenal regeneration. In contrast, it blocked the development of salt hypertension in 80% of his rats. The saline polydipsia of the accelerated salt hypertension was prevented in those treated rats in which captopril was effective in blocking the elevation of blood pressure. He demonstrated that 19-norprogesterone also induced a saline polydipsia and high blood pressure. He observed that the potency of 19-norprogesterone in inducing hypertension was about the same as DOCA or about 2.5–3% as potent as aldosterone. He noted that while testosterone will induce mineralocortocoid-type hypertension, 19-nortestosterone is inert.

Young studied the effect of angiotensin II on sodium excretion in several experimental hypertensive models. His results suggest that angiotensin II has a powerful antinatriuretic effect and may contribute to the development of hypertension in this way. Aldosterone may also induce hypertension by the same mechanism in spite of the fact that there is an escape from the sodium-retaining effect of aldosterone. Young reported that a sustained change in renal function persisted when aldosterone-treatedd dogs returned to daily sodium balance.

McCaa studied the effects of converting enzyme inhibitors on the renin-angiotensin–aldosterone–kinin systems during long-term infusion of dogs with captopril. He also used the new Merck compound, MK-421, with about the same results. He noted that plasma aldosterone concentration was decreased. Plasma renin activity was increased and urinary sodium and potassium excretion increased while arterial pressure decreased. Interestingly, renal blood flow was increased in the animals while glomerular filtration rate (GFR) decreased rather markedly. The urinary kinins increased and the urinary kallikrein concentration decreased as one would expect. When angiotensin II was infused into sodium-deficient dogs treated chronically with captopril, it restored the animal to the pretreatment state within a period of three days.

Fujita studied the role of prostaglandins in salt-sensitive and non-salt-sensitive essential hypertensive humans. The non-salt-sensitive hypertensives excreted more sodium and more prostaglandin E_2 in their urine than did the salt-sensitive patients. With a reduction in dietary sodium alone, or in combination with furosemide, he noted that captopril decreased blood pressure to a greater extent in the salt-sensitive patients.

Reisin studied obese rats. When he produced ventromedial hypothalamic lesions in rats, they became obese. These rats had a contracted blood volume, an increased peripheral vascular resistance index, and a decreased cardiac index to both the kidney and the fat mass. With sodium loading in these rats, he restored the hemodynamic changes without a change in the mean arterial pressure or in the peripheral vascular resistance index. There was no change in renal blood flow when he restored the cardiovascular hemodynamics. He concluded that obesity was responsible for the increase in blood pressure.

Luft and Weinberger and associates have undertaken a series of most interesting studies in normal and hypertensive individuals exposed to a very wide range of sodium intake. Dietary sodium levels in these studies ranged from 1000 to 1500 mEq per day. With one exception, patients submitted to 1500 mEq of sodium per day developed edema and had an increase in blood pressure and cardiac output with an associated decrease in urinary norepinephrine. The blood pressure rise of norepinephrine infusion is enhanced by a high sodium intake. Sodium retention was also enhanced by norepinephrine infusion. Both the adrenergic and dopaminergic systems showed abnormalities in hypertensive subjects included in these studies, and the investigators suggest that this represents a link between these systems and abnormal renal handling of sodium.

Weinberger reported on studies of the adrenergic and dopaminergic systems and showed abnormalities in hypertensive humans. He and his group suggested that there is a link between these systems and the defect in the handling of sodium in these individuals.

Katovich studied β-adrenergic responsiveness in DOCA-sodium hypertensive rats and noted that the chronic administration of DOCA appears to be associated with an increased vascular responsiveness to β-adrenergic agonists. An increased responsiveness of β_2-adrenoreceptors and a decreased responsiveness of β_1-adrenoreceptors was noted in the DOCA-hypertensive animals.

Garay presented studies demonstrating a membrane defect in the red blood cell with respect to the transport of sodium and potassium in hypertensive humans. His studies were particularly concerned with sodium–potassium cotransport. Most hypertensive humans had a delayed efflux. However, 40% of the normotensive Parisians and more than 80% of the Ivory Coast normotensive natives also demonstrated this same delay. This test may well prove to be useful in selecting out of the population those individuals who are destined genetically to become hypertensive. However, more information regarding the genetic linkage of the abnormality of transport is essential, and a study of the natives of the Ivory Coast, representing a more homogenous genetic pool, may be very helpful in this regard.

MacGregor carried this same general concept further and suggested that hypertensives have a circulating sodium transport inhibitor which influences sodium transport from all cell membranes. Using a quantitative cytochemical technique, he found that plasma from normotensive humans inhibits renal Na^+,K^+-ATPase in vitro and stimulates renal glucose-6-phosphate dehydrogenase (G-6-PD) in vitro. Both of these activities are influenced by sodium intake. MacGregor also reported that the plasma from hypertensive patients has a very much greater ability to stimulate renal G-6-PD activity than that of normotensive plasma. Since there appears to be a reciprocal relationship between G-6-PD activity and Na^+,K^+-ATPase activity, MacGregor feels that the results suggest that the plasma of hypertensive patients contains an increased concentration of Na^+,K^+-ATPase inhibitory activity. He also studied the total leukocyte sodium efflux rate constant in hypertensives and reported that it was reduced compared to normotensives. The reduction was due to a decrease in the ouabain-sensitive component. These results suggest that there may be a rise in a circulating sodium transport inhibitor in hypertensive subjects that may serve as an important link between salt intake and the development of hypertension.

Bolton reviewed the effect of changing the frequency of discharge of action potentials of smooth muscles from small blood vessels on the modulation of their resistance to blood flow and their development of tension. In the case of smooth muscle of larger blood vessels, which have less of a tendency to discharge action potentials, he pointed out that resistance and tension are dependent on changes in intracellular calcium concentration. The opening of receptor-operated ion channels for calcium in the cell membrane, as well as the release of intracellularly bound calcium, may be important to initiate an increase in tension in these smooth muscles. Inhibitory substances may act not only on the permeability of the cell membrane to calcium but may reduce in some fashion the tension developed in response to either an influx or an intracellular release of calcium.

Westfall pointed out to us that sodium is involved in several aspects of adrenergic neuronal function, including release, uptake, and storage of norepinephrine. He presented evidence that increasing the dietary intake of sodium increased the activity of adrenergic nerves and enhanced the normal facilitatory action of angiotensin on adrenergic transmission. He feels that those types of experimentally induced hypertensions that are sodium dependent have an adrenergic component that contributes to the hypertension. Westfall was uncertain whether sodium plays a causative or merely a permissive role in the development of hypertension.

Friedman proposed that ''net sodium pumping activity'' is the central theme of the hypertensive state, whatever its origin. This involves changes in permeability and changes in sodium transport. He believes that the SHR and DOCA-hypertensive rats are examples of hypertension where both factors are increased, although he feels that combinations of these may suffice to produce hypertension.

Haddy reported his experiments on the role of the ouabain-like humoral factor in the genesis of low renin hypertension. He suggested that it is a heat stable factor which depresses the vascular Na^+,K^+-ATPase activity. This factor appears in response to volume expansion, and the AV3V region of the brain seems to influence its production. It has long been known that the suppression of the sodium pump increases both contractile activity and the contractile response to vasoconstrictor agents. Hence, we have evidence from yet another laboratory that an inhibitor of Na^+,K^+-ATPase may play a role in the development of hypertension.

Blaustein reported on the role of the exchange of sodium for calcium ions in the regulation of the intracellular concentration of ionized calcium. The transport system that mediates the exchange of sodium for calcium ions derives energy for calcium extrusion from the electrochemical gradient for sodium. The ionized calcium concentration inside sympathetic neurons as well as vascular smooth muscle cells is visualized to be controlled by changes in sodium transport. Hence, factors interfering with sodium transport, such as natriuretic hormone, will increase intracellular accumulation of both sodium and calcium ions.

Van Breemen performed studies on guinea pig taenia coli and rabbit aorta in which he inhibited the Na/K pump and substituted several substances for external sodium. In guinea pig taenia coli ouabain induced an increase in intracellular sodium concentration, a decrease in intracellular potassium, but no change in intracellular calcium. Removal of external potassium induced similar changes in intracellular sodium and potassium but resulted in a 25% loss of cellular calcium. The results of additional studies in which either sucrose or choline was substituted for sodium suggested to van Breemen that calcium homeostasis in smooth muscle is not maintained by a sodium/calcium exchange carrier. He believes it is more likely to be maintained by an ATP-fueled calcium extrusion pump.

I want to thank all of the participants for making this an informative meeting and particularly for making it exciting for me to try to follow what each of you had to report. It was difficult to pull out the one or two most salient features of each presentation. I hope that I have been able to do this faithfully.

Index

DEVICE FOR DRYING SALT IN SHAKERS OR OTHER RECEPTACLES.

APPLICATION FILED OCT. 6, 1916.

1,252,872. Patented Jan. 8, 1918.

Fig. 1.

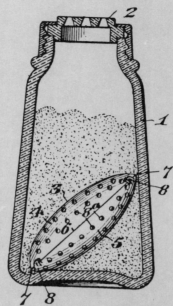

Fig. 3.

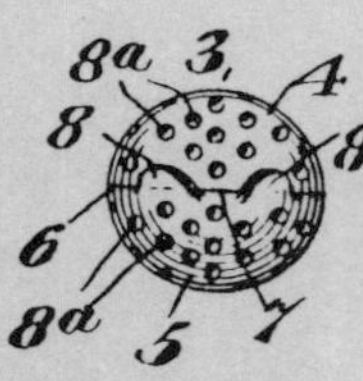

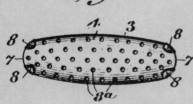

Fig. 7.

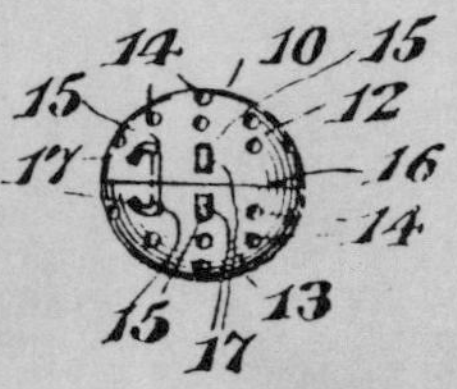

Fig. 2.

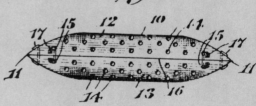

Fig. 6.

Fig. 4.

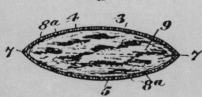

Fig. 5.

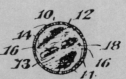

WITNESSES

Jas. K. McCathran

Howard D. Orr

Lawrence G. Yoggerst, INVENTORS
Walter A. Hutchison,

BY E. G. Siggers

ATTORNEY